Nursing Care of Women

Dinah Gould BSc MPhil RGN DN Cert Ed

Course Director, BSc Nursing Studies,
Department of Community Health and Nursing Studies
South Bank Polytechnic, London

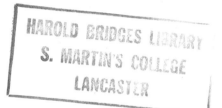

Prentice Hall
New York   London   Toronto   Sydney   Tokyo   Singapore

First published 1990 by
Prentice Hall International (UK) Ltd,
66 Wood Lane End, Hemel Hempstead,
Hertfordshire, HP2 4RG
A division of
Simon & Schuster International Group

Printed and bound in Great Britain at
the University Press, Cambridge

British Library Cataloguing in Publication Data

Gould, Dinah
  Nursing care of women.
  1. Gynaecology & Obstetrics. Nursing
  I. Title
  610.73′678

  ISBN 0-13-629106-6

1 2 3 4 5 94 93 92 91 90

Nursing Care of Women

before

;

Contents

Preface

How to use this book

As this book is about the nursing care of women much of its content relates to gynaecology but material concerned with other aspects of women's health has been included to provide a more comprehensive account of the total health care needs of the client group. Thus, I hope that it will have wide appeal.

The care of women is a responsibility of nurses in a range of specialisms, in hospital and the community not only those on gynaecology wards. Hospital stay is nowadays brief, with growing reliance on day care facilities and a trend towards community care, hence the emphasis on advice/information-giving presented with a minimum of technical language in an attempt to demonstrate how nurses could provide information for patients/clients in terms they can readily understand.

The first chapter opens with a case study showing how knowledge of a woman's social circumstances can affect health, underlining the need for health education and individualised care. Psychological care is emphasised and the role of the biological sciences in nursing care is indicated.

The remaining chapters are concerned with different aspects of health and illness, illustrated with case histories and individualised care plans. Physiology is described at appropriate points in the text, followed by nursing care and treatment. Normal physiology precedes disturbed function to expand and build on previous knowledge. It is important to remember that nursing and medical practice vary between different centres and with increasing knowledge, research findings and available technology. Where variations are particularly likely to occur, this has been indicated in the text. Similarly, nursing models have been used with the care plans, but this is not meant to be prescriptive: the view taken is that no model can be considered ideal for every individual in every situation. Readers are encouraged to consider alternative models for delivering care and to construct care plans for patients presented in the vignettes where this has not been done. The findings of research studies have been presented wherever possible, with some indication of the method used to obtain them, as there is now increasing recognition of the need to use research findings and growing awareness of the need to appraise research reports critically. References are given at the end of every chapter to encourage further reading and a glossary of terms has been provided so the book may be used for reference. However, readers are likely to obtain maximum advantage if they read each chapter, or at least sections of the chapter with related care plans and illustrative case studies, when gathering information about a particular topic. Straightforward facts can be obtained from any standard medical textbook: it is the philosophy of understanding the patient/client as an individual and providing holistic care that differentiates nursing from medicine, and this is the emphasis of this text.

This book is illustrated with numerous care plans and case studies of women in hospital and the community. They are not meant to represent any of the patients I have nursed or met in the course of my research.

    I should like to thank Andrée Thorpe for all the help with typing and preparing the manuscript, and Pam Walter and Ginny Dunn for their help with the care plans.

Dinah Gould

Glossary

Abortion Expulsion of the products of conception before the twenty-eighth week of gestation.

Amenorrhoea Absence of menstruation.

Amniocentesis Removal of some of the fluid surrounding the fetus, to be examined for evidence of genetic or congenital abnormality.

Anovulatory cycle Menstrual cycle in which no egg (ovum) is released.

Anteversion Positioned forwards. Refers to the normal position of the uterus.

Bartholin's glands Paired glands positioned just inside the labia majora. Responsible for secreting a mucoid lubricating substance during sexual arousal.

Biopsy Removal of tissue for histological examination.

Cervicitis Inflammation of the cervix.

Cervix Narrow lower portion of the uterus projecting down into the vagina.

Chorionic villus biopsy Removal of a fragment of the tissues surrounding the fetus to be examined for evidence of genetic or congenital abnormality.

Chromosome Thread-like structures within a cell nucleus, carrying the genes which are the units of heredity.

Climacteric Time around the menopause often referred to as the 'Change of Life'.

Colporrhaphy Repair of the vagina.

Colposcopy Examination of cervix by a low powered magnifying instrument (colposcope).

Combined pill Oral contraceptive containing oestrogens and progestogens.

Cystocele Prolapse of the bladder affecting the anterior wall of the vagina.

Dilatation and curettage (D and C) Diagnostic procedure in which the cervix is dilated with instruments and endometrial fragments obtained for examination in the laboratory.

Dysmenorrhoea Painful menstrual periods.

Dyspareunia Painful or difficult coitus.

Ectopic pregnancy Pregnancy outside the uterine cavity.

Endocrine organ A gland or cell releasing hormone(s) directly into the bloodstream, to be carried to target tissue(s) elsewhere in the body.

Endometriosis Presence of functioning endometrium in a site other than the uterus.

Endometrium Uterine lining.

Enterocele Herniation of the bowel through the upper, posterior vaginal wall.

Fibroid Benign growth arising from myometrium (muscular wall of uterus).

Fundus Top of uterus (the part lying above the insertion of the Fallopian tube).

Gonadotrophins Protein hormones released from the pituitary gland which in the female control ovarian functioning and menstrual cycle.

Haematocolpos Blood in the vagina.

Hormone Chemical messenger released by an endocrine (ductless) gland.

Human Chorionic Gonadotrophin (hCG)   Hormone released during pregnancy. Detection in the urine forms the basis of modern pregnancy tests.

Hydatidiform mole   Benign or malignant growth arising from placental (chorionic) tissues.

Hysterectomy   Removal of the uterus.

Laparoscope   Telescopic, fibre-optic instrument used to examine the contents of the female pelvic cavity.

Menarche   First menstrual period.

Menopause   The last menstrual period.

Menstruation   Periodic loss of blood and endometrial tissue from the functional non-pregnant uterus, occurring approximately every twenty-eight days.

Miscarriage   Termination of pregnancy before the fetus is viable, generally when loss is not therapeutically induced.

Müllerian ducts   Prototypes of the reproductive structures in the female fetus.

Myomectomy   Removal of fibroids.

Myometrium   Muscular wall of the uterus.

Neoplasm   'New growth'. May be malignant or benign.

Oestrogens   Female steroid hormones (three closely related chemicals) produced throughout the menstrual cycle.

Oöphorectomy   Removal of an ovary.

Ovary   Female gonad, producing eggs and hormones.

Ovulation   Release of an ovum (egg) from the ovary.

Ovum   Female germ cell (gamete).

Parametrium   Tissues (blood vessels, nerves, lymphatic and connective tissues) surrounding the uterus.

Postmenopausal bleeding   Bleeding after the menopause.

Procidentia   Complete prolapse of the uterus, so that the fundus (top of the uterus) is visible at the vaginal entrance.

Progestogen   Synthetic progesterone.

Progesterone   Steroid hormone released in the female, mainly during the second part of the menstrual cycle.

Progesterone only pill (POP)   Oral contraceptive containing progesterone, taken every day.

Prolapse   Displacement of the pelvic organs.

Prostaglandins   A large group of locally acting hormones naturally produced by the tissues, some of which have clinical use, e.g. in therapeutic termination of pregnancy.

Puberty   Stage in the life cycle when the reproductive organs mature and the secondary sexual characteristics become apparent.

Pyosalpinx   Pus in the uterine tube (abscess).

Rectocele   Herniatation of the rectum through the posterior vaginal wall.

Retroversion   Tilted backwards. Refers to abnormal position of uterus, bent backwards from the cervix.

Salpingectomy   Surgical removal of uterine tube.

Salpingitis   Inflammation of the uterine tubes.

Salpingo oöphorectomy   Surgical removal of uterine tube and ovary. May be uni or bilateral.

Sterility   Absolute infertility.

Steroid   Chemical substance in the body, often important as a hormone, e.g. oestrogen and progesterone.

Subfertility   Impaired fertility.

Trachelorrhaphy   Surgical repair of the cervix.

Urethrocele   Prolapse of urethra through anterior vaginal wall.

Uterine tube (Fallopian tube, oviduct)   Fine tube via which the egg (ovum) travels from the ovary to the uterus.

Vulva   External female genitals.

Vulvectomy   Removal of vulva.

Wolffian ducts   Prototypes of the reproductive structures in the male fetus.

1   Women, Health and Illness

Introduction

■   Sally met Errol when she was 17 years old. When they married, two years
later, she continued to work in a shop until the birth of their first baby.

Initially Sally and Errol Carder lived in a one-bedroom flat but, with the
baby's arrival, the family was rehoused by the council. Sally was pleased as
she now lived near her mother, whom she visited several times each week.
She derived a great deal of support from her mother, her sister and other
female friends. Errol worked as a deckhand aboard ship and was at sea much
of the time; left alone with the baby, Sally often felt isolated. Her health
visitor advised her to take the baby to a playgroup but, as Sally did not have
access to a car and public transport was unreliable, she became discouraged.
Bus journeys with a small child proved tiring. This accounted for Sally missing
several ante-natal appointments throughout her second pregnancy. She
worried about the cost of transport too.

The house was damp and expensive to heat. Sometimes Sally found it
necessary to economise on food to meet bills. The eldest child had a series of
chest infections and she knew this was made worse by their living conditions.

Although she was pleased at the arrival of her two older children, Sally was
distressed to find herself pregnant again. She wished that Errol need not be
absent for such long periods, as she found coping with two toddlers exhaust-
ing despite the help of her mother and sister, now divorced.

Sally became depressed. Even before the third pregnancy was confirmed,
her GP prescribed tranquillisers (diazepam) which helped her to get through
the day, although they did nothing to tackle the real problems.

The time to which she looked forward was the evening when both children
were in bed and she was able to relax and smoke a cigarette. She had been
warned about the dangers of smoking during her earlier pregnancies but
could not contemplate giving up altogether, although she had cut down.

Sally found the health visitor and midwife helpful because they allowed her
to talk about her worries without trying to find 'magic' solutions to a difficult
and inter-connected series of problems. After the birth of the third baby the
health visitor explained different methods of birth control, and Sally eventually decided to take oral contraceptives because she felt she definitely could

not cope with another child. She was continually anxious about the new baby, mainly because she felt so guilty about smoking during pregnancy. However, the little girl was well, although rather small, and Sally gradually felt better herself, especially as Errol had managed to take extended leave when she came out of hospital. Sally's sister, bringing up two small children alone, could not understand what all the fuss was about, for Errol was always ready to help in the home. However, Sally pointed out that he would only undertake certain tasks: most of the responsibilities for housework and childcare devolved upon herself.

When the youngest child reached school age, Sally found a part-time job as a nursing auxiliary. She particularly valued companionship from the other women, but the money was also an important incentive as Errol had never earned a great deal. Sally's two main regrets about her work were that she developed backache and that she had no access to childcare facilities. She would have gone to work sooner if a crèche had been provided.

As Sally's children grew older her financial position eased to some extent and, when she had more time to herself, she began to feel happier. She went through a worrying time when her mother had a stroke but, fortunately, she and her sister were able to work as a team until the old lady was sufficiently recovered to cope. During this time Sally had to take considerable time from work and the family income suffered. However, to Sally and her sister the main concern was obtaining information about their mother's progress while she was in hospital. The District Nurse provided enormous practical help when she first came home, but Sally sometimes wished that she had given more information about the progress expected.

Now that her children were school age, Sally saw less of the health visitor, but she found support from the school nurse who encouraged her to join a Parents' Group where members occasionally met informally for companionship and discussion. Inevitably the conversation shifted towards plans for the future when children would be independent. Sally found that she had much in common with the other women. She regretted the lack of opportunities for education and career when she was younger which had placed her in a job with modest pay and prospects. She often felt that her life at work mirrored her role at home as a carer on whom the health and welfare of the rest of the family depended.

Social problems

Nurses recognise through use of the nursing process that all people are individuals who need care tailored to meet their particular requirements. The use of vignettes and care plans throughout this book is meant to highlight this need. However, Sally Carder's experiences reflect those of many other women in modern society, and may be used to draw attention to numerous 'typical' women's problems outlined below:

- Many people accept a 'cornflake packet' image of family life – working father, housewife mother and two children. But only 5 per cent of families accord with this ideal (Coussins and Coote 1981) for only a quarter of British households contain any children at all and, in most cases, the mother works in gainful employment outside the home.

- Today one marriage in three ends in divorce, usually leaving the woman to bring up the children. These one-parent families do not, therefore, accord with the ideal model.

- Other family units differ because care is provided to other, often older, members. There are approximately 7 million families in Britain which provide care and accommodation for 26 million individuals – nearly half the total population (Graham 1984).

- Most of the informal care within the community is provided by married or single women. They are therefore the greatest consumers of the health care services, which they receive not only on their own behalf but on behalf of their dependents (Hart 1982).

- Women experience more chronic ill health than men and visit the GP more often for themselves (Graham 1984).

- The rate of psychiatric illness is higher among women than men, especially for depression and neurosis. Admission rates to psychiatric hospitals are three times higher for women, who are also more likely to be prescribed tranquillisers (Weissman and Klerman 1977). However, this may reflect the attitudes of doctors rather than women's needs and treatment may not tackle the real problems.

- Sally Carder was typical in that her chronic mental health problem stemmed, at least to some extent, from her unfavourable home environment. Women living in poor social conditions with dependent children are at particular risk, especially if they lack a close relationship with their partner (Brown and Harris 1978). Financial problems and isolation with pre-school children may help to fuel depressive illness (Richman et al. 1982).

- Women who work outside the home appear to be protected against psychiatric illness (Weissman and Klerman 1977).

- Most women in Britain today (approximately 60 per cent) are in paid employment outside the home, mainly in service employment (cleaning, catering, nursing, teaching or clerical work) rather than industry. Most work part-time to fit in with family needs and tend to be less well paid than men (Rimmer and Popay 1982). Women's activities outside the home tend to be similar in nature to those within it.

- Women have traditionally lacked the range of occupational and educational opportunities open to men (Sharpe 1976) and they face a variety of problems, particularly lack of childcare facilities (Sharpe 1984). Faced with these difficulties most women with children (70 per cent) abandon work until the youngest goes to school.

- Like men, women encounter a number of occupational hazards. Among nurses and nursing auxiliaries, the chief physical problem is backache (Stellman 1977).

- Although men help in the home, they are unlikely to relieve their partners of childcare and housework, even when unemployed (Land 1983).
- Despite working fewer hours on average than men and having lower incomes, women's earnings are often crucial to family economy (Graham 1984). This may be because money is unequally divided between members: for example, the man may retain a disproportionate amount to spend on himself.
- Most women with children work extremely hard within the home: in one study up to sixty hours were spent cleaning every week (Oakley 1974). These unpaid activities are generally invisible. Results are observable only when household and childcare tasks are *not* performed (Graham 1984).
- Conditions within the home may contribute to chronic stress resulting in physical and mental health problems. Dampness, over-crowding and lack of basic amenities create problems for everyone but particularly for those most tied to the home – women and young children (Doyal 1983).
- Transport problems often prevent women using health care facilities such as ante-natal classes (Perkins 1979). Carrying shopping may also be a problem (Hunt 1985) for men usually have first claim to the family car to travel to work (Hillman *et al*. 1974). The woman's sense of isolation is therefore increased.
- Health is inevitably related to social class. The Black Report on *Inequalities in Health* (1982) showed morbidity and mortality to be higher among lower socio-economic groups. Even the Western 'diseases of affluence' (cardiovascular conditions, many types of malignancy) occur more often in the lower socioeconomic groups. There is a wealth of evidence to suggest that those who need health care services most, especially preventative services, make least use of them (Townsend and Davidson 1982).
- Despite increased risk of developing chronic ill health, women tend to live longer than men. The structure of the population in Western society is changing; people survive longer, and most of these survivors are women who in turn require care, delivered mainly in the community by other women.
- Despite all that has been written about the breakdown of family networks and the increasing geographical mobility of the nuclear family unit, women still rely heavily on their female relatives for help and support (Argyle 1983).
- There is regional variation in health throughout the country, with most affluence concentrated in the South East. The underprivileged tend to live in inner city areas with inferior conditions and amenities.
- When money is short women often impose sacrifices upon themselves to prevent suffering by other family members. The woman herself may then experience ill-health (Burghes 1980).

The combined evidence of the research studies cited above suggests that large numbers of women face a lifetime of caring for children, partners and often for elderly relatives. In doing so their personal needs may become overlooked and their health may suffer. However, many mental and physical health problems are preventable and health education is today regarded as an important aspect of the nurse's role. Those who work with women are in a key position to promote health, for it is the woman who makes the greatest use of the services available and who provides care for the rest of the family: if she is made health conscious other family members are likely to benefit directly.

Health education and health promotion

Nearly a decade ago Smith (1979) defined the goal of health education as helping the individual achieve optimal physical, social and mental well-being, not just avoiding disease or infirmity. Three main phases were outlined:

- Giving knowledge;
- Changing attitudes;
- Changing behaviour.

Health education therefore comprises much more than giving people the facts and exhorting them to behave sensibly. It demands an understanding of the circumstances of the individual patient or client, and of those factors likely to help promote behaviour change. Clearly it is hopeless to blame an individual for a damp home resulting in her child's chest infections when she is not directly responsible for the condition of her house and, apart from stating her case to the council, remains powerless. In such a case, help may only be provided by ensuring that clients know their rights. Urging a woman to attend ante-natal classes and make use of other health services is not likely to meet with success unless the reasons for previous lack of interest are explored.

■   Sally felt able to make up her own mind about two important aspects of health once she had been given sufficient information: choice of suitable contraception and reduction in daily consumption of cigarettes. (For information about oral contraceptives and smoking see Chapter 2.) She did not feel able to give up cigarettes altogether, a decision respected by her health visitor who recognised the sometimes negative image of health education campaigns in the public mind.

Health professionals have a responsibility to provide information so clients are given the opportunity to make informed choice. Explanations do much more to generate effective interest and co-operation than orders (Faulkner 1984). The health visitor also recognised that aims for health education will be achieved only if they are intentional, planned, methodical and therefore open to evaluation; sporadic attempts are not likely to succeed.

■   Sally's changes of behaviour were the result of joint planning with her health visitor, so that she was made a partner in her own care. This was possible because of their relationship, which was based on mutual respect. It was therefore her health visitor from whom Sally sought help when she developed an alarming symptom – vaginal bleeding.

The Outpatient Department

■   The health visitor persuaded Sally to see her GP who suggested that she should have an appointment with a gynaecologist. Sally was nervous, although she had worked in a different department of the same hospital for several years. She was relieved when the sister greeted her by name and promised that she would not have long to wait. A group of student nurses were visiting the department that day, and the Sister explained what happens during a gynaecological examination, taking care to emphasise the importance of psychological care to reassure the woman during an experience that may be perceived as embarrassing or threatening.

At the initial visit the gynaecologist will follow these procedures:

* Take a careful history from the patient;
* Perform a full physical examination, including the entire body not just the re-productive organs;
* Perform a bimanual pelvic examination and a speculum examination.

The supportive presence of a nurse throughout the examination may be helpful to the woman.

History taking

The gynaecologist will ask the patient about the following:

* Her age and age at the menarche (first menstrual period);
* The amount, duration and frequency of her menstrual periods, and episodes of intermenstrual bleeding;
* Previous gynaecological, general medical and obstetric history (including any tendency to bleeding disorders);
* Drugs;
* Contraception.

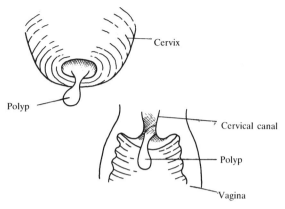

Figure 1.1 Cervical polyps.

■   It is unusual for a woman taking the combined contraceptive pill to complain of intermenstrual bleeding, and the gynaecologist thought that Sally might have polyps. These are small benign growths arising from the uterine wall or cervix (see Fig. 1.1) which often cause irregular bleeding. The gynaecologist reassured Sally that cervical polyps do not undergo malignant change.

Vaginal examination

During bimanual pelvic examination the woman is required to lie in the dorsal position. The gynaecologist uses one hand to examine the vagina and cervix while gently pressing the top (fundus) of the uterus downwards with the other. This ensures that the cervix comes within reach of the examining fingers.

Bimanual examination helps the gynaecologist to estimate the size of the uterus which increases during pregnancy (never returning to its nulliparous size) and in some pathological states, to detect whether it is in the correct position and whether it is free

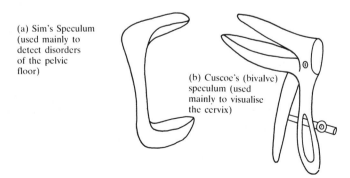

(a) Sim's Speculum (used mainly to detect disorders of the pelvic floor)

(b) Cuscoe's (bivalve) speculum (used mainly to visualise the cervix)

Figure 1.2 Vaginal speculae.

of the other pelvic structures, as it should be. Abnormalities such as cervical polyps are detectable.

Speculum examination permits the gynaecologists to visualise the cervix directly, confirming the presence of lesions such as a polyp. Several different types of speculum are commercially available, some made of metal, others of plastic, to be used only once. The two most commonly used are Cuscoe's speculum and Sim's speculum (see Fig. 1.2).

Figure 1.3 shows two other positions commonly used during gynaecological examinations.

Sim's position can be used routinely instead of the dorsal position. The lithotomy position is employed mainly in theatre when the woman is anaesthetised. If the lithotomy position must be adopted when the woman is awake, she is liable to feel very exposed, so draping must be arranged carefully and promptly.

Day care

■   The gynaecologist explained to Sally that a polyp had been found which should be removed to stop the bleeding. This would take place under a general anaesthetic in the operating theatre. It is a minor procedure, so she would be required to come to the ward the afternoon before the operation and would probably be able to go home the day afterwards.

      The nurse noticed that Sally was looking rather upset and, when she emerged from the changing room, it was evident that she had been crying. She explained to the nurse that she did not want to be away from her children during the night because she had recently had to stay several times overnight with her mother who had had a stroke. The children's routine had been upset and the youngest had been most distressed. The nurse realised from Sally's notes that her husband was not available to provide support. Instead she suggested that Sally should be admitted as a day patient. It was agreed that she should come to the ward on the morning of the operation and would go home in the evening providing she felt well.

The nurse knew that, when women come into hospital for investigations or treatment, this new worry is added to all those they may already have. To understand their patients' worries, nurses must have some information about their social background, particularly as this may have some bearing on their health and social problems. This information must be collected during the initial nursing assessment, which is just as important for women having a short hospital stay as for those who will be away from home longer. One of the main problems facing nurses working on gynaecology wards is the very short period of hospital admission, which reduces the amount of time available to get to know their patients. Since much information is collected in the outpatient department, the nurse working there may begin the assessment. Good liaison with the ward staff is therefore essential.

(a) Sim's position

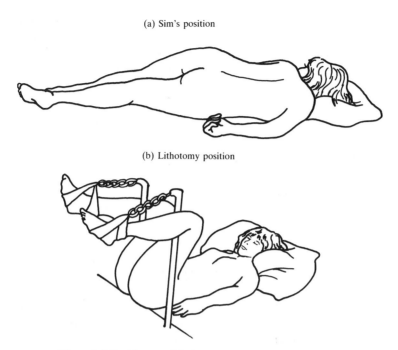

(b) Lithotomy position

Figure 1.3 Positions used during gynaecological examinations.

Day surgery is acceptable to many people because it involves minimal disruption of their circumstances, and to cost-conscious hospital managers because it permits maximum use of hospital facilities, but it is only suitable if the patient's home circumstances allow adequate rest afterwards and if she understands and is sufficiently responsible to follow medical and nursing instructions precisely. Before the patient leaves the hospital, the nurse explains what she should do before admission and what to expect afterwards. She should provide her with a leaflet of instructions as research evidence suggests that women find written information a useful adjunct to verbal instructions (Steele and Goodwin 1975).

■   The nurse gave the following information to Sally:

- She must fast for at least six hours before coming into hospital, as her operation would take place early in the morning allowing maximum opportunity to recover during the day. Food can remain in the stomach for up to six hours and may be aspirated into the respiratory passages, causing obstruction if vomiting occurs during anaesthesia.
- She should arrive on the ward promptly at the time stated on the admission form, as she would have to be prepared for theatre quickly. Failure to do so could hold up her operation and might mean that she was insufficiently recovered to go home as planned.

- She would be seen by the gynaecologist in the evening and, if sufficiently well, would be able to go home providing she was accompanied by a responsible adult and did not have to use public transport. She should bring overnight requirements in case she was not well enough to go home.
- She was told how to contact the hospital social worker in case of problems, and her attention was drawn to the ward telephone number in case further information was required.

Patients receiving day surgery may not receive pre-medication and receive very light anaesthesia so they recover swiftly. As pre-medication invariably contains drugs to help alleviate anxiety, this approach is not suitable for those who feel particularly nervous.

Investigations in the Outpatient Department

Some women receive all or most of their gynaecological investigations and treatment in the outpatient clinic. The nurse has an important role supporting the woman, providing explanations and acting as the co-ordinator of care.

■   Gloria Henry, aged 43, was married with four children. Her periods had always been heavy and recently they had become much worse, although not painful. Bimanual and speculum examinations failed to reveal any obvious problem but a blood test showed that Gloria's haemoglobin was 10 gms/dl (normal female range 12–14 gm/dl), suggesting that she had developed anaemia as a result of heavy bleeding. The gynaecologist decided to perform *vabra curettage* to take a biopsy of the lining of the uterus (*endometrium*) to try and determine the cause.

The vabra apparatus consists of a small suction pump attached to a fine aspirator that can be passed through the opening of the cervix without dilation. When suction is applied, a small quantity of endometrium can be obtained for microscopic examination. Vabra aspiration can be performed in the outpatient department, but it may be painful. The nurse, who was present throughout the procedure, warned Gloria that the sensation would resemble moderately severe period pains, and that she would probably wish to rest afterwards.

Vabra aspiration is not considered adequate as a method of investigating possible malignancy by some gynaecologists and, if the uterus is enlarged, it may be thought preferable to perform curettage under anaesthesia when the cervix can be more fully dilated. It is then possible to obtain more tissue for biopsy.

Care plan 1.1 Pre-operative care for gynaecology patients

Nursing Intervention	Rationale
(1) Record vital signs (pulse, temperature, blood pressure, rate and depth of respirations)	To establish a baseline for post-operative observations
(2) Record weight	Used by anaesthetist to calculate drug dosages
(3) Perform urinalysis	To detect possible abnormality
(4) Obtain a clean catch specimen of urine (not all hospitals)	To detect possible urinary tract infection – these often co-exist with gynaecological conditions
(5) Give aperients, suppositories or enema as prescribed (often not considered necessary for minor surgery, e.g. D and C)	– To empty bowels and reduce the chance of damage during surgery – To avoid post-operative constipation when diet and mobility are reduced
(6) Check special pre-operative instructions, e.g. vaginal douching with topical antiseptics	To reduce the risk of post-operative sepsis
(7) Shave pubic hair (no longer considered necessary for minor procedures)	Believed to reduce the risk of post-operative sepsis
(8) Teach chest and leg exercises (often done by physiotherapist)	– To reduce the risks of pulmonary complications – To prevent venous stasis and deep venous thrombosis
(9) Ensure that the patient fasts for 4–6 hours	– To ensure that the stomach is empty and the gastric contents cannot be aspirated into the lungs
Approximately one hour before theatre	
(10) Ensure that the patient has had a bath or shower and is wearing nothing but an operating gown	To reduce the risks of post-operative sepsis. (In some hospitals patients are requested to use a topical disinfectant such as chlorhexidine, but the evidence that it reduces post-operative sepsis is mixed (Gould 1987))
(11) Ask the patient to empty her bladder	A full bladder may be damaged during pelvic procedures
(12) Ensure that the patient has removed all cosmetics including coloured nail varnish	– Cosmetics obscure cyanosis – The nail beds are one of the sites frequently checked during anaesthesia to ensure adequate tissue perfusion

Nursing Intervention	Rationale
(13) Check that the patient's notes are available, with the results of all investigations (X-rays, ECG, blood tests etc)*	These must accompany the patient to theatre
(14) Ensure that all jewellery, prostheses, hairgrips, dentures have been removed. Wedding rings may be worn but must be completely covered by adhesive tape. Dental crowns must be reported to the anaesthetist	Failure to so so could result in damage when the patient is unconscious (e.g. asphyxia from dentures obstructing the airways during induction of anaesthesia, diathermy burns from metal)
(15) Record any allergies reported by the patient	To avoid use of materials causing allergies. Many people are allergic to elastoplast, a component of numerous dressing materials, and to iodine which is often used routinely as a topical disinfectant
(16) Ensure that the consent form has been signed	Legal requirement
(17) Ensure that the patient is identified correctly by details on a wristband	Safety
(18) Give pre-medication as prescribed. This may consist of: • A sedative or narcotic • An anticholinergic agent Other drugs often included with pre-medication: • Antibiotics • Heparin	 – To allay anxiety – To dry secretions – Prophylaxsis against infection – To avoid venous thrombosis post-operatively following major surgery when mobility is restricted
(19) Instruct the patient not to get out of bed once the pre-medication has been given	The drugs may induce dizziness, with loss of balance
(20) Show the patient how to summon a nurse if necessary and leave her to rest while the pre-medication takes effect	

* Although it is the doctor's responsibility to perform or to request these tests to be performed, the nurse should know which ones are likely to be required in a given situation as it is her responsibility to check that all documentation is complete. It is customary for all patients to have the following:
• Haemoglobin estimation;
• Leucocyte count;
• Blood grouping and cross matching;
• Sickling of red blood cells for women of Afro-Caribbean origin.

Care plan 1.2 Post-operative care for gynaecology patients

Nursing Intervention	Rationale
On return from theatre	
(1) Record vital signs (pulse, blood pressure, rate and depth of respirations) at least half hourly until stable	To detect post-operative shock and haemorrhage
(2) Check warmth and colour at least half hourly until condition is stable	As above
(3) Check the wound site for oozing blood and serous fluid	– To detect blood loss promptly – To detect 'strike through' of tissue fluid, which increases the risks of wound infection and environmental contamination, leading to cross-infection
(4) Check vaginal loss at least half hourly until condition is stable	To detect excessive blood loss promptly (NB blood may 'pool' in the vagina as long as the patient is supine)
(5) Record temperature: • On arrival in the ward • Four hourly for 5–7 days after surgery	 – To detect circulatory shock – To detect infection
(6) Check the patency and optimal functioning of all drains and intravenous infusions when monitoring vital signs (NB care of fluid balance charts)	To monitor correct functioning of equipment
(7) Check all charts and casenotes to ensure they are up to date. Ensure that anti-emetics, analgesia and other appropriate drugs have been prescribed. Note any special instructions, e.g. care of vaginal packs, clamping and release of urinary catheters	
(8) Ask the patient whether she is in pain or nauseated	Analgesics or antiemetics may be given as appropriate (NB powerful analgesia are hypotensive, and are contraindicated if the patient is in shock)
As drowsiness wears off	
(9) Ask the patient to empty her bladder, preferably using a commode or the WC	– To ensure that the bladder and ureters are patent – To reduce urinary stasis and risks of urinary tract infection
(10) Help the patient to wash and to brush her hair	

Nursing Intervention	Rationale
(11) Encourage mouth washes and dental hygiene	To reduce the risks of oral infection following the use of drugs that diminish oral secretions
(12) Encourage chest and leg exercises	To reduce the risks of chest infections and venous stasis leading to deep venous thrombosis
(13) Patients who have had minor procedures may eat and drink as soon as they wish. Those who have had major operations may take sips when they are no longer nauseated and eat a normal diet when bowel sounds are established	Paralytic ileus is not a common problem after gynaecological operations because the gut is not handled, although its activity may be reduced by anaesthetic agents

Note: Specific post-operative care is discussed in relation to particular operations in later chapters.

■ Gloria Henry was inconvenienced by heavy periods, but put up with them for a long time before seeking help. She knew that many women with this problem end up having a hysterectomy and regarded this as unacceptable. The results of her investigations suggested that she had dysfunctional uterine bleeding, a condition which may be treated by hormones rather than surgery if this is more acceptable to the woman (see Chapter 7). In this situation nurses must provide support, information and the opportunity for the woman to explore her feelings. Discussing how she would feel in the same situation herself is *not* part of the nurse's role for this does not help the woman to make decisions.

■ Sally Carder found her health visitor and midwife helpful because they allowed her to talk about her problems without trying to find instant solutions where none existed. She found the nurses caring for her mother less helpful because they provided so little information about the old lady's progress and did not reveal whether it was taking the expected course.

One of the main complaints levelled against health care provision in this country is lack of communication, and it is often regarded as a major dissatisfaction with care. This omission is particularly unfortunate in view of research evidence to suggest that by providing information in terms that patients can understand anxiety is decreased and recovery is enhanced (Hayward 1975, Boore 1978).

In order to provide information, nurses need a knowledge not only of hospital routines and available services but of the biological sciences in relation to gynaecology,

Table 1.1 Biological/medical aspects of gynaecology

Anatomy
Physiology
Pathology
Pharmacology
Immunology
Biochemistry
Epidemiology
Microbiology

particularly as women may ask for clarification or for further explanations of what the doctor has said. A list of the biological sciences most helpful to nurses working with gynaecology patients is shown in Table 1.1.

Biological science and nursing care of women

Anatomy and physiology

Anatomy is the study of body structure. It is an important area of knowledge for nurses because the design of the human body directly affects its function (physiology). Knowledge of normal structure and function is essential before it is possible to understand the changes that accompany disease.

The organs making up the female reproductive system permit the following:

- Sexual arousal by lubrication of the female genitalia;
- Coitus;
- Conception;
- Safe development of the embryo and fetus;
- Expulsion of the fetus by muscular uterine contractions during labour;
- Protection from invading micro-organisms.

The external female genitalia
The description given here refers to the adult female throughout reproductive life. Changes taking place at puberty and the menopause are discussed in Chapters 14 and 9 respectively.

The vulva
The *vulva* (from the Latin 'cover') is the collective name given to the external female reproductive organs (see Fig. 1.4). Anteriorly it extends from the *mons pubis* to the *perineum*, and is bounded on each side by the *labia majora*. The following structures are enclosed by the labia majora:

- Labia minora;
- Clitoris;

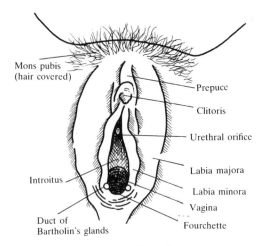

Figure 1.4 The vulva.

- Vestibule;
- Fourchette.

The mons pubis
The mons pubis is a pad of fatty tissue lying immediately above the *symphysis pubis* (pelvic bones). It is covered with skin, which gives rise to the pubic hair, and large numbers of specially modified sebaceous glands. The mons pubis acts as a cushion during sexual intercourse.

The labia majora (Latin: labium, *lip)*
The labia majora are two folds of skin with an underlying layer of fat extending downwards as extensions of the mons pubis until they merge into the perineum. The outer surfaces are covered with hair, but they are smooth on the inner surfaces where sebaceous glands are abundant. The function of the labia majora is to protect the vaginal opening. They are homologous to the scrotum in the male, and Fig. 14.8 (page 392) shows that in the developing fetus they look very similar, although the two structures appear to bear little resemblance in adult males and females.

The labia minora
These are the two much smaller inner folds of skin closely guarding the vaginal opening. They are smooth, hairless and contain sebaceous glands. Anteriorly the labia minora fuse to form the hood-like *prepuce* over the clitoris. Posteriorly they reunite to form the fourchette.

The clitoris
The *clitoris* is a small projection of highly vascular, erectile tissue homologous to the penis in the male. Situated at the junction of the labia minora, it has a very good nerve supply and is extremely sensitive.

The practice of female circumcision, which involves removing the clitoris and suturing together the labia minora, has received considerable attention in both the nursing and medical press (Cox 1985, Cranfield and Cranfield 1983, Nursing Times News Focus 1989). It is still practised by several religious and ethnic minority groups residing in Great Britain so nurses working in some localities may meet women who have been circumcised, and should be prepared for this. Numerous side effects have been documented, the chief ones being recurrent urinary tract and vaginal infections. Female circumcision is also reported to result in scarring which may make intercourse and childbirth difficult. It is undertaken mainly in the Sudan.

The vestibule
The space enclosed by the labia minora is called the *vestibule*. Four different structures open onto its surface:

- The urethra;
- The vagina;
- Bartholin's glands;
- The paraurethral (Skene's) glands.

Bartholin's glands
The ducts of these two glands open on either side of the vaginal orifice. Their function is to provide lubrication during sexual stimulation (see Chapter 6).

The paraurethral glands
The ducts of these two rudimentary structures open onto the *urethral meatus*, representing the vestigial remains of the prostate gland of the male.

The hymen
The *hymen* is a membrane which covers the vaginal orifice, with a small perforation allowing menstrual flow to escape. It is stretched by the use of tampons and during intercourse, and is finally obliterated during childbirth to leave only skin tags called the *carunculae myrtiformes*. An intact hymen cannot be regarded as conclusive evidence of virginity (Underhill and Dewhurst 1978).

The perineum
The perineal body is formed by the junction of the muscles making up the pelvic floor, plus an external covering of skin. It extends from the fourchette to the anus. The significance of the perineum is discussed in relation to pelvic support (see Chapter 10).

The internal female genitalia (see Fig. 1.5)

The vagina
The vagina is a fibromuscular canal extending upwards and backwards from the vulva to the uterus. The anterior wall is approximately 7.5 cm long, the posterior wall about 9 cm. Normally both walls are in close contact with one another. They lie in folds

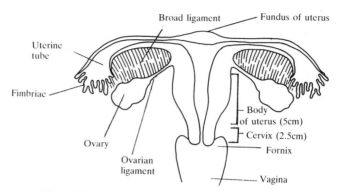

Figure 1.5 Organs of the adult female reproductive tract.

called *rugae* permitting expansion during intercourse. The rugae are obliterated during the enormous expansion required during childbirth.

The vaginal wall consists of four layers, as shown in Fig. 1.6. They include the following:

- A lining of tough, stratified squamous epithelium. This contains no glands, but some fluid may seep through the vaginal walls as transudation to lubricate.
- A layer of areolar connective tissue carrying blood vessels and nerves.
- A layer of circular and longitudinal smooth (involuntary) muscle fibres.
- An outer coat of tough, fibrous connective tissue blending with the pelvic fascia.

The cervix dips down into the vagina, forming a gutter called the fornices. The posterior fornix is deeper than the anterior fornix because of the sloping position of

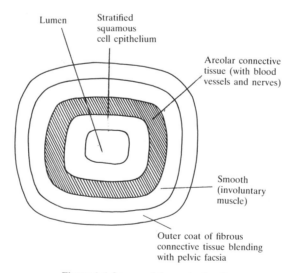

Figure 1.6 Layers of the vaginal wall.

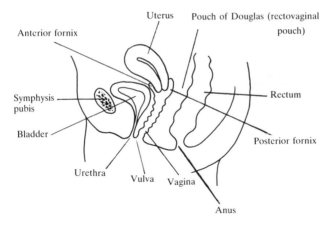

Figure 1.7 Sagittal section of the female pelvic organs.

the vaginal vault. Semen is deposited mainly into the posterior fornix where the sperm may live for several days in the alkaline environment provided by mucus secreted from the cervical glands. The vaginal environment does not favour the survival of sperm because it is acidic owing to the action of bacteria living there, which produce lactic acid as part of their normal metabolic processes. Lactic acid helps to prevent invasion by other, potentially harmful micro-organisms.

It is important for nurses to appreciate the anatomical relations of the vagina and cervix, as conditions which affect both these organs can affect related pelvic structures:

- The upper part of the anterior vaginal wall lies against the bladder (see Fig. 1.7).
- The lower part of the anterior vaginal wall is adjacent to the urethra.
- The upper two thirds of the posterior vaginal wall lie directly in front of the *Pouch of Douglas* (rectovaginal pouch). Behind this is the rectum.
- The lower third of the posterior vaginal wall lies in front of the perineal body.

The uterus
The *uterus* (see Fig. 1.8) is a hollow, thick-walled muscular organ, lying between the bladder (in front) and the rectum (behind). It is divided into a *corpus* (body) and *cervix* (neck) projecting down into the vagina. In the healthy, non-pregnant state the entire uterus is approximately 7.5 cm long and 5.5 cm wide. Its walls have a thickness of about 1.2 cm, almost obliterating the inner cavity. The two uterine (Fallopian) tubes (oviducts) project laterally from the upper part of the uterus. Their points of insertion are called the *cornuae*, and the area above them is the *fundus* (top) of the uterus.

The thick muscular wall of the uterus is called the *myometrium*. It consists of a system of tightly interlacing circular, longitudinal and oblique muscle fibres which contract tightly after childbirth to reduce bleeding from the raw placental site (living ligatures). Some fibres are present in the myometrium of the body of the uterus, but towards the cervix fibrous tissue gradually becomes the predominant tissue, so the cervix is structurally different from the corpus.

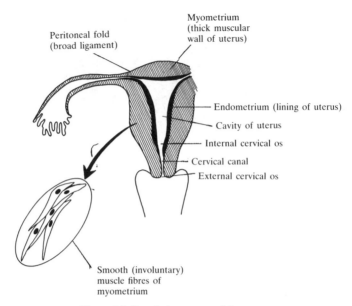

Figure 1.8 Detailed structure of the uterus.

The cervix is lined with columnar epithelium containing glands which secrete mucus. This forms a protective plug throughout pregnancy and during those parts of the menstrual cycle when the woman is not fertile. During the fertile phase the mucus changes character, becoming copious and slippery to allow the passage of sperm.

The body of the uterus is lined with *endometrium*, an epithelial tissue also containing glands. The endometrium consists of two layers, a basal layer and an upper layer which is shed and regenerated approximately every 28 days. The menstrual cycle is discussed in more detail in Chapter 7.

The outer coat of the uterus is formed by a layer of peritoneum called the *perimetrium*. It covers the anterior and posterior surfaces of the body of the uterus, then the posterior fold dips down, forming a cul-de-sac in the Pouch of Douglas close to the posterior vaginal fornix. Peritoneum extends in a fold laterally as *the broad ligament*.

The endometrium provides the site of implantation for the fertilised egg and the protective, nourishing environment required for embryonic and fetal development. The thick, muscular myometrium contracts during labour to expel the fetus. The uterus and other pelvic organs are held in position by a series of ligaments and muscles, including those of the pelvic floor (see Chapter 10).

The uterine (Fallopian) tubes
The two uterine tubes extend from the uterus laterally towards the pelvic walls. They are approximately 10 cm long and very narrow in diameter, ending as a series of fine fimbriae closely applied to the surface of each ovary, though not in direct contact with it. They are extremely delicate, highly specialised structures designed to carry sperm towards the ovary, while conveying the egg from the ovary towards the

uterus. The structure and functions of the uterine tubes are described more fully in Chapter 5.

The ovaries

The two ovaries are the female *gonads* (sex glands) responsible for producing hormones as well as eggs. They lie on either side of the pelvic cavity. They are situated behind the broad ligament, with their surfaces closely applied to the fimbriae of the uterine tubes. The structure function of the ovaries is discussed in greater detail in Chapter 7.

The pelvic blood supply

The blood brings oxygen and nutrients to the tissues and removes the toxic waste products of cellular metabolism. Tissues which have a high rate of metabolic activity consequently receive a generous blood supply because their demands for oxygen and nutrients are considerable.

Not surprisingly, the uterus commands a good blood supply to meet the demands of pregnancy. Two uterine arteries, one on each side of the uterus, branch off from the internal iliac artery running through the base of the broad ligament (see Fig. 1.9). The uterine arteries divide at the level of the internal os (the opening between the uterus and cervix), one branch running up to the uterine fundus, the other down to supply the cervix and vagina. The small vessels supplying the body of the uterus are highly coiled to allow for expansion during pregnancy.

The ovarian arteries branch directly from the abdominal aorta. The veins carrying blood away from the pelvic organs travel along the same pathways as the arteries.

Lymphatic supply to the pelvic tissues

Lymphatic vessels drain tissue fluid which has escaped from the capillary network. Along their length are structures called lymph nodes which act as the sites of storage for white blood cells of the immune system (*lymphocytes*). The lymph nodes help to filter bacteria and other foreign particles from the body. They may trap malignant cells, becoming the secondary sites of spread when cancer develops.

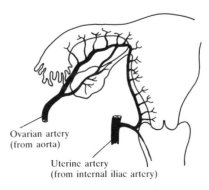

Ovarian artery
(from aorta)

Uterine artery
(from internal iliac artery)

Figure 1.9 Blood supply to the pelvic organs.

Lymph channels drain tissue fluid into lymph nodes in the groin from the major pelvic arteries. Collateral drainage occurs from one side of the pelvis to the other so that if one ovary or one lymph node cluster is affected by the spread of malignant disease, the corresponding organ on the other side is also likely to become involved.

The pelvic nervous supply
The vulva, perineum and vagina are all innervated by the *pudendal nerve* which forms part of the somatic (voluntary) nervous system.

The vulva is a highly sensitive area with many nerve endings. The perineum also has a good nervous supply; lacerations during childbirth and episiotomy wounds are usually painful. The lower part of the vagina is pain sensitive, but the upper vagina, cervix and uterus, all innervated by the sympathetic (autonomic) nervous system, are not. Lacerations and other injuries, including malignant growths, are not therefore painful. Diathermy of the cervix does not usually cause discomfort if performed without anaesthesia. However, the cervix is exquisitely sensitive to stretch, contributing to the pain of labour. Any surgical procedure involving cervical dilation must be performed under local or general anaesthesia.

The uterine tubes are highly sensitive, as are the ovaries. Palpation of the ovaries during bimanual pelvic examination can be painful.

Pathology

Pathology is the study of disease. Pathological processes fall into nine main categories:

- Congenital;
- Traumatic;
- Infections;
- Neoplasms;
- Metabolic disorders;
- Allergies;
- Degenerative changes (not including normal ageing);
- Iatrogenic;
- Idiopathic.

Infections and neoplastic diseases are particularly likely to affect the female reproductive organs, but congenital problems are quite rare. Many conditions affecting women reflect changes that occur with ageing – such as menopausal problems – or are disorders of early pregnancy, so they do not fit neatly into the classification shown above. Others can be considered metabolic because they develop when some factor interferes with the function of the endocrine organs, the ductless glands which empty their secretions, the *hormones*, directly into the bloodstream.

Hormones

Hormones are chemical messengers which enter the bloodstream directly from the glands or cells producing them, exerting their effects at distant sites in the body. Their molecules are usually small, so they can be rapidly broken down once their effects are no longer required, and they are usually excreted in the urine or the faeces which they enter via the biliary system. Chemical degradation of most hormones, including the female sex hormones, is by enzymes in the liver.

Endocrinology provides the key to understanding normal reproductive physiology as well as the changes occurring with disease: for example, the effects of the oral contraceptive pill, the control mechanisms of the menstrual cycle, fertility problems and the hormonal changes of puberty and the menopause.

Research techniques are now so refined that it is possible to study hormonal effects not merely on organ systems and tissues, but on individual cells at the molecular level. Nurses whose work demands an understanding of endocrinology therefore need to know about the biochemical aspects of hormone action.

Biochemistry

Hormones fall into two main categories:

- Steroids;
- Proteins.

These differ in their modes of synthesis, the manner in which they enter their target cells across the barrier afforded by the cell membrane and their mechanisms of action.

The sex steroids

The female (and male) sex hormones are steroids synthesised from cholesterol in the cells of the ovary (Fig. 1.10). The two female sex hormones are progesterone and oestrogen. Progesterone is released mainly during the second half of the menstrual cycle to prepare for pregnancy and lactation in the event of conception. Its actions are shown in Table 1.2.

Oestrogen is really a combination of three hormones:

- β oestrone;
- Oestrone;
- Oestriol.

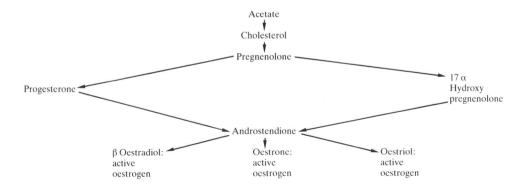

Figure 1.10 Biosynthetic pathway for production of the sex steroids.

Table 1.2 Action of progesterone

Target organ	Action of progesterone
Uterus	Promotes secretory changes in the endometrium preparing the uterus for the implantation of a fertilised egg each month
Uterine tubes	Stimulates secretory changes in the mucosal lining each month to nourish the egg
Breasts	1. Promotes development of the ducts and glandular system and prepares the breasts for lactation (milk is only secreted after stimulation by another hormone, prolactin, from the anterior pituitary) 2. Causes additional enlargement of the breasts every month by increasing fluid retention in the subcutaneous tissue

β oestrone is the most abundant and biologically the most active.

The main actions of the oestrogens are shown in Table 1.3. Unlike progesterone, the oestrogens are produced in significant quantities during the first as well as the second half of the menstrual cycle. They have a mildly anabolic action, and are responsible for the female secondary sexual characteristics developing at puberty. These include the following:

- The typical curved female shape. This is due to fat deposition on the buttocks, thighs and breasts. Women's bodies generally contain more adipose tissue than men's in proportion to their weight.
- The typical female distribution of body hair.
- Skeletal development. On average women are shorter in stature than men, and have a wide pelvis to accommodate pregnancy.
- Higher pitch of the female voice, due to thinner vocal chords.

Tables 1.2 and 1.3 show that the oestrogens and progesterone exert their effects on a wide variety of different target tissues throughout the body. It is known that both hormones operate on their target cells in a very similar, possibly identical, fashion, but they cause their different target cells to perform quite different functions.

Mechanisms of steroid hormone action

The sex steroids are carried to all the cells in the body by blood and tissue fluids. Because they are soluble in fat (*lipid*), one of the main components of cell membranes, they are able to enter all cells, not just their target cells. However, only the target cells contain special receptor molecules allowing them to respond to specific hormones.

When a molecule of sex steroid hormone has entered a target cell, it is able to travel freely through the cytoplasm into the nucleus, where it combines with its special receptor, a protein molecule attached to the chromosomes. Each hormone will bind

Table 1.3 Action of oestrogen

Target organ	Action of oestrogen
Breasts	1. Increases fat deposition 2. Stimulates development of the ducts. Both these actions are initiated at puberty. Oestrogen maintains the state of development of the breasts until the menopause, but does *not* initiate lactation
Skeleton/Muscles	1. Increases the activity of osteoblast cells which build up bone as the girl enters puberty, therefore increasing skeletal growth and increase in height 2. Stimulates closure of the epiphyses at the tips of the long bones towards the end of the growth spurt of puberty 3. Broadens the pelvic outlet. Parturition is therefore easier. Increases the deposition of fat in: (a) subcutaneous tissues (b) breasts (c) thighs (d) This results in the typical, curved female shape and higher fat content compared to the male
Skin	Increases vascularity. Female skin is often warmer than that of the male, and cut surfaces bleed more easily
Reproductive organs	1. Increases the size of the external and internal genitalia at puberty, and maintains their functional state of development until the menopause 2. Changes the vaginal epithelium from the cuboidal cells of the prepubertal girl to the stratified epithelium of adulthood 3. Promotes the cyclical endometrial and vaginal changes of the menstrual cycle

only to its own receptor because it has a special shape allowing it to fit exactly, like a key in a lock (see Fig. 1.11). Once the hormone and receptor are united the hormone stimulates the cell's *deoxyribonucleic acid* (DNA) stored on the chromosomes to release a chemical called *ribonucleic acid* (RNA). DNA controls all cellular activities, including the type and number of new protein molecules that it is able to make via the actions of RNA. As soon as the formation of new RNA has been triggered by the binding of the hormone to the receptor, RNA moves into the cytoplasm and new protein molecules are synthesised according to the dictates of DNA (see Fig. 1.12).

All cells contain the same DNA, but its ability to be stimulated varies according to

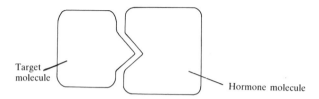

Figure 1.11 Lock and key hypothesis for hormone action.

the type of cell it occupies: the DNA in endometrial cells is able to control the synthesis of proteins that will nourish the fertilised egg when it is 'switched on' by progesterone at the appropriate stage in the menstrual cycle. The same cells contain DNA which *could* promote milk secretion but this DNA is never activated by progesterone (although in theory the hormone would be able to do so) because the DNA responsible for milk production is permanently 'switched off' in endometrial cells.

Many synthetic hormones resembling oestrogen and progesterone have been developed in recent years. Clinically they are used as contraceptives and to help relieve heavy menstrual bleeding due to an imbalance of the naturally occurring hormones (*dysfunctional uterine bleeding*). They operate by binding to the specific hormone receptors in the appropriate target cells because of their very similar, though not identical, molecular shapes. They may be considered to 'force the lock' of the lock and key mechanism (see Fig. 1.13). Their effects are generally more potent than those of naturally occurring hormones and they may produce a range of side effects. In most cases the long term effects of continuous therapy are not known, although they are

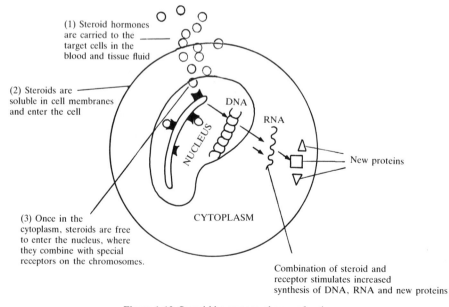

Figure 1.12 Steroid hormones: theory of action.

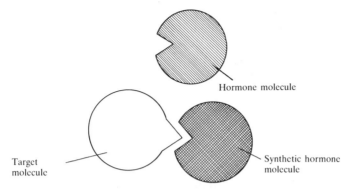

Figure 1.13 'Forcing the lock'.

evidently able to influence many organ systems in addition to the reproductive structures. Clearly, an understanding of endocrinology and the biochemistry of the sex
hormones is needed to appreciate pharmacological aspects of gynaecology.

Protein hormones
The sex steroids are released from the ovary under the control of two further hormones, *follicle stimulating hormone* (FSH) and *luteinising hormone* (LH). These are
synthesised in the anterior pituitary gland at the base of the brain. The control
mechanism is described in Chapter 7.

FSH and LH are both protein hormones. They enter their target cells via a complicated series of steps as they are not readily soluble in cell membranes, and their
mode of action is much less perfectly comprehended than that of the sex steroids.
Nevertheless, synthetic FSH and LH can be used to treat women who have fertility
problems.

Microbiology and immunology

Many women develop infections or inflammations of the genitourinary tract, hence
microbiology is an important discipline related to gynaecology. Sexually transmitted
diseases have long been regarded as an unglamorous medical specialty, although these
conditions are known to affect large numbers of women (see Chapter 6). Two particularly worrying problems have emerged in recent years: *toxic shock syndrome* and
the *acquired immune deficiency syndrome* (AIDS).

Toxic shock syndrome

■   Gloria Henry had read about toxic shock syndrome in the newspapers. She
       was particularly concerned as her teenage daughters insisted on using internal

sanitary protection which she knew to be associated with the disease. When she was waiting for an appointment to see the gynaecologist she took the opportunity to ask the nurse for some more information.

Gloria's nurse reassured her that despite all the publicity, toxic shock syndrome is a rare disease which, although associated with the use of tampons, is not caused by them.

Toxic shock syndrome is caused by toxins from the bacterium *Staphylococcus aureus* entering the bloodstream. *Staph. aureus* is carried harmlessly by large numbers of the population in the nose, axillae and perineal area. It produces toxins which may result in food poisoning if swallowed or, more rarely, a severe generalised illness if it gains access to the bloodstream. The following symptoms develop:

- High temperature;
- Rash;
- Vomiting;
- Headache;
- Diarrhoea;
- Sore throat.

In severe cases dehydration and hypotension lead rapidly to shock. Treatment is supportive, aimed at relieving symptoms and curative by eradicating the source of toxin production, including antibiotic therapy. Diagnosis is by obtaining vaginal swabs containing *Staph. aureus*.

It is thought that bacteria are transferred to the tampon on the hands and, as the tampon absorbs menstrual flow, ideal conditions are provided for bacterial multiplication. Toxins gain access to the bloodstream via minute ulcerations in the vaginal mucosa caused by the tampon, especially the super-absorbent varieties which have a drying effect. Several brands have been withdrawn from the market.

■   Gloria's nurse explained that the following precautions can do much to reduce the chances of developing infection:

- Washing the hands thoroughly before as well as after inserting a tampon;
- Using only one tampon at a time;
- Using a tampon of the absorbency necessary to absorb the flow only – super absorbency tampons should not be used when bleeding is moderate or slight;
- Changing the tampon frequently (every 4–6 hours);
- Taking care not to forget tampons, especially when bleeding has stopped.

Women who are very concerned may feel happier restricting the use of tampons to the day, and switching to sanitary towels at night.

Staph. aureus may gain access to the bloodstream via other routes, accounting for cases of toxic shock syndrome reported in women who are not menstruating and in men.

AIDS and other immunological problems

The problem presented by AIDS has focused greater attention on the needs of people who have long-term infectious conditions, and nurses and doctors are now much more aware of the special needs of infected and infectious patients.

Although women can develop AIDS as a result of vaginal intercourse, most victims in this country so far have been homosexuals or intravenous drug abusers. The nature of the disease has drawn attention to the important role of the immune system in protecting the body from harmful substances (micro-organisms, allergens). It is now believed that the immune system may play a part in the control of malignant disease. It has also been implicated in early miscarriage and is thought to be responsible for some fertility problems. This is a rapidly expanding area which nurses involved in the care of women cannot afford to ignore.

In the case of AIDS, and most other diseases, it is known that many people exposed to the risk of a particular disease do not actually develop it. In many cases, especially with infections, modern medicine has reduced the risk or provided a cure. Often this has been the result of epidemiological research.

Epidemiology

Epidemiology is the study of disease in defined populations. It is concerned with the distribution and aetiology (causes) of ill health and provides the scientific basis for much of community medicine. By identifying people who are at particular risk of developing a given disease, public health measures may be taken to help prevent or reduce it.

Traditionally epidemiology has been concerned with infectious diseases, which were the major cause of death until the beginning of the century. Today, the development of immunisation programmes to eliminate childhood infections and the inspection of shops and factories to ensure safe hygienic practice still form an important part of the work. However, epidemiology is now also concerned with disease that is not communicable, and epidemiologists are concerned with the natural history and prevention of disease in general.

When reading the results of epidemiological reports it is vital to distinguish between two important terms which are sometimes confused:

- Incidence, and
- Prevalence.

The *incidence* of a disease is the number of new cases detected over a given period of time, while *prevalence* refers to the total number of cases in the community at any

Table 1.4 Criteria to be considered before the development of a screening programme (from Wilson and Jungner 1968 for the World Health Organisation)

The condition should:

1. Pose an important problem
2. Have a natural history that is well understood
3. Have a recognisable early stage
4. Be better treated at an early stage than at a later one
5. Be detectable by a suitable test acceptable to the population, that is not physically or psychologically harmful even if repeated at regular intervals (determined by the natural history of the disease)

The cost of any screening programme must be balanced aganst its benefit

single point in time. Unless a disease is very rapidly fatal it therefore follows that its prevalence on any one occasion will be higher than its incidence, illustrating that even though the two terms are sometimes used interchangeably, for the sake of clarity they should not be.

One of the diseases presently receiving a great deal of attention from epidemiologists is cervical cancer and, at the present time, the early detection and prevention of this disease represents an important public health endeavour.

Screening for carcinoma of the cervix

The purpose of screening to detect disease is to separate from a large group of apparently well people those who have a high risk of having the particular condition, so they may be more firmly identified and treated early if necessary. It is not feasible or even desirable to screen for all known diseases; for screening to be possible or worthwhile it is necessary for the disease in question to meet the criteria shown in Table 1.4.

An understanding of the natural history of cervical cancer shows that it is potentially an avoidable disease and that women derive benefit from regular screening:

- Cancer of the cervix ranks as the eighth most commonly occurring malignancy in the female population. In 1983, 4,400 new cases were diagnosed and 2,200 women died of it (see Table 12.1, page 290).
- Cancer of the cervix is curable if early treatment is provided. Experts have calculated that with very early detection recovery would be 100 per cent following effective treatment (see Chapter 12).
- The screening test is cheap, reasonably accurate and has proved acceptable to thousands of women. (Screening itself cannot be equated with diagnosis as false negative and positive results occur. Its purpose is to select subjects who would benefit from more intensive investigation with more reliable and possibly more expensive tests.)

There is however, some evidence that those women who would benefit most from

cervical screening do not have access to it (Broadley 1986). This problem is discuss
further in Chapter 12.

Cervical cytology
The practice of *exfoliative cytology* was developed in the 1840s, but the technique of
cervical cytology perfected by Papanicolaou did not gain popularity in Britain until the
1940s. Its purpose is to detect pre-malignant changes restricted to the surface of the
cervix which could lead to cancer if neglected. Cervical cells are shed just as cells are
normally lost from the surface of the skin, and can be collected by a nurse or doctor
and sent for microscope examination in the cytology department. A new technique
called *cervicography* has now been developed. A *cervigram* is a photograph of the
cervix after it has been painted with a solution of iodine and acetic acid to show up
abnormal cells. It is said to be a more accurate technique, producing fewer false
negative results (Holmes 1988).

■ Sally Carder had her first smear test at the ante-natal clinic. The midwife
explained the purpose of the test and, with Sally in the dorsal position, passed
a Cuscoe's speculum to visualise the cervix. A wooden (Ayre's) spatula was
gently rotated around the external os to collect exfoliated cells (see Fig. 1.14).
These were smeared over the surface of a glass microscope slide and immediately placed in fixative to prevent deterioration before the slide reached
the laboratory. Unless fixative is used and the slide is immersed at once, the
result may be inconclusive and the test may have to be repeated. Smears are
best obtained half way through the menstrual cycle; near the beginning results
may be obscured by endometrial tissue and towards the end by leucocytes.

At present the DHSS recommends routine cervical screening only for those women
aged 35 years and older, but there is evidence that the disease is beginning to occur
among younger women and may progress rapidly in this age group. The service is also

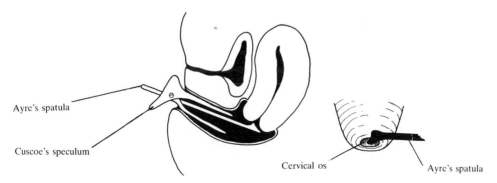

Figure 1.14 Cuscoe's speculum used to separate vaginal walls while a cervical smear is taken.

rather unco-ordinated, as those attending family planning, ante-natal and special clinics may also be tested, sometimes without their knowledge.

■   Sally had repeated smear tests each time she was pregnant, then routinely when she went to the family planning clinic. She did not worry about them, regarding them as routine. She was very disturbed, however, when her GP's receptionist telephoned to ask her to come to the health centre to discuss the results of a recent smear, which was indicative of early malignant change.

An appointment was made for Sally to undergo *colposcopy*. This investigation helps to assess the size, site and extent of the lesion, so that biopsies can be taken. Colposcopy is an accurate, reliable method of diagnosis, but too expensive and time consuming for routine screening.

Risk factors for cancer of the cervix

A number of risk factors predispose certain women to the disease. If nurses are to fulfil their role as health educators, they must be able to identify women most at risk and explain the value of screening. Those at particular risk may fall into the following categories:

- Women who are members of a low socioeconomic group;
- Women who have multiple sexual partners (Harris *et al.* 1980);
- Women who first have coitus at an early age (Nelson 1967);
- Women who have several children;
- Women who have had a sexually transmitted disease;
- Women whose partners belong to occupational groups in which they may often be away from home – for example, long distance lorry drivers, or sailors (Buckley *et al.* 1981);
- Women whose partners work in dusty occupations;
- Women whose husbands have not been circumcised (Wakenfield *et al.* 1973);
- Women who smoke (Trevathan *et al.* 1983);
- Women who take the oral contraceptive pill (Yule 1984, Vessey *et al.* 1983);
- Women who are widowed or divorced (Sibary *et al.* 1977).

Some women have a very *low* risk of developing cancer of the cervix and may fall into one of the following categories:

- Jewish women (whose husbands are circumcised);
- Virgins.

Evidence suggests that cancer of the cervix may be caused by an agent transmissible during sexual intercourse, and there is a suggestion that at least two viruses, the herpes simplex type 2 virus and the papilloma virus (which causes genital warts) may be involved. Male behaviour may also be influential. Possibly some carcinogenic factor may be carried beneath the foreskin of uncircumcised males, especially if hygienic practices are not good. The semen of certain men seems to spark off

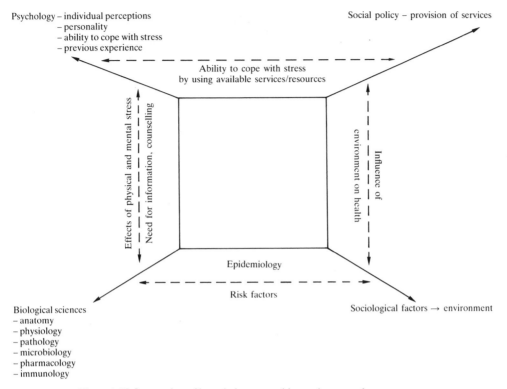

Figure 1.15 Integration of knowledge to provide nursing care of women.

malignant changes in cervical tissue. However, 'labelling' women as a particular type because they develop the disease is not helpful, and may be misleading: although some women may have several obvious risk factors, others may have few or none. People are individuals and do not always appear as classic textbook presentations.

Discussion of risk factors in relation to health problems and disease brings us back to the main point introduced earlier in the chapter: women are individuals who require individual consideration whether they receive most of their care in hospital or as outpatients. To provide this care effectively nurses need to integrate knowledge from many different subject areas, as shown in Fig. 1.15.

References

Argyle, M. (1983) 'What use are relatives?', *New Society* 64 (1071), pp. 293–4.
Boore, J. (1978) *Prescription for Recovery*, London: Royal College of Nursing.
Broadley, K. (1986) 'Cervical cancer', *Nursing Times* 82 (24), pp. 29–32.
Brown, G. and Harris, T. (1978) *The Social Origins of Depression*, London: Tavistock Publications.

Buckley, J.D. *et al.* (1981) 'Case control study of the husbands of women with dysplasia or carcinoma of the cervix uteri', *Lancet* 2, pp. 1010–5.

Burghes, L. (1980) 'Living from hand to mouth: a study of 65 families living on supplementary benefit', *Poverty Pamphlet 50*, London: Family Service Units and Child Poverty Action Group.

Coussins, J. and Coote, A. (1981) 'The family in the firing line: a discussion document on family policy', *Poverty Pamphlet 51*, London: National Council for Civil Liberties and Child Poverty Action Group.

Cox, C. (1985) 'Outlawing a barbaric practice' (Female Circumcision Bill), *Nursing Times* 81 (7), p. 20.

Cranfield, R. and Cranfield, E. (1983) 'Female circumcision: an assault?', *Practitioner* 227, pp. 816–17.

Doyal, L. (1983) 'Women's health and the sexual division of labour', *Critical Social Policy* 7, summer, pp. 21–33.

Faulkner, A. (1984) 'Health education and nursing', *Nursing Times* 80 (9), pp. 45–6.

Franklin, B.L. (1974) *Patient Anxiety on Admission to Hospital*, London: Royal College of Nursing.

Gould, D.J. (1987) *Infection and Patient Care: A Guide for Nurses*, London: Heinemann, p. 146.

Gould, D.J. (1982) 'Recovery from hysterectomy', *Nursing Times* 78 (42), pp. 1769–71.

Gould, D.J. (1986) 'Hidden problems after a hysterectomy', *Nursing Times* 82 (23), pp. 43–5.

Graham, H. (1984) *Women, Health and the Family*, Brighton: Wheatsheaf Books.

Harris, R. *et al.* (1980) 'Characteristics of women with dysplasia or carcinoma *in situ* of the cervix uteri', *British Journal of Cancer* 42, pp. 359–69.

Hart, N. (1982) 'Explaining health inequality between the sexes', *Radical Community Medicine* 11/12, pp. 25–34.

Hayward, J. (1975) *Information – Prescription against Pain*, London: Royal College of Nursing.

Holmes, P. (1988) 'Cervicography in the picture', *Nursing Times* 84 (9), pp. 20–1.

Hillman, M. *et al.* (1974) *Mobility and Accessibility in the Outer Metropolitan Area*, Report of the Department of Environment: Political and Economic Planning.

Hunt, S. (1985) 'Below the breadline', *Nursing Times Community Outlook* (October), pp. 19–21.

Land, H. (1983) 'Poverty and gender: the distribution of resources within the family' In: Brown, M. (ed.) *The Structure of Disadvantage*, London: Heinemann.

Nelson, J.H. (1967) 'The relationship of coitus to carcinoma of the cervix', *American Journal of Public Health* 57, pp. 840–7.

Nursing Times News Focus (1989) *Nursing Times* 85 (15), pp. 16–17.

Oakley, A. (1974) *The Sociology of Housework*, Bath: Martin Robertson.

Perkins, E.R. (1979) 'Defining the need. An analysis of varying teaching goals in ante-natal classes', *International Journal of Nursing Studies* 16 (3), pp. 275–82.

Richman, N. *et al.* (1982) *Preschool to School: A Behavioural Study*, London: Academic Press.

Rimmer, L. and Popay, J. (1982) *Employment Trends and the Family*, London: Study Commission of the Family.

Sharpe, S. (1976) *Just like a Girl*, London: Pelican.

Sharpe, S. (1984) *Double Identity: the Lives of Working Mothers*, London: Pelican.

Sibary, K. *et al.* (1977) 'Women with cervical cancer detected through population screening: implications for health education', *International Journal of Health Education* 20 (3), pp. 205–11.

Smith, J.P. (1979) 'The challenge of health education for nurses in the 1980s', *Journal of Advanced Nursing* 4, pp. 531–43.

Steele, S.J. and Goodwin, M.F. (1975) 'A pamphlet to answer the patient's questions before hysterectomy', *Lancet* 2, pp. 492–3.

Stellman, J. (1977) *Women's Work, Women's Health*, New York: Pantheon Books.

Townsend, P. and Davidson, N. (1982) *Inequalities in Health: the Black Report*, Harmondsworth: Penguin.

Trevathan, E. *et al.* (1983) 'Cigarette smoking and dysplasia and carcinoma *in situ* of the uterine cervix', *Journal of the American Medical Association* 250, pp. 499–502.

Underhill, R.A. and Dewhurst, J. (1978) 'The doctor cannot always tell', *Lancet* 1, pp. 375–6.

Vessey, M.P. *et al.* (1983) 'Neoplasia of the cervix uteri and contraception: a possible adverse effect of the pill', *Lancet* 2, pp. 930–4.

Wakenfield, J. *et al.* (1973) 'Relation of abnormal cytological smears and carcinoma of the cervix uteri to husband's occupation', *British Medical Journal* 280, pp. 142–4.

Weissman, M. and Klerman, G. (1977) 'Symptom patterns in primary and secondary depression: a comparison', *Archives of General Psychiatry* 34, pp. 854–6.

Wilson-Barnett, J. (1975) 'Factors affecting patients' response to hospitalisation', *Journal of Advanced Nursing* 3, pp. 221–8.

Wilson-Barnett, J. (1979) *Stress in Hospital*, Edinburgh: Churchill Livingstone.

Wilson, J.M.G. and Jungner, G. (1968) *Principles and Practice of Screening for Disease*, World Health Organisation WHO Public Health Paper 34.

Yule, R. (1984) 'Cervical cancer 2. Screening and prevention', *Nursing Mirror* 159 (13), pp. 37–9.

2   Controlling Fertility

Choice of contraception, a problem facing most sexually active women during their fertile years, will depend on a range of factors – particularly the existence or otherwise of a permanent partner, and the stage in the lifespan of the family. Advice given to a couple in a stable relationship may be quite inappropriate for a single girl or older people who feel they definitely could not cope with another baby. Parity may be more important than age. A couple in their twenties may request sterilisation because they judge their family to be complete while others, already in their late thirties, may decide to have a baby. Other influential factors include religious or cultural beliefs, social class, financial circumstances and existing medical or gynaecological conditions. The purpose of this chapter is to illustrate the services available and the different methods of birth control which suit the needs of different people.

Provision of the Family Planning Services

Although contraceptives are supplied free of charge under the National Health Service, provision of the service is not uniform across the country (Leathard 1980). Women may obtain advice and supplies from a family planning clinic organised by the health authority, from a GP who has received appropriate training, or from one of the private or charitable organisations, e.g. the Marie Stopes Clinics, the British Pregnancy Advisory Service (BPAS), or the Brook Clinics which are geared to the needs of young people.

The nurse's role

Nurses who work in family planning clinics, health centres and gynaecology departments can take a special course organised by the English National Board. They are then in a position to provide guidance and to fit contraceptive devices, but not to prescribe oral contraceptives.

Family planning nurses sometimes argue that these restrictions prevent them using all the skills they have acquired (Cowper 1984). However, the success of the family planning service depends upon other important nursing skills, especially those of communication and counselling, not just ability to prescribe the pill. Most people have some idea about the type of contraception they wish to use but need health professionals to provide detailed information. General knowledge about success rates and side effects is quite different from information needed when a woman contemplates using a particular contraceptive herself. Having heard about possible advantages and disadvantages, she will want to know 'Will this apply to me?'.

Clients must feel comfortable talking to the nurse about one of the most private aspects of their lives. Details of how often they have intercourse will probably influence choice – a woman who has sex infrequently is unlikely to choose the pill. There may be reluctance to share this information with doctors, who are often perceived as being 'too busy' and concerned mainly with health problems.

The role of the non-specialist nurse
The need for contraception is not connected with illness, but with normal, everyday life. The nurse, in her role as a health educator, is often regarded as the most appropriate source of advice, especially if she has already established a relationship with the woman. It is evident that opportunities are needed for nurses who work outside family planning and gynaecology departments to update their knowledge in this sphere. Any nurse may be approached by a woman requesting information. Those working in the community (midwives, health visitors, school and occupational health nurses) may provide information informally and as a part of health education programmes.

In hospital, women may worry that their own or partner's illness may alter the suitability of their existing contraception. Sometimes the nurse may be asked a question about contraception because the individual really wants some information about another related issue.

■   Janet Reid was in hospital during an exacerbation of acute rheumatoid arthritis. Although she was looking forward to going home, her nurse sensed that something was worrying her.

Janet's hands had now become so badly affected by the disease that she retained little manual dexterity. She had come to terms with many aspects of her disability (not being able to sew or knit) but was distressed that she might no longer be able to fit her vaginal diaphragm. The nurse encouraged Janet to express *all* that was worrying her. This included fears about contraception, and her sex life in general. Janet experienced considerable pain and was distressed about the deformity associated with arthritis. She did not like her husband to see her undressed.

The nurse was able to explore a number of different coping strategies. These included possible methods of pain control long-term at home, and approaching the topic of sexual needs as well as the more practical aspects of contraception with her husband.

Sexual attractiveness and the need to express sexuality are not the exclusive province of the young; they extend to people in all age groups, with and without disabilities. After illness or surgery (colostomy formation, mastectomy, amputation) individuals may need special help to come to terms with altered body image and encouragement to broach this topic.

Advice relating to young people
Although teenage motherhood is a subject often exploited in the media, the number of young girls who have babies is decreasing (Sharpe 1987). This is undoubtedly due to the availability of legal abortion since 1968, and may also be related to increased usage of contraceptives by young people, a situation challenged by the Gillick campaign in Britain in 1984–85.

Under Section 5 of the Sexual Offences Act (1956), it is unlawful for a man to have sexual intercourse with a girl under the age of 13. Under Section 6 of the same Act, it is also an offence if the girl is between 13 and 16 years. However, health care professionals have long accepted that some girls do become sexually active at an early age and should, in their own best interests, receive contraceptive advice. It was felt that young girls determined to have sexual relations need protection from the physical and emotional effects of pregnancy, and contraception could be lawfully provided. Although the written consent of parents is preferred, it has always been recognised that girls may not receive their support or wish to discuss these issues with them.

Victoria Gillick was initially successful in obtaining a ban on the provision of contraceptive advice and prescriptions to girls under 16 without parental consent. This ruling was overturned by the House of Lords in October 1985. However, the Gillick campaign resulted in a great deal of confusion, both among young people and health care professionals concerned about their emotional and physical welfare.

Evaluating effectiveness

Contraceptive services in Britain gained legitimate recognition as part of preventative medicine in 1930 when local authorities were empowered for the first time to provide birth control to women under 'necessary medical circumstances'. No further legislation was passed until the Abortion Laws in 1967 (see Chapter 3). Potts and Diggory (1983), in their comprehensive account of contraceptive methods, explain that deliberate prevention of conception has traditionally received condemnation. Such attitudes were widespread among health care professionals and lay people until comparatively recently. Information about contraception was disseminated slowly and most available methods were welcomed uncritically by grateful people desperate to avoid yet another baby. Scientific studies of effectiveness were relatively few and not conducted rigorously.

The popularity of different methods relative to one another has changed over the years (see Table 2.1). This is reflected in the amount of scientific interest that has been invested in them, some methods having been subject to more rigorous scrutiny than others. More trials have been conducted with marketable products than with 'natural' methods which nobody is trying to sell. Marketed products have been subject to quality control procedures by the British Institute of Standards since 1927. However,

Table 2.1 Popularity of methods of contraception for women aged 15–44 in Britain and Northern Ireland (based on FPA estimates, early 1980s)

Method	Percentage (%)
Combined pill	26
Condom	25
Infertile	10
Sterilised	7
Pregnant/Trying to become pregnant	5
IUCD	4.5
Cap/Vaginal diaphragm	4
Natural methods	2
POP	1.5
Not sexually active/Other method/None	15

Note: Number of women in survey = 11.5 million

no method of contraception is more efficient than the individual using it, so the client's motivation must form an important part of the assessment when choice is made.

Two different measures are used to evaluate the effectiveness of contraceptives: theoretical effectiveness and use effectiveness. It is important to distinguish between the two, because results are not interchangeable.

Theoretical effectiveness is the rate of pregnancies experienced when a contraceptive is used under *ideal* conditions. It does *not* include mistakes or omissions on the part of the consumer.

Use effectiveness is the rate of pregnancies experienced when the contraceptive is used in the real-life situation. Mistakes and omissions are taken into consideration in the results.

Studies of theoretical effectiveness are performed under controlled conditions in the laboratory, while use effectiveness studies are epidemiological and employ a survey approach, gathering information by interviews or questionnaires. There are a number of problems attached to obtaining detailed, accurate and reliable information from the general public in this way.

Individuals may need some persuasion to take part, especially if the method of data collection is time consuming or inconvenient. They may not understand what is required or be unable to recall past events. Problems are magnified when the topic, like sex or contraception, is of a deeply personal nature. Some methods may appear more effective than they really are because individuals may not wish to admit 'failure', choose to forget that a much-loved child was unplanned or that an abortion was necessary. Spontaneous abortions must be accounted for when calculating failure rate, a difficulty hard to overcome since women may not realise when a very early miscarriage has occurred. Results may be confounded because people willing to take part may already be unusually careful, or become so in the knowledge that they are being monitored. Obtaining a sample can be extremely difficult. When supplies or prescriptions are necessary subjects can be recruited from clinics or health centres, but this is not possible when the method does not involve medical intervention.

Calculating failure rates

The comparative effectiveness of different methods are calculated by the *PEARL formula*, which bases failure rate on the number of pregnancies per hundred women using the method per year (see Table 2.2 for use effectiveness). Much depends on the motivation and perseverance of the couple concerned, and the skill of the researcher when data are gathered. Using the information generated from these studies requires an understanding of the research process because of the limitations of the methods used.

Helping clients to choose a method

Nurses can do much to help clients make informed decisions if they can recommend written information as well as giving verbal advice. Many books about contraception have been designed specifically for lay people. They provide a valuable source of information, since clients are more likely to assimilate knowledge if they are able to read at their own pace and discuss matters with their partner at home.

Suggesting that clients can be advised to read about health care themselves is not meant to imply that nurses or doctors should not provide information, but to point out that much is available to help ordinary people understand their bodies, including the effects of contraception. To make suitable recommendations, nurses need to understand the individual needs of clients, sources of information available, and content, so they can prevent or dispel misconceptions. The quality of books and magazine articles is variable. A reading list with comments is provided at the end of the chapter. Factors likely to influence choice (see page 38) must be taken into consideration.

■   Amanda and Frank Driver were anxious to start a family as soon as their income improved. The occupational health nurse at Amanda's workplace advised against barrier methods because of their relative ineffectiveness compared to the pill and the intrauterine contraceptive device (IUCD). Amanda and Frank felt that a simple reversible method would suit them best. By reading numerous books and articles they soon realised that the effectiveness of barrier methods is enhanced if they are carefully used, in conjunction with spermicide. A study cited by Potts and Diggory (1983, page 64) revealed that failure rate had been as low as 3.9 per cent in a group of newly married couples followed up over a five year period in the North of England. For those who were very highly motivated, the rate was 1.6 per cent. Amanda and Frank used barrier methods with confidence and success until they were able to plan their first pregnancy.

Table 2.2 Comparison failure rates of different methods of contraceptives based on the PEARL formula (all figures are approximate)

Method	Estimated failure rate (use effectiveness)
Oral contraceptives	1%
Vasectomy	1%
Tubal ligation	4%
IUCD	3%
Condom	13%
Diaphragm	14%
'Natural' methods	38%

Methods of contraception

This account begins by describing non-invasive methods which do not disrupt normal physiological processes, moving on to the IUCD, oral contraception and sterilisation.

Coitus interruptus

As far as it is possible to tell, *coitus interruptus*, practised since biblical times, is still popular today. It is referred to by a variety of euphemisms: 'Being careful', 'Taking him to church but not letting him sing in the choir', are two such examples. Unfamiliarity with these terms on the part of health care professionals may have underestimated the extent to which it is practised.

Coitus interruptus has several drawbacks: skill is necessary since the penis must be withdrawn from the vagina before ejaculation (most sperm are liberated in the first part of the ejaculate), it is messy, and it is said to be a cause of psychological upset in one or both partners although hard evidence for this is lacking. Discovery that sperm begin to escape before ejaculation has cast doubts on reliability. However, it is known that coitus interruptus was practised by the upper social classes throughout Europe in the sixteenth and seventeenth centuries. Their families were consistently smaller than those of peasants to whom the practice was unknown, suggesting that it is at least reasonably effective.

Today, it is accepted that sperm do not remain viable long unless deposited directly into the vagina so, in an emergency, coitus interruptus is probably better than taking no precautions at all. After all, it costs nothing, requires no prescription and cannot be left at home.

The main disadvantage of coitus interruptus is that withdrawal can come too late. Once they have entered the female genital tract, sperm remain viable for between three and five days, and in every millilitre of semen there are approximately one million sperm.

Natural methods of contraception

Women can learn to recognise the fertile phase of the menstrual cycle so that intercourse can be avoided when conception is possible. The two main methods, which involve detecting temperature changes at ovulation or variations in the cervical mucus (*Billings Method*), are discussed in Chapter 7 because they depend on sound understanding of the menstrual cycle.

Douching

The use of fluid to wash semen out of the vagina is another old method which, depending on the solution employed, may have been responsible for more harm than good. Soap solutions and many other easily obtainable fluids have been recommended, particularly those believed to have disinfectant properties. In 1842, Charles Knowlton, one of the foremost pioneers of contraception, advocated douching with alum, green tea and vinegar. All these substances exposed the vaginal mucosa to varying degrees of trauma and changes in pH. Sperm can penetrate the cervical canal within 90 seconds of ejaculation; attempts to dislodge them a few minutes later are futile, and may even wash them higher.

Douching gained widespread popularity in the USA where several commercial preparations are still available, but has always been discouraged in Britain. It is not recommended today.

Other ideas current at the time when douching was commonly practised included beliefs that violent activity (jumping backwards, running or shouting) could dislodge semen. Some myths are still with us: it is commonly held, for example, that conception cannot occur the first time intercourse happens, or without female orgasm. Orgasm encourages conception because negative pressure is set up in the uterus as it contracts, helping to draw sperm up the genital tract, but it is not essential.

Barrier methods

Spermicides
The use of chemicals to occlude the cervix and destroy sperm stretches into antiquity. Ancient Egyptians used a variety of materials, including herbs and honey, as mechanical barriers. Francis Place (1771–1854) advised women to insert sponges soaked in vinegar before intercourse. Although the vagina is mildly acidic throughout the reproductive years, semen is alkaline, and conception is favoured in a mildly alkaline environment. Therefore, vinegar, a weak acid, has contraceptive properties.

Modern spermicides (available with or without prescription) are marketed as foams, gels or pessaries (see Fig. 2.1) exerting their effect only when melted or evaporated. Clients should be instructed to insert them *before* intercourse and repeat the application if intercourse occurs again. Vaginal diaphragms and caps are not reliable without spermicide. C film, an advance on some of the older preparations, is a

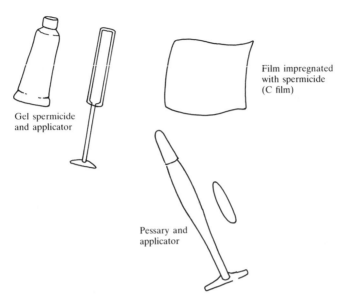

Gel spermicide
and applicator

Film impregnated
with spermicide
(C film)

Pessary and
applicator

Figure 2.1 Spermicides and applicators.

soluble film of dried polyvinyl alcohol which melts without liquefying. It is more likely to stay in place.

Spermicides work by breaking down the surface tension of semen or acting as enzyme inhibitors immobilising sperm. Most modern preparations still contain quinine, one of the earliest substances used. Quality control estimates the number of active sperm in cervical mucus aspirated several hours after intercourse. Anxious clients seeking a non-invasive form of contraception can be reassured that allergic reactions are seldom reported. Spermicides are not absorbed from the vaginal mucosa and are therefore unlikely to result in systemic side effects.

People who find discussion of their sex lives an invasion of privacy may find spermicides an attractive option, yet the extent to which they are used alone has never been estimated. This is an option open to women nearing the menopause who perceive fertility to be declining, especially if their partners experience problems with sheaths or withdrawal as they get older. Even in these circumstances, however, there is sometimes a need for professional guidance.

■   Sarah Cohen was 52 and had not had a period for two years. She and her husband had always relied on condoms and spermicides. As they grew older, using a condom became a nuisance. Eventually Sarah used pessaries. She was alarmed when an acquaintance only a few years younger than herself became pregnant and was persuaded to go to a family planning clinic. A test to measure plasma hormone levels revealed that Sarah had had the change of life (see Chapter 9). Contraception could now be safely abandoned.

Condoms (sheaths, French letters)

Condoms, supposedly invented by a doctor of that name during the seventeenth century, date from an earlier time when they were intended mainly to avoid infection. Traditionally a method favoured among the lower socio-economic groups, they reached the height of popularity in the 1950s. Recently, interest has been renewed. Condoms are recommended as a means of preventing the spread of sexually transmitted disease, especially AIDS.

Used conscientiously, condoms are a reliable form of birth control. Again, they are cheap and available without prescription. Most people choosing this method do not seek professional advice. However, much could be done to promote effective use to avoid conception and infection during health education programmes, especially with young people. They need to be told that the key to success is applying the fine latex sheath over the *full* length of the erect penis, excluding air to minimise risk of bursting. Removal must occur without spillage. Clients should be advised to purchase condoms bearing the kite mark of the British Institute of Standards. These are of approved length and thickness (see Fig. 2.2). Different styles are available. With novelties obtained from mail order suppliers, safety may be of a secondary consideration. Consumers can be reassured that reputable brands are unlikely to rupture since quality control involves rigorous testing and expiry dating.

Condoms reduce sensation, although modern fine gauge varieties are less intrusive. A second criticism is that application disrupts sexual activity.

There have been few studies of use effectiveness, but it is generally accepted that most failures are related to consumer error. At one time, it was suggested that for maximum effectiveness condoms should be worn whenever intercourse took place, but a more liberal view is now emerging. Spencer (1986) writing in the popular nursing press, argues that in the past many couples have been discouraged because of the rigorous stipulations associated with all barrier methods. She argues that condoms or vaginal diaphragms could in theory be effective without spermicide except during the highly fertile phase of the menstrual cycle. Trials to investigate safety are currently underway. Until more is known advice to clients must be cautious, since appropriateness and acceptability are likely to vary between individuals and to change over time for the same couple.

■   Jane and Martin Bishop had two children, four years apart in age. When the second baby arrived, Jane told her health visitor that she did not wish to take oral contraceptives, but was not keen to try a vaginal diaphragm either. The health visitor knew that Jane was not planning to work until both children were at school. The family was financially stable, and Jane and Martin would not be distressed if they had a third child. At the health visitor's suggestion, they used condoms in the fertile part of the cycle only. When, two years later, Jane became pregnant again both were pleased, although the pregnancy had not in the strictest sense been planned.

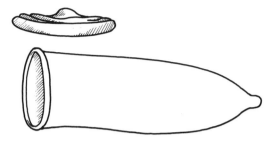

Figure 2.2 Condom.

Vaginal diaphragms and caps

Different styles of diaphragm and cap have been developed (see Fig. 2.3), although diaphragms tend to be tried first on the grounds that they are easier to use.

Female barrier methods have traditionally found favour with women belonging to the upper socio-economic groups. They attained greatest popularity in the 1960s until oral contraceptives became widely available. With the current emphasis on 'natural' and 'healthy' lifestyles, interest has been renewed. Lack of acceptance may again be related to instructions for effectiveness. For the best results, the Family Planning Association advises women take the following measures:

- Smear spermicide around the rim;
- Apply more spermicide if intercourse occurs more than three hours after insertion;
- Add more spermicide if intercourse is repeated;
- Leave the diaphragm in place for at least six but no longer than 24 hours.

Diaphragms and caps can be placed in position to occlude the cervix before intercourse (see Fig. 2.4). Though not disruptive, they are messy. Insertion can be time

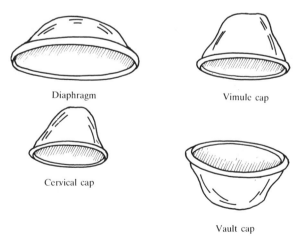

Diaphragm   Vimule cap

Cervical cap

Vault cap

Figure 2.3 Types of vaginal caps and diaphragms available.

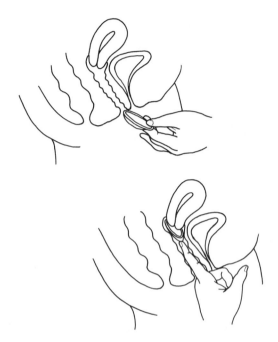

Figure 2.4 Inserting a vaginal diaphragm.

consuming and the woman must be able to locate her cervix: some may be discouraged through dislike of handling their own genitals.

Caps and diaphragms must be fitted by a trained doctor or nurse, and skill is necessary on the part of the woman if the method is to be reliable. Women must first learn
to use a 'practice' cap while not depending on it for contraception, returning to the
clinic to ensure that it is properly in place. If she loses weight, she will require a *larger*
size because fatty tissue will be lost making the cap unstable. She must examine the
cap for flaws or signs of damage, wash it in soap and water after use and store it dry.

Table 2.2 suggests that female barrier methods are slightly less effective than
condoms, but this can be misleading as much depends on the individual concerned.
Failure rate can be as low as 2 per cent (Vessey *et al.* 1982). The nurse plays a crucial
role in assessing the individual woman's suitability to use the cap and motivation to
continue. Time must be taken to explore feelings; minor dissatisfactions may betray
underlying disenchantment, opening the way for carelessness and unplanned pregnancy.

Side effects are few. Isolated instances of toxic shock syndrome have been reported,
but a definite relationship has never been established. Cap users may complain slightly
more often of urinary tract infections, but have some protection against sexually
transmitted disease.

Sponges
Historically natural sponges, impregnated with a variety of different substances, were
used to avoid conception. Synthetic sponges treated with spermicide have recently

been marketed in Britain and are finding favour because they can be purchased without prescription, fitted and removed more easily than caps, although they are less reliable. They are a reasonably effective option for some women during the 'safer' part of the cycle.

The femshield or 'female condom'
The femshield is a newly developed method of contraception which consists of a blind-ended hollow tube 15 cm long and about 7 cm in diameter, with a soft ring at the open end to hold it in place against the vulva. A separate, slightly firmer ring is provided to aid insertion and hold the device in place. It is made of robust elastic polyurethane (similar to the material from which colostomy bags are manufactured) and is said to interfere less with sensation than the male condom. Studies in Denmark suggest that this may prove an effective and acceptable method (Richardson 1988).

The intrauterine contraceptive device (IUCD, coil)

It has been known for many years that a foreign body inserted into the uterus can prevent conception. Medical interest was kindled in the 1950s, when it became apparent that women fitted with vaginal pessaries to correct genital prolapse would rarely conceive. Today, a wide range of IUCDs are available, manufactured from polythene or a combination of polythene and copper (see Fig. 2.5). Some are impregnated with hormones to enhance contraceptive effect. Mode of action is still not fully established, although some effects are exerted after conception (see Chapter 3). It has been demonstrated that the IUCD sets up an inflammatory response in the endometrium. Leucocytes have been isolated from the surface of coils and the cervix in large numbers. These may destroy the implanting blastocyst. Plasma antibody levels increase, suggesting an immune response. This is the only evidence of systemic rather than local effect. Endocrine function is unchanged, although the secretory phase (second half) of the menstrual cycle is shortened. Women may notice their periods becoming more frequent. Locally acting hormones called prostaglandins increase contractability of the uterus and uterine tubes, explaining some of the side effects of the IUCD heard so often by nurses working in gynaecology departments.

Disadvantages and advantages of the IUCD
The main problems are summarised below.

Method of insertion
An IUCD can only be fitted after special training. A Cuscoe's speculum holds the vaginal walls apart while the cervix is grasped with forceps. The introducer containing the device is passed through the cervical canal, and the IUCD is expelled into the uterus, where it assumes its final shape (see Fig. 2.6).

Insertion can be painful, especially in nulliparous women. It must take place in a clinic or hospital department. On a few, very rare, occasions cardiac arrest has occurred so equipment for resuscitation must always be available.

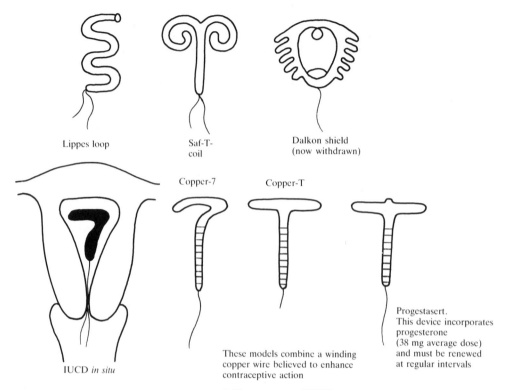

Figure 2.5 Different types of IUCD.

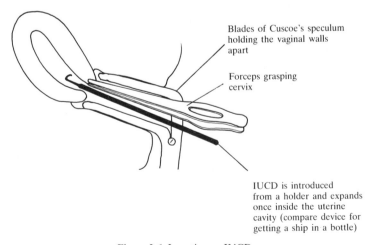

Figure 2.6 Inserting an IUCD.

Expulsion
Five to ten per cent of IUCDs are spontaneously expelled, usually soon after insertion. Fitting is best just after menstruation because the uterus is less likely to contract and there is little chance of pregnancy having occurred earlier in the cycle.

Periodic checking
It is necessary to ensure periodically that the IUCD is still in position. Once it has been fitted, two strings hang down into the vagina. Women should be taught to feel that they are still there. Checking is most convenient after menstruation but some women dislike doing this.

Regular check-ups are necessary to ensure that all is well. Copper devices are usually replaced every 2–4 years, but plastic ones can remain *in situ* indefinitely providing check-ups, are normal. Removal is usually quick and painless.

Occasionally partners complain about the strings, which may need trimming, but sometimes complaints reported by women reflect underlying disenchantment with the method.

Translocation
Very rarely an IUCD may pass through the wall of the uterus into the pelvic cavity, usually because of faulty insertion. Modern IUCDs are impregnated with radio opaque material so they can be located by X-ray. If translocated, an IUCD must be removed via laparoscopic incision.

Increased menstrual loss
As well as stimulating release of prostaglandins, coils may cause the uterus to synthesise more of its natural anti-coagulant substances, which normally help prevent menstrual loss clotting.

Infection
Coils increase risk of pelvic infection and are unsuitable for women with a history of pelvic inflammatory disease. If infection occurs once a coil has been fitted, it must be removed.

Ectopic pregnancy
There is increased risk, probably because the IUCD affects tubal motility. Complaints of pelvic pain should never be dismissed.

Because these side effects may be serious enough to bring women into hospital, nurses working on gynaecology wards may conclude that little can be said in favour of the IUCD. However, their colleagues in the community may disagree. Complaints or hospital treatment occur when something has gone wrong. There are many women, especially those unable, unwilling or too forgetful to take the pill, who need a highly reliable form of contraception and find the coil acceptable. Theoretical failure rate is low and consumer error impossible. For those few failures reported, congenital abnormality is very low.

Table 2.3 Effects of oral contraceptives

Effect	Combined Pill	Progesterone only pill (POP)
1. Reduces FSH released from anterior pituitary so prevents eggs from maturing	X X X X	X
2. Prevents the mid-cycle LH surge, so no eggs can be released from the ovary	X X X X	X X
3. Makes the uterine lining hostile to an implanting blastocyst	X X X	X X
4. Thickens cervical mucus so that it cannot be penetrated by sperm	X X X	X X X
5. Alters motility of the uterine tubes so that the egg arrives at the uterus too immature to be implanted	?	X

Oral contraception

Oral contraceptives are synthetic steroid hormones which disrupt normal endocrine function. They are the only genuinely modern methods, although down the centuries women have taken many different oral preparations hoping to avoid pregnancy.

Two types are available, the combined pill containing oestrogen and progesterone, and the progesterone only pill (*POP*). Effectiveness and mode of action are compared in Table 2.3.

Before the pill is prescribed the following routine investigations are necessary:

- Complete physical examination to ensure the woman is in good health and may safely take steroid hormones (see Table 2.4). Blood pressure and weight are checked and a medical history is taken to rule out cardiovascular disease, diabetes, and other endocrine disorders. Women who smoke are advised not to take the pill, especially after their mid-thirties.
- Bimanual and speculum examination to check for gynaecological abnormalities.
- A cervical smear to detect any abnormal cells.

Client teaching is a very important aspect of the family planning nurse's role. Clients considering the pill need to be informed of the following:

- How it works;
- Why it may very occasionally fail;
- Possible side effects and the action which should be taken if they occur.

Table 2.4 Contraindications against the combined oral pill

Category 1 (Women for whom the combined pill would definitely not be a good choice)
  Evidence of cardiovascular disease
  Family history of cardiovascular disease
  Hypertension
  Heavy smoking
  Obesity
  Migraine
  Liver disease
  Severe depression

Category 2 (Women who require special surveillance)
  Collagen disease
  Otosclerosis
  Diabetes mellitus
  Sickle cell anaemia and other blood disorders
  Severe varicose veins
  Mild to moderate depression
  Women reaching their mid-thirties

Taking the combined pill

Synthetic hormones in the combined pill block the release of natural oestrogen and progesterone so that no egg can be released half way through the menstrual cycle. The first day of bleeding is regarded as Day One of the cycle. One pill is taken every day from Day Five onwards. Each pack contains twenty-one pills. When all have been taken, a seven day break from pill-taking will follow. During this time, bleeding will occur. The new packet of pills must be started again on Day Five of the cycle, regardless of whether bleeding has stopped. This bleeding is not true menstruation, however, for the pill hormones prevent the endometrium developing fully. Periods will be light and probably pain free; the pill is often given for menstrual problems. Another advantage is that the pill regulates the cycle so precisely that women taking it know exactly when they will start to bleed.

Pill failure

For every hundred women taking the pill for one year, 0.1–1.1 per cent failures are reported, almost entirely due to user error. Oral contraception may fail in the following circumstances:

- If intercourse takes place without additional precautions before the first fourteen days of pill taking are complete, because the hormones will not have had time to exert full effect. Women may be given a supply of condoms and pessaries for the first fourteen days.
- If the woman forgets to take one or more pills. Pharmaceutical companies have devised ingenious packaging (see Fig. 2.7), but forgotten pills are still probably the main reason for failure. If the missed pill is taken within twelve hours all will be well. If delay exceeds twelve hours, the remaining pills in the packet should

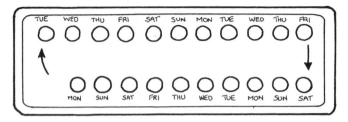

Figure 2.7 Oral contraceptives.

be taken as usual but the woman should consider herself unprotected during this time (*the fourteen day rule*). Modern ultra low dose pills are highly reliable, but there is less margin for error than with older brands containing more oestrogen.

- If the woman has a stomach upset, with vomiting or diarrhoea. The hormones may not be fully absorbed from the gastro-intestinal tract, so the fourteen day rule must be observed.
- If the woman takes drugs which interfere with absorption of the hormones in the pill. Like many hormones and drugs, oral contraceptives are metabolised in the liver, then excreted in bile entering the duodenum from the liver via the common bile duct. Some of the pill hormones are then re-absorbed. If the activity of hepatic enzymes is interrupted by certain groups of drugs, including phenytoin and phenobarbitone, the rate of excretion of oral contraceptives is increased. Antibiotics which destroy normal gut bacteria may cause diarrhoea, so oral contraceptives may not be fully absorbed. Pregnancies have occurred during treatment with ampicillin and erythromycin. Women should be asked about drugs they are taking and specifically warned about antibiotics because these are so often prescribed.

'Breakthrough bleeding'

Although there are several reasons for 'breakthrough bleeding', the most likely is that plasma steroid hormone levels have become very low, so that too little reaches the uterus. If this happens because pills have been forgotten or not properly absorbed, there is a danger of pregnancy and the fourteen day rule must be observed. However, bleeding may be a problem of very low dose pills and, if it becomes a nuisance, the woman may feel happier with a brand containing more oestrogen.

Sometimes intermenstrual bleeding indicates an underlying gynaecological problem. Although this is less likely in young women, it is wise to seek medical advice promptly. All women who take the pill must be followed up regularly.

Health and the combined pill

Despite the possible inconvenience of breakthrough bleeding and narrower safety limits, most doctors now prescribe low dose pills because of side effects reported over the years by women taking higher doses of oestrogen.

Neither the combined pill nor POP are the wonder drugs they were once thought to be. Stimulus for development came in the 1950s, mainly due to rapid population expansion. The earliest trials were conducted among deprived populations in Puerto Rico before cautious introduction to the USA, then Britain. The earliest synthetic progesterone, extracted from vegetables by Russell and Marks in 1943, were hailed as a new and effective form of treatment for menstrual disorders, but it was not long before their contraceptive effects were recognised and found to be enhanced by oestrogen. Pincus, who developed the pill and conducted the earliest trials in Puerto Rico, believed the side effects would prove unacceptable, but the women were remarkably uncomplaining. Possibly their poor standard of living and low expectancy of health care inclined them to be uncritical of any measure guaranteed to free them from additional, unwanted pregnancies. Nevertheless, manufacturers were amazed at the ready acceptance of the pill throughout the Western world.

It has been claimed that oral contraception has been responsible for a revolutionary change in lifestyle, especially for women. This is not exaggerated. Freedom from the worry of unwanted pregnancy is probably one of the main factors which made the emergence of the permissive society possible in the 1960s. More than thirty years later women are beginning to raise the doubts anticipated then. Balanced against this are the considerable benefits of pill taking. Even today in Britain, pregnancy carries some health risks. These are greater in developing countries. Anxious women, nevertheless convinced they need the pill, may keep their fears in proportion if it is pointed out that to exist in the twentieth century at all is to take risks.

Oral contraceptives have been the subject of more rigorous pharmaceutical investigation than any other drug in history (Vaughan 1972). If research with other drugs had been as intensive, the number of side effects reported would increase proportionately. However, the pill differs from other drugs because *healthy* women take it continuously, sometimes for years, for social rather than medical reasons. The synthetic hormones it contains are more potent than natural oestrogen or progesterone, and require detoxification in the liver. Despite all the research so far conducted, more follow-up studies are necessary before the long term effects of the pill become apparent.

Research and the pill
Many of the studies so far undertaken have involved large numbers of women, matched for previous levels of fitness, age and other socio-demographic variables with control subjects, so that health can be compared. However, many of these studies were initiated at a time when higher dosages of oestrogen were used and, in practice, 'matching' has not always been perfect. Three major studies were initiated in 1968 (Guillebaud 1984, page 88). Two of these took place in Britain (*The Oral Contraception Study* by the Royal College of General Practitioners and *The Oxford Study* by the British Family Planning Association). The *Walnut Greek Study* took place in California. The results of all three were similar. They suggested that combined pills affect virtually every organ in the body, with effects so complicated that early comparisons to pregnancy have long since been abandoned. Side effects may represent a serious threat to health or be considered trivial (see Table 2.5), although in practice what a doctor may regard as a nuisance can be a valid reason to a woman for abandoning the method. In view of the many brands available (see Table 2.6), it should be possible to select one most suited to the needs of the individual, but in

Table 2.5 Changes in body chemistry, resulting with use of combined oral contraceptives

Liver metabolism	Generally altered in all pill takers, apparently causing no harm to the liver itself. However, as the biggest gland and major manufacturing unit in the body, the liver is involved in the biosynthesis of *all* the other substances in this table
Blood glucose levels	Tend to be increased, especially immediately after eating. Some pill takers have fasting glucose problems similar to those in mild diabetes mellitus
Blood lipid levels	Tend to be increased, but effects are greatly reduced with modern low dose pills. The increased risk of thrombosis, especially with older pills, was probably due to this
Blood albumin levels	Albumin is the main plasma protein in the blood. Its levels decrease in pill takers. Significance is unknown
Clotting factors	Oestrogen increases blood levels of most of the clotting factors and reduces the levels of anti-thrombin III, the main anti-clotting factor, so it enhances blood coagulability
Platelets	Aggregation of platelets increases, further enhancing the tendency of the blood to clot. (Smoking is also responsible for this effect, but the mechanism is probably different)
Fibrinolysis	The body's mechanism for removing unwanted clots is increased. This explains why so few pill-takers actually develop thrombosis despite their increased tendency to clot
Hormones: Hormones insulin	Levels increase, explaining the increased blood sugar levels of pill-takers, and increased blood lipid levels
Growth hormone	Levels increase. Growth hormone increases blood glucose and lipid levels, potentiating the effects of insulin
Adrenal steroid hormones	Levels of cortisol and other adrenal cortex steroids increase. These have the effect of increasing blood glucose and lipid levels
Blood viscosity	Increases (blood becomes more thick and sticky) due to increase in coagulability
Fluid retention	This effect of the pill is due to a complex series of metabolic interactions. It is much more marked for some women than others, and less likely with modern low dose pills
Factors affecting blood pressure	In many women who take the pill there is a slight, demonstrable increase in blood pressure. Factors which affect this include increased cardiac output and increased levels of the hormones **renin** and **angiotensin**, which help to increase blood pressure by acting on the kidney
Immune system	The pill increases leucocyte and the number of circulating plasma antibodies. It alters behaviour of the lymphocytes, the group of white blood cells specifically concerned with the function of the immune system. Evidence is mixed; it appears that some women taking the pill, who already have allergic or auto-immune diseases, find their symptoms worse, while for others they are improved

Table 2.6 Oral contraceptives–some of the brands available

'Ordinary' low dose pills containing
50 micrograms of oestrogen

Ovran
Eugynon 50

Norinyl-1
Norinyl-1/28
Ortho-Novin 1/50

Anovular 21
Gynovlar 21
Norlestrin
Orlest 21
Minovlar

Ovulen 50

Ultra low dose pills containing less
than 50 micrograms available oestrogen

Ovran 30
Eugynon 30
Ovranette

Microgynon 30

Marvelon

Norimin
Neocon 1/35
Binovum

Trinovum
Brevinor
Ovysmen

Loestrin 30
Loestrin 20

Conova 30

Progesterone only pills

Neogest
Microval
Norgeston
Micronor
Noriday
Femulen

Note: The combined pills in the two groups differ mainly in
their progestogen content. Those grouped together have the
same formula but are marketed by different companies.

practice there is no 'ideal' pill for any woman. Matters are further complicated since the effect of one pill on the unique endocrine system of one particular woman may not be the same as its effects upon another.

Endocrinologists have known for some years that breast cancers have receptors for steroid sex hormones on their cell membranes (see Chapter 1;). Such cancers grow more readily when levels of circulating oestrogens are high. Women with a history of breast or ovarian cancer should *never* be given the pill, and in the past the ovaries were sometimes removed to try and prevent metastases. A possible link between the combined pill and subsequent breast cancer in young women was suggested by Pike *et al.* (1983). Several control studies (matching pill takers with non-pill takers) soon afterwards tended to support this finding, but recently a major study from the USA has negated these results for women up to forty-five years of age taking oral contraceptives for more than four years (Stadel *et al.* 1985). The possible relationship between breast cancer and the pill is now confused although risk may be slightly increased according to the most recent evidence (UK National Case-Control Study Group 1989).

A recent update on the 1968 study supported by the Medical Research Council suggests that the incidence of cervical cancer is increased for women who have taken the combined pill at some time in their lives (Beral *et al.* 1988). This study, conducted among 47,000 women followed up for twenty years, showed that after standardisation by age, parity, smoking, social class and history of sexually transmitted disease, cancer of the cervix was more likely to develop in pill takers, rising to four times the rate recorded for non-users among women who had taken the pill for more than ten years. Standardised mortality rates were the same because, in most cases, malignancy was detected at an early stage. The study cannot, of course, take into account risk factors other than oral contraceptives of which nothing is known at present. Among its other findings, the study suggests that a woman who has ever taken the pill is less likely to develop carcinoma of the ovary.

As well as being able to evaluate scientific reports, nurses must be aware of the image of the pill portrayed in the media. It is likely that women and their partners will be swayed by it.

The progesterone-only pill
Clients considering the progesterone-only pill (mini-pill, POP) should be informed of the following facts:

- The POP works mainly by causing the cervical os to become occluded by a thick plug of sticky mucus so that it cannot be penetrated by sperm. (The POP has been described as a 'barrier contraception taken orally.)
- Because it contains a synthetic progesterone with no oestrogen, the POP avoids the side effects of combined pills.
- The POP is slightly less reliable than combined pills. For every 1,000 women taking the POP for one year, the expected theoretical failure rate is 0.5–4 per cent.
- For maximal effectiveness, the POP *must* be taken at *exactly the same time* every

day. If a missed pill is not taken within three hours, the fourteen day rule must be observed.

- The POP must be taken continuously, from the beginning of one cycle to the next, without a break.
- Because the method depends mainly on cervical occlusion by mucus, the POP is best taken a few hours before bed, so it has exerted maximum effect by the time intercourse is most likely.
- Change from the combined pill to the POP should be made without a break, but the fourteen day rule does not apply as there is some 'carry-over' of contraceptive effect.

Many women have taken the POP for years and remained happy with the method, but much less is known about it than about combined pills, partly because it has never been so popular, and partly because much less research has been attempted. It is only fair to point out to women requesting the POP that the possibility of unexpected long-term effects cannot be entirely ruled out. A few side-effects have been well documented:

- *Breakthrough bleeding* can be pronounced. Women vary with the extent they are willing to put up with this.
- *Amenorrhoea*. Some women taking the POP do not bleed at all. To avoid unnecessary worry they *must* be taught to recognise the early symptoms of pregnancy (see Chapter 3).
- The POP has been associated with a slightly increased incidence of ectopic pregnancy, and is not suitable for women with a history of tubal disease.

Injections and implants

Long acting synthetic contraceptive hormones can be injected or implanted subcutaneously. Implants can be removed if there are side effects but, as some of the hormones will already have entered the bloodstream, their effects cannot be eradicated quickly. This is one of the main disadvantages.

One of the drugs most commonly used is *Depo Provera*, sometimes also used to treat endometriosis. In the UK it is mainly used short-term for its contraceptive effects (after Rubella immunisation, or until the disappearance of sperm following vasectomy). It is a synthetic progesterone (progestogen) which works in much the same way as the pill, except that it does not appear to affect lactation and can therefore be used during the post-natal period. Numerous side effects have been reported and, in developing countries, there have occasionally been reports of Depo Provera being used in a racist way to control the fertility of women not fully aware of its effects.

Sterilisation

Sterilisation is becoming an increasingly popular method of contraception among men and women (Shapiro 1986). Despite the obvious advantages of this method once the family is complete, clients should be advised to regard sterilisation of either partner as

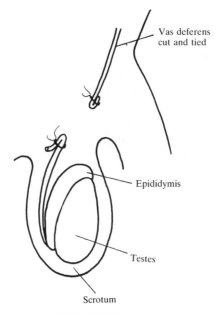

Figure 2.8 Vasectomy.

permanent because reversal cannot be guaranteed. The consent of both partners is often requested before male or female sterilisation is performed.

Vasectomy
Vasectomy was originally used to treat epididymitis but soon gained an enthusiastic following for its supposed ability to diminish the effects of ageing. Attitudes changed during the Second World War when it was reported that both men and women, interred in German concentration camps, were being sterilised against their will. Vasectomy became equated with castration and loss of masculinity. Today, these ideas are fading as its benefits as a method of contraception are becoming apparent.

The operation is usually performed in the outpatient department under local anaesthesia (see Fig. 2.8). The *vasa efferentia* carrying semen from the testes are cut, but the ejaculate looks exactly the same and there is no reported loss of libido. The operation is generally considered safe, although animal experiments have indicated that levels of serum cholesterol become higher even though the male sex steroids, synthesised from cholesterol, continue to be released from the testes. Most researchers dismiss any possible relationship between vasectomy and cardiovascular disease however (Walker 1981). Sperms continue to be made, but are destroyed by leucocytes.

Vasectomy is a highly reliable method of contraception, although failure is occasionally reported because the ends of the vasa efferentia spontaneously re-unite. However, efforts to restore fertility by skilled micro-surgical techniques sometimes fail because the body develops antibodies able to destroy its own sperm (Linnet *et al.* 1981).

Thus Goldstein and Feldberg (1982), providing information to the lay person, urge *both* partners to be sure that sterility is what they want, even though this may involve asking themselves and each other a number of unpalatable questions. What would they feel like if they lost one or all of their existing children? Suppose one partner was killed or they were divorced? These authors argue that sterilisation of either the man or the woman has ramifications beyond contraception, and the self-image of both may be altered when they realise they or their partner are no longer biologically able to have a child. The men and women most likely to regret sterilisation are those who have the operation at a time when they face emotional upheaval (soon after birth, abortion, or because their partner was insistent while they remained ambivalent). There is a clear need for adequate discussion and counselling to both partners before a final decision is taken.

If the couple decide to go ahead with the procedure, it should be emphasised that it will take several months for sperms to leave the storage system in the male genital tract. Unprotected intercourse must be avoided until the ejaculate is free of sperm. Specimens for microscope studies in the laboratory must be provided just before examination, as sperm rapidly lose motility when they fall below body temperature. They cannot be collected in a condom because most brands are treated with spermicidal lubricants.

If the operation is to be performed in the Outpatient Department, the man will probably be requested to make the following preparations:

- To shave the scrotal area, then bath or shower, making sure that all hair is washed away.
- To check there are no pimples or boils in the scrotal area. If there is evidence of sepsis, surgery must be delayed.
- To make arrangements for someone to collect him after the operation, as he is likely to feel shaky and may have received a sedative.
- To wear loose fitting clothes for comfort, and be prepared to spend the day resting, possibly in bed.

Two small incisions are made either side of the scrotum. Careful hygiene is necessary until they heal. Infection can be a problem because of close proximity to the perineal area, where numerous bacteria, including *Staphylococcus aureus*, are carried. It is impossible to prevent bleeding into the surrounding connective tissue because the skin covering the scrotum is loose. Bruising is to be expected. Haematomas develop in about 5 per cent of cases. Clients should be warned about this and know where to seek help if discomfort becomes excessive or if oozing does not stop. The wounds may be closed with absorbable sutures or left to seal. Heavy lifting should be avoided to prevent straining the wound edges. Sperm granulomas (small sperm-filled cysts) occasionally develop at the vasectomy site. They can be painful and sometimes require surgical excision.

Female sterilisation

At one time women wishing to be sterilised had to undergo laparotomy, but today it is possible to occlude the uterine tubes with sutures, diathermy or small plastic rings

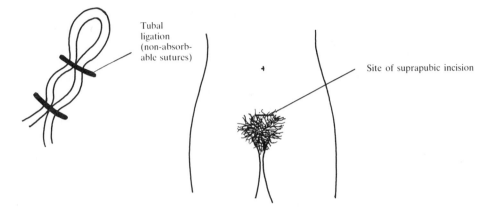

Tubal ligation (non-absorbable sutures)

Site of suprapubic incision

Figure 2.9 Female sterilisation.

(*Yoon's rings*) via the laparoscope (see Fig. 2.9). An increasing number of doctors are now willing to perform this procedure on an outpatient basis, often in a non-NHS clinic, providing the woman has had no previous gynaecological problems and has not undergone previous pelvic surgery. Women admitted to hospital under the NHS are more likely to be given a general anaesthetic and stay overnight.

Although female sterilisation is a more invasive procedure than vasectomy, it is more acceptable to some couples because it is effective immediately. Women lose their fertility as they become older, sometimes as a result of gynaecological surgery before the natural menopause, a fact widely appreciated by the general public.

Female sterilisation must be regarded as permanent. The uterine tubes can be re-anastomosed but, as with vasectomy, fertility cannot be guaranteed, and much will depend on the technique used to perform the first operation. In general, the greater the amount of tissue removed, the safer the contraceptive effect achieved, but the more difficult the operation to reverse.

Before the woman comes in to hospital, the following information may be given:

- She could be admitted the day before the operation, or on the same morning if this is more convenient, but will be asked to have nothing to eat or drink because she may receive a general anaesthetic.
- Her husband will need to give written consent that he is happy for her to undergo sterilisation and fully understands its effects. This is not a legal requirement, but many gynaecologists still ask for it.
- Before the operation the pubic hair, just below the umbilicus, will be shaved since the incision will be made in the suprapubic region. It will probably be invisible once the hair has grown again.
- Under anaesthetic the laparoscope will be inserted through the abdominal wall so that the surgeon can see and divide both uterine tubes. During the operation, the table is tilted downwards to encourage the intestines to fall away from the pelvic area, which is then filled with carbon dioxide to help visualise the pelvic

organs. The gas is absorbed into the blood and excreted via the lungs over the next few days, but causes referred pain to the shoulders.

- D and C will be performed at the same time, so slight bleeding can be expected for the next few days.
- As with all methods of contraception, failure has been reported. The woman should go to her GP if she suspects that she might be pregnant.
- Sutures will be removed the next day, before discharge. Follow up will probably not be required.

A fairly high proportion of women complain of heavy painful periods after sterilisation. The significance of this remains to be established.

The purpose of this chapter is to illustrate the family planning services available in Britain, to describe the different methods of contraception available, and to point out those factors likely to influence choice and suitability of each method. It is aimed at the non-specialist nurse whose daily work is likely to bring her directly into contact with women in hospital and the community who need advice, and perhaps referral. All nurses involved in the care of women need to have some knowledge of the family planning services, and to recognise when specialist help is required.

Resources

Books about contraception for the layperson:

Grant, E. (1985) *The Bitter Pill*, London: Corgi. A rather one-sided account of the oral contraceptive pill, not in its favour. This book could be rather alarming to women who have already taken oral contraceptives, and might dissuade others from trying.

Guillebaud, J. (1984) *The Pill*, Oxford: Oxford University Press. An authoritative and unbiased account of oral contraceptives. Very readable and easily comprehended.

Guillebaud, J. (1986) *Contraception. Your Questions Answered*, Edinburgh: Churchill Livingstone. Intended mainly for GPs, but clear and readable. Sterilisation is not included.

Pauncefoot, Z. (1984) *Choices in Contraception*, London: Pan. A straightforward account of the major methods, including side effects and effectiveness.

References

Beral, V. *et al.* (1988) 'Oral contraceptives and malignancies of the genital tract', *Lancet 2*, pp. 1331–5.

Cowper, A. (1984) 'The present and future role of the nurse in family planning', *Nursing Times* 80 (13), pp. 31–3.

Family Planning Service Information Service *2/81 Method Instruction Sheet. How to Use Your Cap and Spermicide*.

Goldstein, M. and Feldberg, M. (1982) *The Vasectomy Book. A Complete Guide to Decision Making*, Northamptonshire: Turnstone Press.

Guillebaud, J. (1984) *The Pill*, Oxford: Oxford University Press.

Leathard, A. (1980) *The Fight for Family Planning*, London: Macmillan.

Linnet, L. *et al.* (1981) 'Association between failure to impregnant after vasovasostomy and sperm agglutinins in semen', *Lancet* 1, pp. 117–19.

Pike, M.C. *et al.* (1983) 'Breast cancer in young women and the use of oral contraceptives. Possible modifying effect of formulation and use', *Lancet* 2, pp. 926–30.

Potts, M. and Diggory, P. (1983) *Textbook of Contraceptive Practice*, Cambridge: Cambridge University Press.

Renn, M. (1986) 'If the cap fits', *Nursing Times* 82 (4), pp. 22–4.

Richardson, H. (1988) 'Recent developments in contraception', *Midwife, Health Visitor and Community Nurse* 24 (11), pp. 476–9.

Shapiro, R. (1986) 'Fertility rights', *Nursing Times* 82 (4), pp. 24–7.

Sharpe, S. (1987) *Falling for Love. Teenage Mothers Talk*, London: Virago.

Spencer, B. (1986) 'If the cap fits', *Nursing Times* 82 (4), pp. 22–4.

Stadel, B.V. *et al.* (1985) 'Oral contraceptives and breast cancer in young women', *Lancet* 2, pp. 970–3.

UK National Case-Control Study Group (1989) 'Oral contraceptive use and breast cancer risk in young women', *Lancet* 1, pp. 974–82.

Vaughan, P. (1972) *The Pill on Trial*, London: Pelican.

Vessey, M. *et al.* (1982) 'Efficacy of different contraceptive methods', *Lancet* 1, pp. 841–2.

Walker, A.M. *et al.* (1981) 'Vasectomy and non-fatal myocardial infarction', *Lancet* 1, pp. 13–15.

3   Therapeutic Abortion

Although unplanned pregnancy is frequently regarded as unwanted pregnancy, this is not inevitably the case. Women whose lives are already full may find it difficult to make deliberate plans to start or add to a family. If the decision is taken from them, they may find they are pleased to be pregnant after all. For others, however, realisation that they are pregnant will bring dismay. Sometimes there may seem little alternative to therapeutic abortion.

No method of contraception is 100 per cent effective and there are many reasons for failure; nurses who work with women in this situation should not label them as 'careless'.

■   Louise Brown became pregnant because she developed mild gastroenteritis, failing to absorb the hormones in her contraceptive pills. At first she was unsuspecting. Oakley (1979), in her account of women's experiences of first pregnancy, found that early symptoms (see Table 3.1) are often dismissed or overlooked. When her period was two weeks overdue Louise decided to perform a pregnancy test.

Pregnancy tests

Modern pregnancy tests are designed to measure the presence of a hormone, *human chorionic gonadotrophin* (hCG) in urine. This hormone is released by the cells of the developing embryo, enters the maternal bloodstream via the placenta and is extreted in the urine. Figure 3.1 shows that increasing levels of plasma hC G can be detected within eight days of ovulation, when the fertilised egg is implanting, although maximum rate of secretion is not reached until about six weeks later. It is therefore possible to detect pregnancy on the same day that a period was due.

Although pregnancy testing kits afford privacy and yield results rapidly (30–60 minutes, depending on the brand) they have numerous disadvantages:

- Kits are more expensive than the pregnancy testing service available from high street chemists or other agencies (Pregnancy Advisory Service, Brook Clinics).
- In theory kits have an accuracy of 96–99 per cent, but accuracy depends on:

Table 3.1 Signs and symptoms of early pregnancy

Observed by women	⎧ Amenorrhoea ⎪ Sore breasts, with lumpiness or increased vascularity ⎨ Frequency of urine ⎪ Nausea ⎩ Vomiting
Observed by doctor or midwife	⎧ Cervix blue/purple due to increased blood supply ⎨ Uterus enlarged on palpation

(a) adherence to instructions
(b) a steady hand
(c) exact timing.

False negatives or positives *may* occur, and are particularly likely in the hands of an unskilled, highly anxious individual.

Nevertheless an average of 600,000 kits are sold every year, mainly to young women (Renn 1986).

■   Louise was shocked at her positive result for, as far as she was concerned, she had taken her pills exactly as instructed. She and her boyfriend, Mervyn, spent a long time discussing the pregnancy. Both were at college, and could not imagine how they could cope with a baby. Mervyn had heard that very early pregnancy can be terminated by a 'morning after' pill, so Louise went to the family planning clinic resolved to find out about it.

Post-coital contraception

When the egg has been released from the ovary, the cells of the follicle surrounding it persist as a structure called the *corpus luteum* which secretes progesterone (see Chapter 7). This hormone prepares the endometrium to receive a fertilised egg and is essential for the maintenance of pregnancy once fertilisation has occurred. Its secretion from the corpus luteum can be disrupted and preparation for implantation therefore prevented by one of two methods:

● Giving the woman a large oral dose of oestrogen;
● Inserting an IUCD.

Post-coital contraception is extremely effective providing the woman seeks help sufficiently early; oestrogen must be taken within seventy-two hours, while an IUCD is effective if inserted within five days of unprotected intercourse. However, the method of choice is oestrogen which exerts its effect by inhibiting the release of hormones

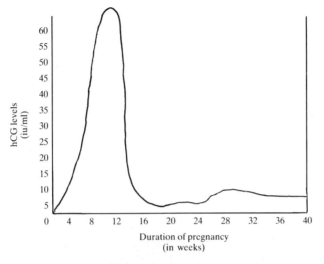

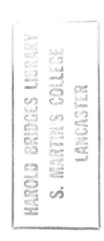

Figure 3.1 hCG secretion throughout pregnancy.

from the anterior pituitary which normally act as the stimulus for progesterone secretion (see Chapter 7).

A woman requesting post-coital contraception will receive the following:

- A general and a gynaecological examination in case there are contraindications against steroid therapy;
- Fifty grams of oestrogen, to be taken immediately;
- A further fifty grams of oestrogen to be taken within twelve hours;
- A second appointment (most clinics) when her period should have arrived to ensure that treatment has been effective and all is well.

She will be given the following information:

- The hormones may induce nausea. Any tablets lost by vomiting must be replaced.
- Although highly reliable, post-coital contraception can occasionally fail and, if this occurs, there is a slightly increased risk of ectopic pregnancy (implantation outside the uterus). If pregnancy is allowed to continue to term, there is a very slight risk that the baby may be affected by the hormones.
- Therapeutic abortion and counselling are available in those cases where failure occurs.

Unprotected intercourse is not a problem for which there are easy solutions as it occurs for a variety of reasons: rape, alcohol or drug abuse, break-up of a previously stable relationship, forgotten pills or other contraceptive failures. However, many of the terminations which follow could be avoided if the availability of post-coital contraception was more widely publicised, both to women and health care professionals who are often poorly informed.

Ethical considerations

Post-coital contraception is not suitable for routine use because of its unpleasant side effects and the potential hazards of repeated exposure to high doses of steroids. It is *not* a suitable 'do it yourself' method. Some people express moral or religious objections on the grounds that it is really abortion in a hidden guise. The view taken depends on the stage at which a new individual is considered to have come into existence – at fertilisation or implantation. Some would argue that, in order to be 'miscarried', the fertilised egg must first be 'carried', and until implantation this has not occurred. Many very early spontaneous abortions take place because the conceptus does not or, for some reason, cannot implant, and go unsuspected by the woman. Variations exist according to culture and religion: in some societies life is thought to commence with conception, while in others a new individual is not thought to exist until much later in pregnancy (Kenyon 1986). Beliefs are likely to change in the same population with the passage of time, depending on the current state of medical knowledge. In our society, the first sign of pregnancy was traditionally regarded as 'quickening' (fetal movements first experienced at about sixteen weeks gestation), but modern technology has reduced this to as little as eight days. When post-coital contraceptive measures are taken, it is never possible to tell whether disruption occurred before or after fertilisation, whereas abortion is presently defined as the interruption of established pregnancy before the twenty-eighth week of gestation.

Termination of pregnancy in the first trimester

■   The family planning nurse asked Louise for the date of her last period and established that she had taken her pills exactly as instructed. The reason for pill failure became apparent when Louise mentioned her recent attack of gastroenteritis. Nevertheless, the nurse repeated the pregnancy test. An early morning sample of urine was used as hCG is more readily detected in concentrated urine stored in the bladder overnight.

Louise's pregnancy test was positive, and the nurse had to explain that it was now far too late for effective post-coital contraception. Unless she wished the pregnancy to continue, she would have to have it terminated surgically.

The 1967 Abortion Act

British Abortion Laws permit termination of pregnancy on the following grounds:

- If allowed to continue, pregnancy would involve greater risks to the woman's health than if it were terminated.
- The pregnancy, if allowed to continue, would risk greater physical or mental damage to the woman than if it were terminated.

- If allowed to continue the pregnancy would be likely to risk mental or physical welfare of any existing children.
- If the baby was born, there would be substantial risk of physical or mental handicap.
- To save the life of the pregnant woman.
- To prevent serious permanent physical or mental health problems to the pregnant woman.

Before an abortion can be performed legally, two doctors must provide signed agreement. One may be the woman's GP or doctor at a family planning clinic; the other, the surgeon who will actually perform the operation.

Early termination of pregnancy

Up to twelve weeks gestation pregnancy can be safely terminated via a curette attached to a suction pump (see Fig. 3.2). Plastic (Karman) curettes are used rather than metal instruments as they are less likely to damage the cervix and uterus since they are more flexible, and less dilation of the cervical os is required. If necessary, the os can be encouraged to open by inserting a prostaglandin pessary just before the operation.

■   Louise was given a letter to take to the gynaecologist. She was very nervous although the family planning nurse had explained what would happen. The gynaecologist agreed that Louise could be admitted as a day patient until he realised that she lived in a student hostel and would have no-one to look after her. She could not go home as she did not wish her parents to know about the pregnancy. Instead, it was arranged for Louise to come to the ward the day before the operation and leave the following morning providing all was well.

Louise was very upset when she arrived on the ward. The nurse checked her personal details and recorded her weight, pulse, temperature and blood pressure explaining that she would be given a mild sedative before she was taken to the anaesthetic room and would probably not remember much until she was back in bed. When she woke up she could expect some pelvic discomfort rather like period pains, and would experience some bleeding, although not much, as she was only seven weeks pregnant. Her pulse, blood pressure and vaginal loss would be observed at regular intervals until her condition was stable.

Short term complications of therapeutic abortion
One of the advantages of legalised abortion has been the development of extremely safe techniques, especially in early pregnancy. The main short term complication is heavy blood loss which is likely to increase as pregnancy advances: by twelve weeks gestation loss of 250–500 ml can be expected. All women must have their blood

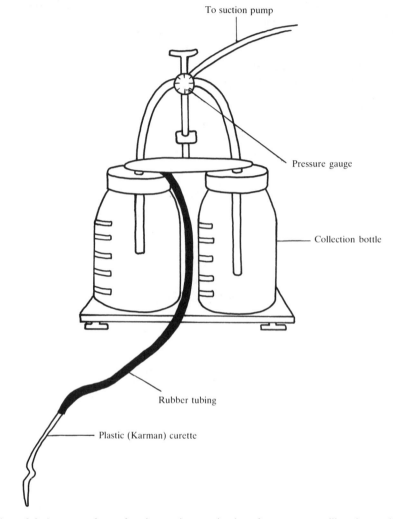

To suction pump

Pressure gauge

Collection bottle

Rubber tubing

Plastic (Karman) curette

Figure 3.2 Apparatus for performing suction termination of pregnancy up till twelve weeks gestation.

grouped and cross-matched. Post-operatively, they must be carefully observed for signs of shock and haemorrhage. The Rhesus blood factor must also be determined as any woman who is Rhesus negative (about 15 per cent of the total British population), having an induced or spontaneous abortion, must receive an injection of *anti D gamma-globulin* within 48 hours. This prevents the development of Rhesus antibodies which could damage the fetus during a future pregnancy.

There is a slight risk that a very early pregnancy may be 'missed' by the curette. The signs and symptoms of pregnancy should disappear within a few days but women whose pregnancies are terminated early should be told to seek medical help if they do not.

Another possible complication is infection. Sepsis is associated with criminal abortion but it can occur when the operation is legally performed if some of the products of conception are retained. This is most likely to happen if pregnancy was further advanced than anticipated. Before discharge the woman's temperature should be checked and she should be asked to wear sanitary towels rather than tampons until the bleeding stops (and for her next period) to reduce the likelihood of bacteria entering the uterus via the cervical os. She can be reassured that bleeding should become darker and stop within a few days. If it becomes bright red or offensive, she should contact the hospital as this could be a sign that infection has occurred.

Septic shock is fortunately a rare complication after abortion today. It is usually caused by bacteria which normally live without causing harm in the vagina or bowel, and is indicated by pyrexia, tachycardia and signs of shock (see Table 5.1, page 108) due to bacterial toxins in the bloodstream causing severe circulatory failure. The woman, who is very ill, requires full nursing care which may be most effectively provided in the intensive care unit. She will also need broad spectrum antibiotics (gentamicin, metronidazole) intravenously.

Longer term risks of therapeutic abortion
A number of longer term complications have been associated with therapeutic abortion but, with safe modern methods, they are rare and the mortality rate is extremely low (Savage and Paterson 1984). In the days of criminal abortion chronic infection, tubal damage and subsequent infertility were common events, but this seldom happens today unless the woman has coincident pelvic inflammatory disease. If the cervix is dilated to more than 12 mm, there is a risk of cervical damage and spontaneous abortions in later pregnancies, but the use of plastic curettes should prevent this. The extensive literature review by Savage and Paterson (1984) strongly suggests that the earlier that termination can be performed the safer it will be.

Contraceptive advice

Ovulation can occur within fourteen days of therapeutic abortion and may result in pregnancy immediately. Women need advice about contraception as soon as, or before, the operation is performed. This can be a sensitive issue for those distressed that a method they trusted has failed. If oral contraceptives are prescribed, careful explanations should be given for taking them. In some centres the woman is advised to take the first pill on the evening of the operation, in others on the fifth post-operative day.

Psychological problems

The psychological effects of therapeutic abortion have been documented by a number of researchers. Conclusions are difficult since the work almost certainly reflects the bias of the particular authors concerned who, like most people, find it difficult to remain impartial about this emotionally, politically and spiritually charged topic. The results of early studies are particularly difficult to interpret. Most are of limited value because data has been collected restrospectively, sometimes years after termination, so the effects of coincident disappointments and problems cannot be ruled out. Although transient unhappiness and guilt appear relatively commonplace (Friedman *et al.* 1974), there is evidence that women become reconciled over time and do not regret their decision (Sloane 1969, Osofsky 1972). Those likely to experience most regret include women with a previous psychiatric history, little social support and those who felt ambivalent about termination, especially if they were sterilised at the same time. However, the results of more recent intervention studies suggest that benefit is gained from explanations and skilled counselling before the ultimate decision is taken (Strassberg and Moore 1985), and from opportunities to discuss feelings in a supportive atmosphere afterwards (Bernstein and Tinkham 1971, Smith 1972, Hardy 1982). Many of the private and charitable abortion agencies provide a follow up service for clients, but this is not so readily available in the NHS at the present time. Women who have supportive partners appear to experience less anxiety (Llewelyn and Pytches 1988).

Provision of the Abortion Service

Greenwood and Young (1976), tracing how the Abortion Act was passed, explain that it was considered necessary to legalise and make safe the illegal abortions already known to take place.

Historical evidence suggests that therapeutic terminations have been performed in virtually every society since time immemorial, irrespective of the attitudes of existing governments, religious bodies or the medical profession, and it is commonly argued that the service has always been available to women who know where to ask and have the means to pay. However, the number of illegal operations actually performed has never been successfully documented, and it is possible that only those resulting in sepsis and haemorrhage came to the attention of the authorities.

Today, therapeutic abortion can be legally performed only in an NHS hospital or approved premises. About 120,000 pregnancies are terminated annually, although since 1977 more have taken place privately than in the NHS, mostly as day cases (Savage and Paterson 1984). In some cases this may be because women and their partners feel that speed and privacy are worth paying for. Information is available in the yellow pages of the telephone directory and clients may sometimes be given the opportunity to pay by instalments if necessary.

Availability of the abortion service under the NHS is unequal across the country and does not match the provision of local gynaecological services (Savage and Paterson 1984). It is known that some family doctors are reluctant to refer women, whether to hospitals within the HNS or private sector (Neustatter 1986), despite persuasive evidence that women forced to have children they do not want are more likely to sustain depression and psychological disturbance than those who succeed in obtaining abortion (Sloane 1969). Neustatter (1986) reports that women, faced with the prospect of 'shopping around' to find sympathetic medical help at a time when they are most vulnerable, may readily agree to private treatment, demonstrating that a double standard still exists between those who know where to seek help and can afford it and those who cannot.

Nursing attitudes

Webb (1985) found strong negative attitudes towards women undergoing therapeutic abortion among nurses on gynaecological wards, sometimes perceived by the women concerned. Kemp (1984) noted that attitudes towards abortion are influenced by age, religious beliefs and the amount of preparation received by nurses before they encounter patients. A study by Such-Baer (1974) revealed that health care professionals were more likely to experience resentment if they were not given choice before caring for women undergoing termination.

Before nurses look after women undergoing therapeutic abortion, it is necessary for them to explore their own attitudes towards this emotionally charged issue and to anticipate how they may feel. Any nurse who registers particular objection to caring for a woman having a termination has a right to refuse, and this is clearly stated in Section 4 of the 1967 British Abortion Act. However, no nurse can decline to participate in treatment necessary to save life or prevent grave permanent mental or physical harm to a pregnant woman, and the Act states this clearly also. Nurses who choose to work where they may encounter women undergoing therapeutic termination of pregnancy should be asked at interview about their feelings and learners should be given an opportunity to discuss this before allocation to gynaecology wards. There is evidence, however, that these measures may not be sufficient. The nurses participating in Webb's study claimed they chose to work in gynaecology wards because they appreciated the special needs of female patients, yet failed to taken these into consideration when describing the care they actually gave. They may have become 'socialised' into overlooking the needs of women undergoing termination for a variety of reasons – lack of opportunity to get to know the individual women concerned, hearing exaggerated accounts of the side effects of abortion or witnessing the distress of women facing miscarriage or fertility investigations. Continual exposure to a problem may dull perception, especially if the nurse believes she can do little to help. Bond (1986), describing 'burnout', the stress syndrome which may develop in health care professionals who feel inadequate because of the demands of their work, points out that symptoms are most likely to develop in those who initially felt most enthusiastic about nursing and were determined to deliver high standards of care.

Like so many issues involving the care of women, the topic of abortion can have implications of a deeply personal nature to nurses. Monitoring feelings may help once the nurse has started to work on the ward. Sometimes it is hard to admit that the challenges of a new job cannot easily be met or that, despite prior consideration, some deep-seated belief has surfaced. In other cases nurses may find satisfaction helping women with this problem yet feel the need to express their feelings with others who will be non-judgemental. Some wards hold support groups for staff, either on a regular basis or as need arises. Special consideration must be given to the feelings of women and the staff caring for them when late abortions are performed.

Second trimester abortion

After twelve weeks gestation the cervix cannot be dilated sufficiently by instruments to allow pregnancy to be terminated. Instead the uterus may be stimulated to contract to expel its content by prostaglandins (PGE2). More rarely hysterotomy is performed. Both methods require a hospital stay over several days.

Hysterotomy

A suprapubic incision is made and uterine contents aspirated via curette. The surgeon must ensure that no endometrial tissue is spilt during the procedure or endometriosis may develop in the scar (see Chapter 7). The risks of hysterotomy are those of any other pelvic operation, and there is also a slight risk of uterine rupture during subsequent pregnancy because suturing weakens the uterine wall. In view of these disadvantages, hysterotomy is seldom performed.

Prostaglandin termination of pregnancy

Details of this procedure vary from one unit to another but there are two main routes of administration, *extra-amniotic instillation* and *intra-amniotic administration*.

Extra-amniotic instillation
A Foley catheter is introduced via the cervical canal so that the balloon, when inflated, lies just above the cervical os. Prostaglandin is injected in solution or allowed to enter via a syringe pump. About 80 per cent of women abort within twenty-four hours.

Intra-amniotic administration
A local anaesthetic is injected into the abdominal wall, then a fine needle is passed into the amniotic sac and prostaglandin inserted (solutions of prostaglandin with saline or urea are generally used). With this method abortion is usually secured more swiftly.

In both cases *syntocinon* may be given to help the uterus contract.

Whichever method is used, it is difficult to detect whether any of the products of conception have been retained in the uterus, so it is usual for the woman to go to theatre for evacuation of retained products of conception (ERPC) under general anaesthesia.
    The whole issue of late abortion has generated heated debate and, at the present time, there are attempts to reduce the time limit to eighteen or twenty-four weeks gestation, although some congenital defects are not apparent until later during pregnancy. In the study by Webb (1985) prostaglandin terminations were the source of

nurses' strongest negative comments, mainly because it was distressing to handle the fetus at the end of the procedure. Nurses were keenly aware that with improved technology it has become feasible to keep alive prematurely born infants, sometimes even those born before the twenty-eighth week of gestation. In practice, however, relatively few very late abortions are performed. Savage and Paterson (1984), in their extensive review of the literature, point to four instances of live births when late abortions have been performed, all reported in the press. When the period of gestation is uncertain, as it was in these cases, ultrasonography should be performed to confirm dates.

The Royal College of Nusing advises its members to ensure that staff on the hospital's obstetric unit are warned well before the procedure to secure a late abortion is initiated, and to have a mucus extractor and resuscitation equipment available in case the fetus is viable. The RCN guidelines point out that if the fetus is still attached to the mother by the umbilical cord it is protected by the Infant Life Preservation Act (1929) which makes it an offence to destroy any fetus born alive. If it is no longer attached to the mother but showing signs of life, under the Children and Young Persons Act (1933) failure to resuscitate could be construed as wilful neglect. According to the RCN, decision to resuscitate is based on clinical assessment but the decision to continue treatment thereafter is a moral one, which should be made jointly among all staff concerned.

■   Maria Grey's third pregnancy had been planned. All seemed well until a discussion with friends drew Maria's attention to the high rate of congenital abnormality among babies born to women of increasing maternal age. Maria, who was 39, and her husband Tom, decided they would like to know more, so they went to see their GP. He explained that some (but not all) congenital abnormalities can be detected pre-natally by a procedure called *amniocentesis*.

Amniocentesis

After a local anaesthetic has been injected into the abdominal wall, a fine needle is inserted into the amniotic sac to withdraw a small quantity of fluid which will contain cells shed from the growing fetus (see Fig. 3.3). Some fetal abnormalities can be detected by the presence of metabolites in the amniotic fluid; spina bifida, for example, is associated with an unusual protein called *alpha feta protein*. Cells can be grown in tissue culture and examined under the microscope to reveal genetic abnormalities such as Down's syndrome, in which there is an extra chromosome (*trisomy*). Ultrasonography can sometimes help confirm diagnosis. The disadvantage of amniocentesis is that it is most safely and effectively performed around fourteen to sixteen weeks gestation. Results are not available for several weeks since the cells need time to grow in the tissue culture. By the time tests are complete, the fetus may have reached twenty

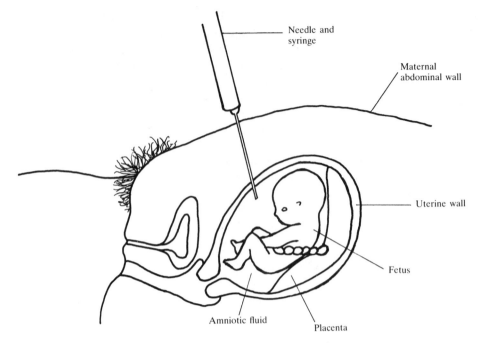

Figure 3.3 Amniocentesis.

or more weeks gestation. The woman will be visibly pregnant and will have felt the baby move. Under these circumstances she may feel differently towards abortion, even if abnormality is detected, so it is necessary for the couple to explore their feelings before even deciding whether or not amniocentesis should be performed. Results are not infallible: it is not possible to detect all kinds of fetal abnormality, and false negative and positive results have been known. Occasionally the cells may not grow in tissue culture so the procedure must be repeated. The decision to perform amniocentesis is never taken lightly as it is associated with a slight risk of spontaneous abortion.

Chorionic villus biopsy

There is a second method of pre-natal diagnosis called *chorionic villus biopsy* which does not seem to carry any greater risk than amniocentesis to the viability of the fetus. Tissue from the placenta is obtained via an incision made through the roof of the vagina (see Fig. 3.4). As this tissue is derived from fetal not maternal cells, it contains the genetic material of the fetus.

Chorionic villus biopsy can be performed as early as the sixth week of gestation, but at present it is only available at a few specialist centres in Britain. If it becomes more widely available, genetic abnormalities will be detectable at a much earlier stage of pregnancy.

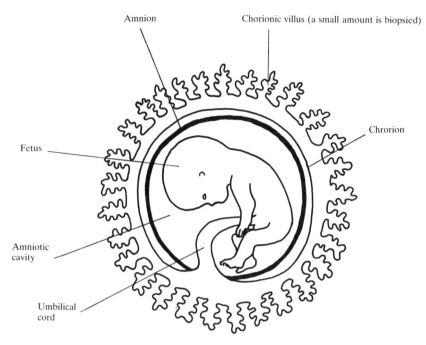

Figure 3.4 Chorionic villus biopsy at eight weeks gestation.

■ Maria was only twelve weeks pregnant so the GP advised the couple to consider carefully whether amniocentesis would be appropriate for them. They had two children, aged six and ten. Although their income was modest, they hoped to give them every opportunity to continue to higher education because they had not had the same option. They had delayed this third pregnancy until their financial prospects improved. Maria thought of all the problems generated by a handicapped child and how these might disrupt the lives of the two children they already had. She and Tom agreed that they would be unfair to their son and daughter if they allowed this to happen, and planned that Maria should have amniocentesis and terminate the pregnancy if anything was seriously wrong.

   Although Maria and Tom both felt they had made the correct decision, they were shocked when they received a telephone call asking them to make an appointment to discuss the findings of amniocentesis.

   It appeared that the fetus was affected by Edward's syndrome, a genetic defect resulting in mental retardation more severe than Down's syndrome and accompanied by characteristic physical defects. The life expectancy of such children is at present severely limited.

   After they had seen the consultant, Maria and Tom spent most of the night talking. They discussed the hazards of late termination which they had been told about, and the way they might feel after the termination. They thought they might experience guilt but perhaps also relief and recognised that they would grieve over the loss of the child they had planned. They also remembered their earlier conversations about the quality of life they felt they could provide for all their children if one was handicapped, and decided that the pregnancy would be best terminated. Under these circumstances, the woman may be considered to undergo abortion for 'altruistic' reasons to spare greater distress to her existing children – as would occur if the baby was actually born (Neustatter 1986). Unfortunately, there is evidence that women who choose abortion because of the risk of congenital disease may suffer more serious emotional trauma than those who do so for purely socioeconomic reasons, perhaps because the pre-natal diagnosis and the long wait for results generate so much additional stress (Beeson *et al*. 1983). The care plan developed for Maria is shown in Care Plan 3.1 (on page 79).

Maria was admitted to hospital later the same week for her pregnancy to be terminated by the intra-amniotic instillation of prostaglandin. Ultrasonography revealed that she was now eighteen weeks pregnant.

The ward to which she had been admitted was rather traditional in its approach and, although the care plan employed the nursing process to identify problems that Maria might experience, it did not incorporate a nursing model. Inevitably care was based on the biomedical model which focuses on people as physical beings, concentrating heavily on fulfilling their physical needs (Pearson and Vaughan 1986). Although Maria's nurse was pleasant and caring, she did not spend much time discussing the couple's emotional needs and, perhaps because of this, did not identify all their needs for information. Although Maria was warned that she would find the contractions painful, for example, she was surprised that they developed so swiftly and were equally, if not more, painful than her previous experiences of labour at full term. Her evaluation of care was different from the nurse's perception (see Care Plan 3.1).

It has been suggested (Menzies 1960) that in the past nurses organised their care along routine, task-oriented lines to protect themselves from the distress that may accompany the development of close relationships with their patients. Unless careful thought is given to the operation of the nursing process and individual patient care, the nurse may still need to distance herself but ultimately this will not allow her to cope with her own feelings or her patient's needs. Women like Maria are particularly likely to encounter this problem because of the nature of their treatment and because they are generally nursed in single rooms and may be unintentionally avoided. Maria and Tom needed privacy to cope with their grief, but might have benefited from the approach to care suggested for women experiencing miscarriage described in Chapter 4.

Care plan 3.1 (Biomedical model)

Name: Maria Grey

Treatment/condition: Intra-amniotic instillation of prostaglandin for termination of pregnancy in the second trimester

Nursing assessment: 20.02.89

11.15 am: Confined to bed
11.30 am: Prostaglandin inserted. Fasting. Distressed because husband has left for work

Vital signs: Temperature: 37°C
Pulse: 76 beats/minute
Respirations: 16 per minute
BP: 110/80
Vaginal loss: slight, bloodstained
Contractions: not yet established
Pain: none yet reported

Problem	Aim	Nursing action	Evaluation
(1) Painful uterine contractions Abdominal discomfort (potential)	(1) Anticipate pain and give analgesia 4 hourly (omnopon 20 mg IM)	(1) Analgesia given 4 hourly until delivery of products of conception	(1) Maria reports that analgesia diminished but did not obliterate pain She feels drowsy
(2) Anxiety due to pain (potential)	(2) Anticipate to alleviate anxiety	(2) Explain action of analgesia to allay anxiety and reduce Maria's pain Pain should subside when products of conception are delivered	See overall comment, p. 81
(3) Nausea/vomiting (potential – effect of prostaglandin)	– Prevent nausea – Alleviate anxiety	– Antiemetic given 4 hourly (metochlorpropamide 10 mg IM)	– Nausea reduced, but persisted until contractions ceased – No vomiting

Problem	Aim	Nursing action	Evaluation
(4) Dry mouth/thirst (actual) NB oral fluids and food are withheld in case of the need for surgical intervention and anaesthesia	Prevent dry mouth	– Effects of prostaglandin and action of antiemetic explained Offer mouth washes 2 hourly and allow Maria to clean her teeth whenever she requests	Maria says that mouthwashes have helped to keep her oral mucosa moist and reduced discomfort
(5) Pyrexia (potential – effect of prostaglandin)	– Reduce pyrogenic effects of prostaglandin – Help Maria remain cool and comfortable	– Monitor temperature 4 hourly provide fan and remove blankets – If it rises above 37.8°C – Change bedclothes when necessary – Offer to help wash frequently – Cool ambient temperature with fan	– Maria's temperature did not rise above 37.3°C – Maria did not report discomfort
(6) Elimination (potential)	Keep bladder empty to maintain Maria's comfort and reduce pressure on the contracting uterus	– Monitor urinary output – Offer bedpans 2 hourly while Maria is confined to bed – Provide privacy while Maria is using bedpan	Urinary output is 800 ml in 7 hours, concentrated in appearance but not offensive. Maria dislikes using a bedpan, but manages to do so
(7) Vaginal loss (actual)	– Prevent haemorrhage	– Observe vaginal loss and vital signs hourly so that medical staff can be alerted promptly if necessary – Summon medical help when products of conception are delivered. Clamp umbilical cord to prevent further blood loss and remain with Maria until doctor arrives	– Vital signs stable and within normal limits. Vaginal loss moderate – Products of conception delivered at 4 pm
	– Provide emotional support	– Spend time with Maria. Do not leave once delivery of products of conception is imminent	

Problem	Goal	Nursing action	Evaluation
(8) Ascending infection from vagina to endometrium (potential) See also 'Pyrexia' (problem 5)	Prevent infection	– Provide sterile sanitary towels – Perform vaginal/vulval toilet as necessary – Change bedlinen as soon as it becomes soiled	All nursing actions performed. Maria remains comfortable NB Evidence of endometrial infection will not be apparent until days or weeks after termination. Maria must be taught the signs and symptoms before she goes home
(9) Distress at loss of baby (actual)	Maria will voice her feelings to her nurse and show her emotions	– Remain with Maria as much as possible – Give her opportunity to talk about this pregnancy and the future – Answer questions honestly	*Nurse* Time spent with Maria every hour when vital signs recorded. No question asked. Maria was not left alone when products of conception were passed. She did not want to see the baby but asked its sex *Maria* Frightened. Lonely. Perceived nurse as very busy, no time to talk, only for specific tasks. Wanted to ask questions about procedure and amount of pain regarded as 'normal', but felt she had no opportunity

The *biomedical model* was chosen here to illustrate the rationale behind prostaglandin termination of pregnancy and the physical aspects of nursing care. Some attempt was made to meet Maria's emotional needs, but overall she received little psychological support and did not perceive the nurse as a possible source of support. The model did not take into account the emotional care required by Maria's husband, and little information was given to the couple by the nurses. No real attempt was made at patient teaching as the need was not identified. Although the biomedical model makes provision for evaluation of nursing actions, Maria's thoughts about her care were not taken into consideration.

Overall
Physical needs are identified and met. There was little provision for psychological care. How could this approach to care be improved? Do you know of any nursing model that might be more appropriate? Give reasons.

Planning discharge and rehabilitation

■   Maria left hospital the day after the procedure. She and Tom were seen by the gynaecologist who knew that the pregnancy had been planned. He enquired whether they had decided to try and conceive again. Maria and Tom were pleased to be asked this. They had always wanted a third child and felt that, as Maria was now 39, they should not leave things too long, especially in view of the risks associated with increasing maternal age. Their main worry was that the same thing would happen again. Frankle (1980), describing the possible reactions of women who feel ambivalent about abortion, suggests that women may become anxious to have another child to replace the one they have lost. In the case of Maria and Tom, genetic counselling was considered advisable.

Genetic counselling
The aim of genetic counselling is to explain to the couple as far as possible the likelihood of their having a handicapped child, and to provide a supportive atmosphere in which they may come to a decision about what they should do. The service is generally provided on a regional basis, and a specialist nurse or health visitor may be involved in counselling.

Although a wide range of genetic diseases are known to exist, some are much more serious than others. In some cases the possibility of having a handicapped child is relatively easy to determine (for example, in cases of Mendelian inheritance, such as Huntingdon's chorea, and sex-linked disorders like classic haemophilia). In other cases, where the disease is multifactorial in origin (resulting through the interaction of several genes with the environment), it is much more difficult to make an accurate prediction. Sometimes genetic defects arise spontaneously through mutation and are not likely to be repeated (most cases of Down's syndrome). In others geneticists themselves are not agreed about the relative contributions of heredity and environment (schizophrenia, spina bifida).

Whether or not prediction is easy, the decision to establish another pregnancy, go through pre-natal testing and face the possibility of abortion, is not easy for prospective parents, especially if it is not the first time that this has happened.

Resources

Abortion Counselling Service Phone In
7.00 pm–9.00 pm   Monday–Friday
01–350   2229

SAFTA   c/o Association for Spina Bifida and Hydrocephalus
22 Upper Woburn Place
London WC1 OPE
01–388 1382 – in cases of termination for fetal abnormality only

References

Beeson, D. *et al.* (1983) 'Prenatal diagnosis of fetal disorders: II Issues and implications', *Issues in Perinatal Care and Education* 10 (4), pp. 233–41.

Bernstein, N.R. and Tinkham, C.B. (1971) 'Group therapy following abortion', *Journal of Nervous and Mental Disease* 152 (5), pp. 303–14.

Bond, M. (1986) *Stress and Self-Awareness: A Guide for the Nurse*, London: Heinemann.

Frankle, L.B. (1980) *The Ambivalence of Abortion*. Harmondsworth: Penguin.

Friedman, C.M. *et al.* (1974) 'The decision making process and the outlook of therapeutic abortion', *American Journal of Psychiatry* 131 (2), pp. 1332–7.

Greenwood, V. and Young, J. (1976) *Abortion on Demand*, London: Pluto Press.

Handy, (1982) J.A. 'Psychological and social aspects of induced abortion', *British Journal of Clinical Psychology* 21(1), pp. 29–41.

Kemp, J. (1984) 'Attitudes to abortion', *Nursing Mirror* 158 (17), pp. 34–5.

Kenyon, E. (1986) *The Dilemma of Abortion*, London: Faber.

Llewelyn, S.P. and Pytches, R. (1988) 'An investigation of anxiety following termination of pregnancy', *Journal of Advanced Nursing* 13, pp. 468–71.

Menzies, I.E.P. (1960) 'Nurses under stress: a social system functioning as a defence against anxiety', *International Nursing Review* 7 (6), pp. 9–16.

Neustatter, A. (1986) *Mixed Feelings. The Experience of Abortion*, London: Pluto Press.

Oakley, A. (1979) *From Here to Maternity*, London: Pelican.

Osofsky, J.D. (1972) 'The psychological reaction of patients to legalised Abortion', *American Journal of Orthopsychiatry* 42 (1), pp. 48–60.

Pearson, A. and Vaughan, B. (1986) *Nursing Models for Practice*, London, Heinemann.

Renn, M. (1986) 'Accurate predictions', *Nursing Times* 82 (4), pp. 22–4.

Savage, W. and Paterson, I. (1984) 'Therapeutic abortion. Methods and sequelae' In: Chamberlain, G. (ed.) *Contemporary Gynaecology*, London: Butterworths, pp. 220–46.

Sloane, R.B. (1969) 'The unwanted pregnancy', *New England Journal of Medicine* 280 (22), pp. 1206–13.

Smith, E.M. (1972) 'Counselling for women who seek abortion', *Social Work* 17 (2), pp. 62–8.

Strassberg, D. and Moore, M.R. (1985) 'Effects of a film model on the psychological and physical stress of abortion', Special Issue – Sex Education: Past Present and Future, *Journal of Sex Education and Therapy* 11 (2), pp. 46–50.

Such-Baer, M. (1974) 'Professional staff reaction to abortion work', *Social Casework* 55 (7), pp. 435–41.

Webb, C. (1985) 'Barriers to sympathy', *Nursing Mirror* 160 (1), Research Forum v–vii.

4   Miscarriage

The word 'abortion' has unpleasant connotations for many people. 'Miscarriage', the layperson's term for interrupted pregnancy, has been used throughout this chapter to emphasise the sensitivity surrounding this issue.

■   When Colin Peters rushed his wife, eleven weeks pregnant and bleeding, to the Accident and Emergency Department, he was perturbed to hear the nurse mention the words 'threatened abortion' during a conversation with the doctor. Colin and Judith had planned the pregnancy and were looking forward to their first baby.

Legal definitions

Abortion is defined as the expulsion of the fetus before the twenty-eighth week of pregnancy, whether naturally occuring or induced. The same definition is not used in all countries, however. This reflects the moral and ethical dilemmas surrounding fetal rights and the time at which different authorities consider the fetus capable of independent existence. The World Health Organisation recommends that the fetus should be considered viable when it reaches more than twenty weeks gestation or weighs at least 500 g. These criteria have been adopted in Australia and some of the States of America, but in Britain and most other nations the fetus is not considered viable until the twenty-eighth week, or until it weighs at least 1,000 g. After this time, it is considered stillborn and its birth is recorded on the official statistics of the Registrar General. However a fetus of less than twenty-eight weeks gestation may also be designated viable if it shows signs of life, which can result in anomalies when nurses rush a fetus breathing spasmodically to neonatal intensive care.

Threatened abortion

When threatened abortion occurs, bleeding from the placental site is slight, the cervix is closed, pelvic pain or backache is mild and pregnancy may continue (see Fig. 4.1).

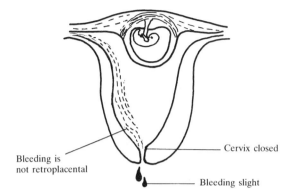

Bleeding is
not retroplacental

Cervix closed

Bleeding slight

Figure 4.1 Threatened abortion.

However, until she has been examined the woman will not know the probable outcome and her most likely emotional reactions will be distress and anxiety.

Treatment of threatened abortion

Although threatened and spontaneous abortions are matters of obstetric concern, women usually receive treatment on gynaecology wards where others having therapeutic abortions may be admitted. This situation is potentially difficult for all concerned. So, whenever possible, it is advisable to ensure that women who are likely to miscarry and those who are admitted for therapeutic abortions are admitted to different ward areas.

■ As soon as Judith had been made comfortable in bed, she was seen by the doctor who performed a gentle pelvic and speculum examination, revealing a closed cervix. Judith had mild backache and little bleeding so it was likely that pregnancy would continue. If bleeding is heavy, there is a greater chance of the pregnancy being lost.

While the doctor was examining Judith, the sister asked Colin about their domestic responsibilities, particularly other young children at home.

Threatened and spontaneous abortion are problems encountered at a time of life when the couple may have small children, and it occurs suddenly. The woman is admitted to hospital quickly, without time to make plans. It is important to consider the feelings of *both* partners, although there appear to be few studies of men's feelings towards very early pregnancy (May 1982). However, partners are bound to feel worried, may have to return alone to an empty house or make arrangements at short notice for the care of other children. They may also have to explain the situation to others recently told about the pregnancy.

Both partners may worry about being responsible in some way. The woman may wonder whether she failed to take adequate care of herself, perhaps not eating or resting properly. Her partner may remember the time he did *not* help to carry the heavy shopping. There is an idea that intercourse during pregnancy may result in spontaneous abortion, but little evidence to support it. Health care professionals emphasise that physiologically pregnancy is a normal event. Most women who give birth to healthy babies have remained active and there is little to suggest that slowing down may avert spontaneous abortion once the embryo has embedded firmly in the uterine wall. Despite early bleeding, many pregnancies continue safely. However the only treatment for threatened abortion presently available is rest, although the literature available does not suggest whether it is genuinely helpful. Success or otherwise probably depends at least to some extent on the reason for bleeding (Pizer and Palinski 1981). Women who have had vaginal bleeding in pregnancy are usually advised not to have intercourse but, again, there is no real evidence to suggest whether this is helpful.

A model for care
Orem's *Self-Care Model* (1985) was used to help plan care for Judith (see Care Plan 4.1 on page 88). This model seems particularly suitable for women with gynaecological conditions as Orem takes the view that people should be allowed to take responsibility for their own health needs. The model therefore envisages that the woman will be a partner in her own care, capable of taking her own decisions after discussion with those offering to provide it. This approach demands that patients and clients are kept well informed about their nursing and medical treatments and progress.

Orem outlines a number of self care requisites (needs) universal to human beings everywhere:

- Maintenance of sufficient oxygen;
- Maintenance of sufficient intake of water;
- Maintenance of sufficient intake of food;
- Provision of care associated with elimination;
- Maintenance of an appropriate balance between activity and rest;
- Maintenance of an appropriate balance between solitude and social interaction;
- Prevention of hazards to human life, functioning and well-being;
- Promotion of human functioning and development within social groups (taking into consideration the potential and known limitations of the individual).

Two further categories of self care needs are also described in Orem's model:

- *Developmental self care requisites*, which occur according to the individual's stage of development and the environment in terms of its effects on development;
- *Health Deviation selfcare requisites*, which arise out of ill health, or because the

effects of illness or disability demand changes in self care behaviour. According to Orem, self care deficits occur when the individual becomes unable to meet his or her own health needs and requires nursing care.

The goals of nursing therefore involve any of the following, chosen for appropriateness in a given situation:

- To reduce self care demand to a level which the patient/client is able to meet;
- To enable the patient/client to increase ability to meet the self care demand;
- To enable another carer (partner/parent) to provide care;
- To meet the individual's needs directly if none of the above is feasible.

■   Before decisions about nursing care could be taken, it was necessary for Judith to undergo investigations to determine whether the fetus was still viable.

Ultrasonography
Ultrasonography is a diagnostic procedure for determining size and position of a mass (pregnancy, tumour, etc.) from the sound echo evoked from the density of the mass. It can be used to diagnose pregnancy since a gestational sac will show up as a very small but characteristic white ring with a dark centre after five weeks amenorrhoea. If the fetus is no longer viable, ultrasound may help to demonstrate the presence of retained products of conception. After twelve weeks gestation, measurement of the fetal head is possible.

The apparatus transmits a beam of ultrasonic energy generated by an electrical current. When this beam strikes the junction between objects of different densities (e.g. fetal limbs, placenta or amniotic fluid) the returning echoes are displayed on a screen.

Ultrasound is performed in a special hospital department by a trained technician. The same investigation is used to monitor progress of normal pregnancy as well as to detect problems. It is likely, therefore, that other women may be waiting in the department to have ultrasonographic examination as part of routine ante-natal care. If possible women with threatened abortion should visit the department before or after the ante-natal clinic is open. Those who have not had this examination before can be reassured that ultrasonic scanning is painless and can do no harm (Proud 1988). However, the investigation may be uncomfortable as it is best performed when the woman has a full bladder.

Ultrasonography showed that the fetus was viable and, as Judith's bleeding was diminishing, it seemed unlikely that any permanent damage had been done.

As well as performing ultrasonography, the viability of pregnancy can be checked by sending urine to the laboratory for a pregnancy test but the result is often unhelpful since it may be positive for some time after fetal death. A positive result is also obtained in cases of *hydatidiform mole* (see page 101).

Care plan 4.1 (Orem's Self Care model)

Name: Judith Peters

Treatment/condition: Threatened abortion at eleven weeks gestation

Universal Self Care Requisites	Therapeutic Self Care Requisites	Self Care Agency	Self Care Deficits	Nursing Systems	Nursing Agency	Future
Maintain sufficient intake of oxygen	Breathing unassisted. Skin warm and well perfused. *Respiratory rate*: 16 breaths/minute		None at present	Supportive	Monitor respiratory rate 4 hourly	Self caring
Maintain sufficient fluid intake	May drink freely (drank copiously for ultrasonography examination)	Understands rationale for high fluid intake before ultrasonography. Knows that she can now drink as desired	Needs to be supplied with fluids of choice while confined to bed	Partially compensatory	Supply fluids: encourage Judith to drink at least 2 litres daily	Self caring
Maintain sufficient food intake	Nutritious well balanced diet required for pregnancy	Eating normal diet before admission Appears adequately nourished	Will rely on nurses to supply food. Doubtful about ability to tolerate hospital food	Supportive/ educative	Provide dietary advice	Husband may bring in favourite foods *On discharge*: Self caring
Provision of care associated with elimination	Receive necessary help with elimination while confined to bed. At risk of constipation due to	*Bowels*: usual pattern once daily in morning. Understands expected constipation	Reliant on nurses at present	Supportive	Monitor bowel pattern and urinary output. Ensure privacy	Self caring

Goal	Assessment	Related factors	Problem	Nursing system	Nursing action	Outcome
	Bladder: urinary frequency since seventh week of gestation. No dysuria or nocturia. Knows she will be reliant on nurses' help with elimination while confined to bed. Vaginal loss: slight, pink	lack of mobility. Aperients not permitted to avoid stimulation of uterine contractions			Monitor vaginal loss four hourly. when using commode.	Self caring
Maintain balance between rest and activity	Understands and accepts need for bedrest, but anxious about restricted activity. Understands that she must move legs while in bed	Bedrest to avert loss of pregnancy until vaginal bleeding ceases. Advice about leg exercises to prevent deep venous thrombosis	Restricted activity	Supportive/ educative	Explore ways of passing the time and diverting anxiety, including husband in discussions. Spend as much time with Judith as possible	Self caring
Maintain balance between solitude and social interaction	Understands temporary limitations but resentful of them	Alteration in usual activities and reduced social interaction by confinement to bed in ward (single room not available). Says she dreads questions from other women about her possible loss of pregnancy. Feels helpless	Cannot seek privacy when desired. Normal social interaction disrupted	Supportive	Discuss likely length of time necessary bedresting. Draw curtains round bed when Judith wishes to be alone	
Prevent hazards to life, well-being and functioning	All vital signs currently within normal limits. Vaginal loss minimal.	At risk of: – Haemorrhage and shock if abortion	Potential hazards of bedrest. Loss	Supportive/ educative	Monitor vital signs four hourly. Monitor vaginal	Probably good. Pregnancy

Universal Self Care Requisites	Therapeutic Self Care Requisites	Self Care Agency	Self Care Deficits	Nursing Systems	Nursing Agency	Future
	becomes inevitable – Deep vein thrombosis – Sore, broken pressure areas – Depression/anxiety due to admission/ possible loss of pregnancy	No pelvic discomfort, no back pain. Pressure areas intact, no inflammation. No calf pain or tenderness. More cheerful than when admitted, but still anxious about admission and possible loss of pregnancy *Ultrasonography:* Pregnancy still viable	of pregnancy. Anxiety		loss. Pressure area care. Advise frequent changes of position. Provide information/ emotional support, include husband, and significant others (mother)	appears viable. Will need emotional support during pregnancy from husband/ midwife/ mother
Promote normality	Altered self concept because of threat to pregnancy	Says she feels inadequate because pregnancy 'should be normal' and the reaction of her body has been 'abnormal'. Knows that miscarriage sometimes occurs 'because something is wrong with the baby' and worries about this	Has difficulty coming to terms with her situation. Pessimistic about outcome of pregnancy	Supportive/ educative	Give Judith and her husband opportunity to voice their fears. Answer all questions honestly	Outcome should be good providing pregnancy continues. Will need continued support throughout pregnancy from husband/ midwife/ mother

Orem's Self Care Model (1985) was chosen for this patient because she was not 'ill' and though confined to bed could to some extent be self caring. The model proved a good choice for Judith because it drew attention to the need for psychological care, including the support required by other members of her family, and the need for information-giving, teaching and preparation for discharge. By the time she was ready to go home Judith's needs had changed, and the care plan could be adapted using the same model to highlight longer term needs (see Care Plan 4.2). The model also serves to draw attention to those aspects of care over which the nurse has little or no control, in other words, the limits of nursing actions. Advice for a healthy lifestyle during pregnancy can be provided but the client will make decisions for herself when she leaves the hospital. The model did not explore social conditions in much depth, beyond documenting that this was a wanted first pregnancy in a stable relationship, and family support appeared adequate. Should nurses spend time documenting problems over which they have little or no control? Another criticism of the model was the difficulty in adapting it to meet physical needs for care in this example. Is this a valid criticism of the model itself or of the way it was used?

Overall

Orem's model was very successful in highlighting psychological needs, adequate in outlining possible social needs (although this aspect could be developed), but less helpful for providing physical care during dependency. The model by Roper *et al.* (1985) is discussed in Chapter 5. You could try to plan Judith's care using this model rather than Orem's. Are there any weaknesses using this approach?

Rehabilitation and planning discharge

■   After Judith had been resting in bed for several days and the bleeding showed
    no sign of recurrence, she was allowed to get up and gradually become more
    independent. After ten days in hospital she was bored and restless. Both she
    and Colin felt that she would be able to rest more effectively at home, and
    arrangements were made for her discharge. Care Plan 4.2 (on page 93) shows
    two nursing interventions performed in preparation for rehabilitation.

Inevitable abortion

Inevitable abortion occurs when there is bleeding from the placental site and the fetus
is dead. Although blood loss is usually slight or moderate depending on the stage of
pregnancy, the cervix is open (see Fig. 4.2) and there is pelvic pain with backache.

Abortion may be complete or incomplete. If it is complete all the products of conception are lost through the vagina. If abortion is incomplete the fetus and membranes
are expelled, but the chorionic tissue remains attached to the uterine wall and
bleeding continues (see Fig. 4.3).

Examination and treatment

The woman is admitted to hospital and ultrasound is performed, if necessary, to
establish whether the fetus is viable. If only part of the products of conception are
passed, or if the fetus has already been expelled, the abortion must be completed by
evacuation of the retained products of conception (ERPC) under general anaesthetic.

In practice most spontaneous abortions are regarded as incomplete because there is
risk of sepsis even if a small amount of tissue is retained. Sepsis has been reported
after spontaneous abortion as well as when termination has been induced. A second
complication of incomplete abortion is severe blood loss from the placental site. If
there is *any* possibility of spontaneous abortion, a sample of blood must be sent to the
laboratory to be grouped and cross matched. The Rhesus factor must also be checked
(see Chapter 3).

Unless there has been haemorrhage or evidence of sepsis, most women who have
spontaneous abortion spend a very short time in hospital. However, emotional reaction to the lost pregnancy can be profound.

Considering the number of women admitted to hospital with this problem every
year, spontaneous abortion has attracted remarkably little interest by nurses or
doctors. Only one research study has been conducted in Britain to document women's
emotional reactions (Oakley *et al*. 1984). Although a few studies have been conducted
in the USA, most other literature is concerned with the aetiology and incidence of
spontaneous abortion.

Care plan 4.2 (Orem's Self Care model: longer term care)

Name: Judith Peters

Treatment/condition: After-care following threatened abortion

Universal Self Care Requisites	*Therapeutic Self Care Requisites*	*Self Care Agency*	*Self Care Deficits*	*Nursing Systems*	*Nursing Agency*	*Future*
Maintain balance between rest and activity	Bored in hospital. Unable to sleep and rest. Sedentary lifestyle recommended in view of threat to pregnancy	Hopes/expects to feel less tired and bored at home. Accepts need to rest and knows this would be recommended as pregnancy advances anyway. Knows she must not return to work for several weeks and will need help with heavy housework	In hospital: none *Discharge planning*: Modified activity	Supportive/ educative	Explore ways in which activity must be modified and sources of help available	*Immediate discharge*: Mother will stay, husband will help at weekends *Long-term*: Self caring
Prevention of hazards to life, well-being and functioning	Pregnancy may be at risk. ? reason	Knows date of next ante-natal appointment and understands need for attendance. Demonstrates understanding of what constitutes suitable diet and is aware of need to avoid alcohol. Does not smoke cigarettes	Worried bleeding may resume	Supportive/ educative	Discuss action to take if bleeding/ pain resume (contact hospital at once, then rest)	Outcome should be good

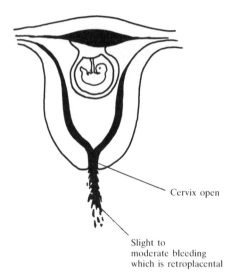

Cervix open

Slight to
moderate bleeding
which is retroplacental

Figure 4.2 Inevitable abortion.

Incidence and aetiology of spontaneous abortion

The number of legal abortions performed annually is officially recorded (see Chapter 3) but no comparable figures are kept for spontaneous abortions. Documentation is not possible because very early spontaneous abortions may occur without the woman ever realising she was pregnant. Edmonds *et al.* (1982) showed that these 'biochemical pregnancies' could be detected by demonstrating raised plasma levels of hCG before the woman exhibited any other signs or symptoms of pregnancy. However incidence may be as high as one in five of all conceptions (Glass and Ericsson 1982).

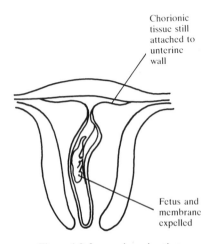

Chorionic
tissue still
attached to
unterine
wall

Fetus and
membrane
expelled

Figure 4.3 Incomplete abortion.

Spontaneous abortions are classified as early (before thirteen weeks gestation) and late (thirteen to twenty-eight weeks). Early abortion seems to occur mainly due to defects in the conceptus, but later abortions more often reflect maternal problems.

Up to 65 per cent of spontaneous abortions occur before the thirteenth week of gestation, mainly between week six and week ten. Although four hormones, oestrogen, progesterone, hCG and human placental lactogen, are essential for the continuance of pregnancy, adequate levels of progesterone appear to be particularly important.

Up to the eleventh week progesterone is secreted mainly by the corpus luteum (cells left behind in the ovary after ovulation). From the eleventh week onwards the placenta is sufficiently developed to take over hormone production, and the corpus luteum gradually regresses. It is thought that spontaneous abortions are particularly likely to occur at the critical time when the site of hormone production is changing. However, low progesterone levels often observed in women at the time of spontaneous abortion may be a consequence rather than a cause of disrupted pregnancy. There is no indication that, once pregnancy has become established, giving hormones is of any help in avoiding spontaneous abortion; in fact hormone therapy may damage the fetus.

It appears that some early pregnancies are lost due to defective gametes. Microscope studies have demonstrated that imperfect sperm are still able to fertilise. A defective ovum or one fertilised by a defective sperm (*blighted ovum*) may not be able to develop properly or implant, resulting in spontaneous abortion.

Although aborted fetuses are not routinely examined unless the woman has lost several pregnancies in succession, it has been estimated that a very high proportion have chromosomal abnormalities. Presumably these are too severe to be compatible with life.

It has been suggested that the uterus somehow recognises the abnormal conceptus and has developed a mechanism, not yet known, to reject it. The body normally recognises tissues distinct from its own (skin grafts, organ transplants) and rejects them. The mechanism which permits the mother to carry a fetus *without* rejection has long puzzled immunologists. Further research in this field would undoubtedly help shed light on the whole area of tissue transplant rejection. At present, understanding is hazy, not least because a proportion of children born each year (one per cent) are genetically or congenitally defective (Weatherall 1985). Presumably these are not sufficiently 'imperfect' to arouse the maternal rejection mechanism. Research with human embryos taking place in conjunction with *in vitro* fertilisation programmes could provide valuable information.

Maternal health and behaviour may help to determine the outcome of early pregnancy. Pyrexial illness appears to trigger abortion. Cigarette smoking during pregnancy is known to influence the baby's health post partum, but there is less evidence to suggest that it may trigger spontaneous abortion (Edwards 1983). Evidence about the effects of alcohol on early pregnancy is more persuasive. Risks seem to increase with frequency of consumption (Kline *et al.* 1980). Moderate drinking (one or two glasses daily) has been reported to double the risk during the second trimester, compared to non-drinkers (Edwards 1983). This study, conducted on 32,000 women, suggested that the fetus is vulnerable to the effects of alcohol at *any* stage, conflicting with earlier findings indicating that harm was most likely to occur during the second trimester (Harlap and Shiono 1980).

The need for health education is clearly demonstrated. Ante-natal classes may be poorly attended for a variety of reasons. Women who participate may receive information at inappropriate times because they are told about classes when the pregnancy is advanced. Opportunities to modify health behaviour are then limited (Perkins 1979). More could be achieved if women and their partners could receive pre-conceptual counselling, especially as environmental damage is most likely to occur during the very early stages of development, before the woman even realises she is pregnant. In some cases this may have legal implications. Kroll (1987) describes how in the United States the first prosecution for misconduct in pregnancy was initiated against a known drug addict whose baby died of brain damage soon after she was born. Placenta praevia had been diagnosed. The woman had been advised to refrain from sexual intercourse, to avoid street drugs and to seek medical help if she began to bleed vaginally. Her prosecutors set out to prove that she ignored these instructions and was therefore legally responsible for her baby's death.

In other cases the working environment can affect the developing fetus, especially exposure to chemicals or radiation. Women who are planning or become pregnant may ask to be moved to another area. Clearly there is a need for health education to be arranged as early as possible. Pre-conceptual counselling deserves recognition as part of the school nurse's role. The effects of blindness and other severe congenital malformations as a result of Rubella, a common virus infection, during the first trimester are well documented. Schoolgirls are offered vaccination against Rubella between the ages of 11 and 15. This occasion could provide an opportunity to begin pre-conceptual teaching.

Stress has sometimes been cited as a possible cause of spontaneous abortion by operating through the higher centres of the brain and influencing the production of hormones from the hypothalamus. These hormones, in turn, affect the uterus. It is difficult to find hard evidence in support of this theory. Most studies have been poorly controlled, relying on the case history reports of only a few women.

Emotional reactions

Although the literature contains several anecdotal accounts of women's grief when miscarriage occurs (Hardin and Urbanus 1986, Procter 1985, Lovell 1983, Moore 1984), there is a clear need for further research to document actual feelings and identify common patterns as a first step before a helping or counselling strategy can be developed. Stack (1984) reports that grieving is common after spontaneous abortion but that it is not generally recognised by family, friends or health care professionals. Standish (1982) interviewed thirty-two women fourteen weeks after miscarriage. She found that women needed to ventilate feelings of grief and loss and, when asked whether anything could have helped, replied that 'being listened to' was the most important unmet need. Nine women in a detailed case history study by Wall-Hass

(1985) were most helped by caring professionals who explained exactly what was happening to them, and by friends and relatives who showed appreciation of their loss by their comments and bringing flowers.

Reactions to stillbirth and perinatal death have been well documented (Lovell 1985). Lack of documentation surrounding spontaneous abortion is sharply contrasted against this. One of the factors reported most helpful to parents who have experienced the tragedy of stillbirth is to see their baby. For women who have miscarried, particularly at a very early stage in pregnancy, there is little to see. The birth is not registered and the event is not formally marked by a funeral or a legitimate period of mourning. In this situation it is perhaps significant that sympathy and the gift of flowers should be particularly valued because they allow the woman to admit to others and to herself that her loss is real.

Berezin's observations (1982) suggest that women who have had a spontaneous abortion experience the classic stages of the grieving process:

- Denial and inability to accept that loss has occurred, often combined with shock;
- Confusion and anger, often directed against health care professionals;
- Bargaining;
- Depression, guilt, tendency to blame self for loss;
- Acceptance.

However, eventual acknowledgment that loss of a baby had occurred still tended to be regarded as unjust and unfair.

Until the results of further research and intervention studies become available, nurses may do much to help their patients by applying some of the strategies which research has demonstrated as helpful to parents experiencing perinatal loss.

Carr and Knupp (1985) report that parents found solace from telephone conversations with their nurses to discuss their feelings, and derived much comfort from follow-up visits at home. A protocol was specially developed to provide guidelines for care.

Beckey et al. (1983) shared their feelings of inadequacy in the face of perinatal death in a workshop held for all nurses working on the same maternity unit. As a result they developed a strategy to help parents and allow the nurses themselves to cope with their own similar, but less intense, grief reactions. A checklist was developed to help parents explore their feelings, to ensure they were informed about helpful agencies and to avoid needless repetition of information at a sensitive time. Nurses needed training to complete the checklist, since a major limitation proved to be a tendency towards completion in a rigid, inflexible manner as though the chief goal was placing a tick in each box. For this reason it was suggested that the checklist should not be taken to the bedside, but completed after an open discussion with the parents. Parents were encouraged to express their sorrows rather than deny or forget them, in the belief that emotional growth can develop through the experience of grief. Referral to support organisations proved especially helpful, perhaps because parents were able to accept that miscarriage is an all too common phenomenon and does not suggest inadequacy on their part. This supports the findings of Oakely et al. (1984) who

Table 4.1 The attachment concept and early pregnancy loss

Before birth	1. Planning pregnancy 2. Confirming pregnancy 3. Accepting pregnancy 4. Experiencing fetal movements 5. Accepting the fetus as an individual
After birth	5. Experiencing the birth 7. Hearing and seeing the baby 8. Touching and holding the baby 9. Caring for the baby

Source: Klaus and Kennell (1976)

observed that many women did not appreciate the high incidence of miscarriage until it happened to them.

Before they were able to help their clients, nurses in Beckey's unit needed to understand the concept of attachment and apply it to perinatal loss. Klaus and Kennell (1976) describe nine steps that occur in the process of attachment to the unborn and newly delivered child. These are outlined in Table 4.1, which shows that the first five steps are experienced *before* birth and are therefore likely to influence loss of the baby in the event of miscarriage. Parents may feel a sense of regret because, in the case of spontaneous abortion, they have not seen, touched or cared for their baby and, in the case of pregnancy loss during the first trimester, the mother will not even have felt her baby move.

Habitual abortion

Habitual abortion is said to occur when the woman has experienced three or more consecutive spontaneous abortions. Investigations have indicated that in approximately eight per cent of cases the fetus is chromosomally abnormal. In others it is expelled prematurely, sometimes because the space inside the uterus is restricted by fibroids (see Chapter 7) or the septum of a bicornuate uterus (see Fig. 4.4). Pregnancy may continue to term once the defect is surgically repaired. In other cases elevated levels of prostaglandins in the uterus may increase contractility of the myometrium, triggering spontaneous abortion or premature birth. The endocrine events triggering normal labour at full term are poorly understood. Maternal events are known to be important: it is only in recent years that scientists have suspected that the fetus itself may have some influence.

Early pregnancies may be lost because of maternal immunological defects. A number of centres in the UK have introduced a programme of immunisation with paternal antibodies to help prevent habitual abortion. Although results of early clinical trials indicate success (Mobray 1983), the reason is unclear. It has been sug-

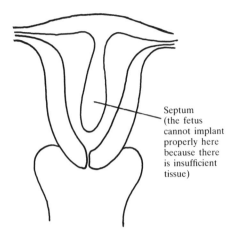

Septum
(the fetus
cannot implant
properly here
because there
is insufficient
tissue)

Figure 4.4 Bicornuate uterus.

gested that during normal pregnancy the maternal immune system recognises the trophoblast of the fetus and responds by producing special 'blocking' antibodies which prevent the normal maternal antibodies from destroying the fetus. This may not happen in women who experience habitual abortion. Injection of paternal antibodies may protect the fetus or stimulate maternal blocking antibodies to form.

Incompetent cervix

Incompetent cervix is said to be one of the major causes of late spontaneous abortion. It may follow a D and C or therapeutic abortion in which the cervix has been over-stretched, although more gentle surgical techniques today have helped to eliminate this problem, especially when very early abortions are performed. In other cases there may be no apparent reasons for incompetent cervix. The weight of the growing fetus may force the cervical os to gape until pregnancy can no longer be maintained (see Fig. 4.5).

If the woman has a history of habitual abortion, particularly during the second trimester, she may be admitted to hospital when she is approximately fourteen weeks pregnant for a *Shirodkar's suture* to be inserted under general anaesthesia (see Fig. 4.6). A non-absorbable suture is inserted like a purse-string at the level of the internal os to hold it closed. The suture is withdrawn just before the onset of labour.

Missed abortion

Missed abortion occurs when the fetus has died but is not expelled. If this happens early in pregnancy (up to twelve weeks), the whole conceptus is gradually re-absorbed. After twelve weeks, bleeding between the chorionic villi and uterine wall results in the

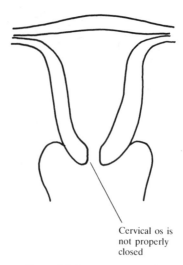

Cervical os is
not properly
closed

Figure 4.5 Incompetent cervix.

formation of a *carneous mole*. After eighteen weeks the dead fetus becomes
mummified if it is not expelled and is macerated by the time it is eventually passed.
The reason why the uterus does not expel the dead fetus in missed abortion is not
known.

Early in pregnancy, the woman may seek medical advice because of unexplained
amenorrhoea or discharge, or the signs and symptoms of pregnancy gradually regress
and the uterus ceases to increase in size. Spontaneous expulsion usually occurs without intervention, but most women feel very distressed at the thought of carrying a

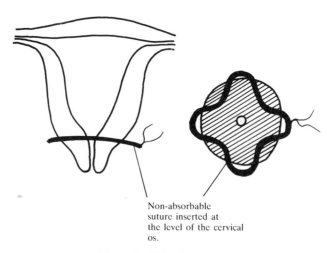

Non-absorbable
suture inserted at
the level of the cervical
os.

Figure 4.6 Shirodkar suture.

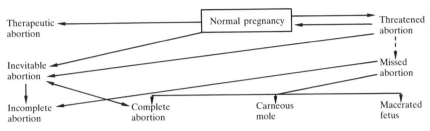

Figure 4.7 Classification of abortion.

dead fetus and it is usual for the products of conception to be removed by suction (before twelve weeks gestation) or prostaglandin induction (after twelve weeks).

The possible outcomes of pregnancy are shown in Fig. 4.7.

Hydatidiform mole

A *hydatidiform mole* is an uncommon, abnormal outcome of pregnancy in which the trophoblast undergoes neoplastic changes. More than 90 per cent of women who develop this condition have no further trouble once it has been diagnosed and the mole has been removed (Crawford and Pettitt 1986). In the remainder, abnormal tissue continues to proliferate. It may invade and perforate the uterus, leading to haemorrhage. Unless emergency hysterectomy is performed this can be fatal. In a further, very small proportion (three per cent), the mole undergoes frankly malignant change. The resulting tumour is called a *choriocarcinoma*.

Diagnosis of hydatidiform mole

Evidence that pregnancy is not progressing normally may be provided by symptoms reported to the doctor, or on the basis of clinical examination. Signs and symptoms are mainly due to abnormally high plasma levels of hCG. This condition is also associated with a clotting deficiency. Elevated hCG levels result in excessive vomiting (*hyperemesis gravidum*). The woman may be anxious and demonstrate features of thyrotoxicosis because hCG is chemically very similar to thyroxine. The coagulation defect may result in uterine bleeding so she may be admitted to hospital with a diagnosis of threatened abortion. On examination, the uterus is usually larger than would be expected for the stage of pregnancy according to dates, and will feel very soft because there are no fetal parts. The characteristic appearance of the mole can be confirmed by ultrasonography while hormone assay will reveal high levels of hCG. Bleeding may result in anaemia and the signs of pre-eclampsic toxaemia (hypertension and pro-teinuria) may be exhibited.

A hydatidiform mole is classified as either *partial* or *complete*. A complete mole consists entirely of chorionic villi enlarged to form fluid filled sacs (*hydropic vesicles*). The outer layer of the sacs is derived from trophoblast. This is the part that can become malignant. Malignancy is much more likely to occur when the mole is complete and there is no evidence of any fetal tissue.

A partial mole is much less likely to become malignant. As well as hydropic vesicles, there is evidence of some normal fetal tissues ranging from a few blood vessels to a complete fetus.

A complete mole results from an abnormal conception in which all the genetic material is derived from the sperm. Partial moles contain one set of maternal chromosomes and two sets of paternal chromosomes.

Like other genetically abnormal conceptions, hydatidiform mole is most likely to occur in women who are at the extremes of their childbearing years, but aetiology is obscure. In Europe it is a rare condition, with an incidence of one in 2,000 pregnancies. In some parts of Asia, incidence may be as high as one in 250, but this may be due to the extended period of childbearing. Dietary deficiency has also been suggested as a possible causal factor.

Various schemes have been suggested for classifying the degrees of malignant change from hydatidiform mole into highly malignant choriocarcinoma, but there is no generally accepted system. In practice all women who develop a mole are followed up by referral to a specialist centre. Choriocarcinoma is a curable disease and, in recent years, nearly every woman who has received treatment has responded.

Follow-up

Women are referred to one of three specialist hospital departments in the UK (Charing Cross London, Jessop Sheffield, or Ninewells Dundee) to monitor plasma and urinary levels of hCG. The main reason for measuring hCG is that its level is an extremely reliable way of assessing how much trophoblastic tissue has been retained. The following patterns are watched for:

- Very high hCG levels within twenty-four hours of evacuation of the mole (by suction up to twelve weeks or otherwise by prostaglandin induction);
- High levels (above 20,000 IU/litre) four weeks after evacuation.

These signs suggest that trophoblastic tissue is invading the uterus, with a risk of severe haemorrhage or perforation. Monitoring is continued since high or unchanged levels four to six months later indicate malignant change with rapid metastases to lungs and brain, or local spread to the vagina, all likely to result in bleeding.

Treatment of invasive mole and choriocarcinoma

The aim of treatment is to eradicate all invasive tissue, avoiding neoplastic spread and haemorrhage while retaining the uterus so that future fertility is not impaired. This is achieved by treatment with the cytotoxic drug methotrexate, an antimetabolite of folic acid, which destroys rapidly dividing cells. Choriocarcinoma is highly susceptible to methotrexate, but as with all neoplastic conditions, success of treatment depends on the extent of the disease. Women whose disease is more extensive require other chemotherapeutic agents used in conjunction with methotrexate, and higher doses, but these have adverse effects including nausea, hair loss and bone marrow suppression. The treatment regime is tailored to the individual needs of the patient by calculating a score based on the interval between pregnancy and treatment, hCG levels and the site and number of metastases. Depending on the score, the woman is assigned to a low, medium or high risk group and treated accordingly.

The physical and psychological care of women undergoing chemotherapy for malignancy of the genital tract is discussed in Chapter 12. It is important to remember that women in this particular client group are young, may already be bringing up a family, and may hope to have other children. More than 80 per cent have successful pregnancies after completing treatment for choriocarcinoma, although they are advised not to start another pregnancy until at least one year later to avoid genetic damage to the fetus by methotrexate which can remain in the body for several months. Hormones can encourage residual disease to persist, so monitoring continues long term. Relapse occurs in only about five per cent of cases, but the use of oral contraceptives is not encouraged, especially during the first six months after treatment.

Resources

The Miscarriage Association
18 Stoney Brook Close
West Breton
Wakefield
West Yorkshire
WF4 4TP
Tel.   0924 885515

In some cases the National Childbirth Trust is willing to provide support to women who have had a miscarriage.

The National Childbirth Trust
5 Queensborough Terrace
London W2 3TB
Tel.   01–221 3833

Booklets of advice on preconceptual care are available from:

The Maternity Alliance
309 Kentish Town
London NW5 2TU
Tel.   01–267 3255

References

Beckey, R.D. *et al.* (1983) 'Development of a perinatal grief checklist', *Journal of Obstetric, Gynaecological and Neonatal Nursing* 12 (3), pp. 194–9.

Berezin, N. (1982) *After a Loss in Pregnancy*, New York: Simon and Schuster.

Carr, D. and Knupp, S.E. (1985) 'Grief and perinatal loss: a community hospital approach to support', *Journal of Obstetric, Gynaecological and Neonatal Nursing* 14 (2), pp. 130–9.

Crawford, M. and Pettit, D. (1986) 'Hydatidiform mole and choriocarcinoma', *Nursing Times* 82 (49), pp. 38–9.

Crawford, M. and Pettit, D. (1986) 'Treatment schedules for hydatidiform mole and chorio-carcinoma', *Nursing Times* 82 (50), pp. 40–2.

Edmonds, D.K. *et al.* (1982) 'Early embryonic mortality in women', *Fertility and Sterility* 38, pp. 447–57.

Edwards, G. (1983) 'Alcohol advice to the pregnant woman', *British Medical Journal* 1 pp. 274–291.

Glass, R.M. and Ericsson, R.J. (1982) *Getting Pregnant in the 1980s, New Advances in Infertility: Treatment and Sex Preselection*. California: University of California Press.

Hardin, S.B. and Urbanus, P. (1986) 'Reflections on a miscarriage', *Maternal and Child Nursing Journal* 15 (1), pp. 23–30.

Harlap, S. and Shiono, P.H. (1980) 'Alcohol, smoking and incidence of spontaneous abortions in the first and second trimester', *Lancet* 2, pp. 173–6.

Klaus, M. and Kennell, J. (1976) *Maternal–Infant Bonding*, St Louis: Mosby.

Kline, J. *et al.* (1980) 'Drinking during pregnancy. Spontaneous abortion', *Lancet* 2, pp. 176–9.

Kroll, D. (1987) 'The consequences of fetal rights', *Nursing Times* 83 (6), pp. 59–60.

Lovell, A. (1983) 'Women's reactions to late miscarriage, stillbirth and perinatal death', *Health Visitor* 56 (9), pp. 325–7.

May, K.A. (1982) 'Three phases of father involvement in pregnancy', *Nursing Research* 31 (6), pp. 337–42.

Mobray, J.F. *et al.* (1983) 'Controlled trial of treatment of recurrent spontaneous abortion by immunisation with paternal cells', *Lancet* 1, p. 994.

Moore, J. (1984) 'Miscarriage: a common tragedy', *Nursing Times: Community Outlook* June, pp. 210–11.

Oakley, A., McPherson, A. and Roberts, H. (1984) *Miscarriage*, Glasgow: Fontana Paperbacks.

Orem, D. (1985) *Nursing: Concepts of Practice* (3rd ed.) New York: McGraw-Hill.

Perkins, E. (1979) 'Defining the need: an analysis of varying teaching goals in antenatal classes', *International Journal of Nursing Studies* 16 (3), pp. 275–82.

Pizer, H. and Palinski, O. (1981) *Coping with a Miscarriage*, London: Jill Norman.

Procter, E. (1985) 'Too young to live', *Nursing Mirror*, 160 (20), p. 31.

Proud, J.P. (1988) 'Sound judgement', *Nursing Times* 84 (29), pp. 70–1.

Stack, J.M. (1984) 'The psychodynamics of spontaneous abortion', *American Journal of Orthopsychiatry* 54 (1), pp. 162–7.

Standish, L. (1982) 'The loss of a baby', *Lancet* 1, pp. 611–12.

Wall-Hass, C. (1985) 'Women's perceptions of first-trimester spontaneous abortion', *Journal of Obstetric, Gynaecological and Neonatal Nursing* 14 (1), pp. 50–3.

Weatherall, D.J. (1985) *The New Genetics and Clinical Practice*, Oxford: Oxford University Press.

Wilson-Barnett, J. (1976) 'Patients' emotional reactions to hospitalisation: an exploratory study', *Journal of Advanced Nursing* 1, pp. 351–8.

5   Ectopic Pregnancy

Ectopic pregnancy (from the Greek *ektopos*, misplaced) occurs when the fertilised egg embeds itself outside the uterine cavity. Possible sites of implantation are shown in Fig. 5.1. Extrauterine implantation occurs most commonly in the uterine tubes, but is also possible on the ovary, cervix or in the pelvic cavity. This is very rare, however. Nash (1974) estimated the incidence of abdominal implanation to be one in 15,000 pregnancies and reported that, over a period spanning fifty years, only two cases had been presented in one of the largest London teaching hospitals.

Successful pregnancy and survival of a healthy baby is rarer still. Even if it is born alive, the baby, lacking uterine protection, will probably be deformed due to pressure from maternal organs.

The uterine tubes: anatomy and physiology

Ectopic pregnancy is an important topic for nurses because its incidence throughout the Western world is increasing (Macafee 1984). Outcome depends on the site of implantation, and the degree of development achieved by the fertilised egg.

Figure 5.2 shows that the uterine tubes are not of uniform diameter along their length. The fimbriae at the ends of the tubes are delicate structures which in health can move about and apply themselves closely to the surface of the ovary. Since they are open-ended, the egg enters soon after it is released and travels down the tube towards the uterus. Fertilisation occurs in the next, slightly expanded, region called the *ampulla*. Passage of the egg is speeded by peristaltic contractions of the muscular walls of the tube and the wafting action of cilia lining its epithelium. Years ago, physiologists believed that the uterine tubes merely acted as pathways, conducting the egg to the uterus, but now it is known that secretory cells scattered between the cilia release substances to nourish the egg before and after it is fertilised.

If, for any reason, the fertilised egg is prevented from reaching the uterus, it will burrow into the wall of the uterine tube (or, rarely, another extrauterine site) instead. The cells continue to divide and the egg enters the trophoblast stage of development, when it increases in size. Meanwhile, the endometrium continues to prepare itself as it would in the case of normal pregnancy, and a pregnancy test performed at this time would be positive.

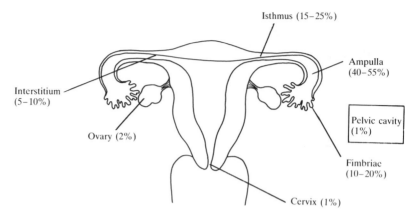

Figure 5.1 Extra-uterine sites for implantation.

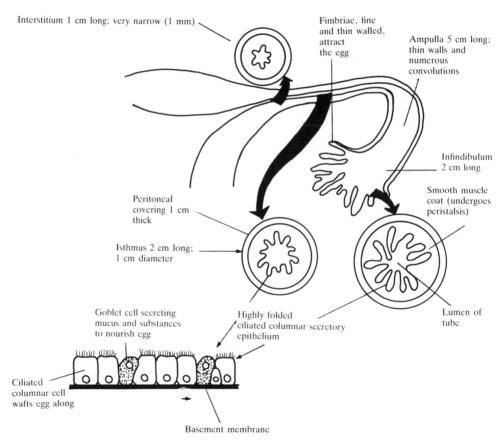

Figure 5.2 Structure of the healthy uterine tube.

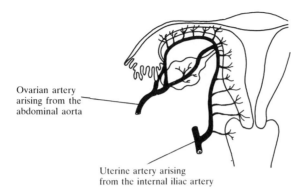

Ovarian artery
arising from the
abdominal aorta

Uterine artery arising
from the internal iliac artery

Figure 5.3 Blood supply to the female reproductive system.

Outcome of ectopic pregnancy

The uterine tubes are highly vascular (see Fig. 5.3) because they contain major tributaries of blood vessels supplying the rest of the female reproductive system, so erosion by the trophoblast soon results in bleeding, but the amount, and symptoms experienced by the patient, will vary according to the degree of damage.

There are three possible consequences:

1. The embryo may die soon after implantation, leading to the formation of a tubal mole. A certain amount of bleeding will occur at the site, causing pain or tenderness if blood escapes into the abdominal cavity. The signs and symptoms of pregnancy regress and a pregnancy test would now be negative. The endometrium is shed. Loss is usually less than with normal menstruation, but darker. The tubal mole may be absorbed, giving rise to no further symptoms, or it may cause tubal abortion or tubal rupture.
2. Development may continue until a slightly later stage, so bleeding will be more profuse. Blood and the products of conception are carried into the pelvic cavity tending to drain to the lowest point (the Pouch of Douglas). A *haematocoele* forms, possibly displacing the pelvic organs. Adhesions may result. There will be more pain, and signs of shock (see Table 5.1). Surgical intervention is necessary.
3. The trophoblast causes marked erosion of the tubal wall, ultimately rupturing it. Profuse bleeding occurs into the pelvic cavity and the patient is shocked, with severe abdominal pain.

Official statistics show that over a two year period twenty-one women in England and Wales died as a consequence of ruptured ectopic pregnancy, five at home, and three on the way to hospital (HMSO 1979). This dramatic picture is only seen in a few cases, however. Patel (1985), conducting a five year study of ectopic pregnancies, showed that only twelve out of sixty-seven cases (18 per cent) gave the classic acute

Table 5.1 Signs and symptoms of hypovolaemic shock (due to diminished blood volume)

1. Falling blood pressure
2. Rapid pulse
3. Deep sighing respirations–air hunger
4. Restlessness
5. Cold, clammy extremities
6. Pallor or cyanosis
7. Confusion, unconsciousness
8. Disordered blood clotting and fluid distribution within the tissues–oedema

picture. Most of the women in his study (55–82 per cent) presented as subacute cases, often not diagnosed until at least twenty-four hours after admission. Other medical authors agree that ectopic pregnancy may be difficult to diagnose (Lucas and Hassim 1970) and patients may be suspected of having appendicitis because their symptoms of abdominal pain are so non-specific.

■   Clare Parry, aged 29, was married with one child. She felt ambivalent about having another baby. Although she had been happy about her first pregnancy, she felt unstimulated at home and was looking forward to returning to work when her daughter started school. She was aware, however, that her husband would welcome another baby.

Clare had been feeling unwell for several days. Her period was due, but it was unusual for her to experience discomfort before menstruation. She was taking the progesterone-only pill (see Chapter 2) and her periods were light and frequently irregular. During the day she developed cramping abdominal pain and started to bleed vaginally, but the discharge was thin and dark, unlike her usual menstrual loss.

Clare's husband drove her to the Health Centre, where the GP performed a full physical and vaginal examination. His findings are shown below:

Temperature: 37°C
Pulse: 100 beats/minute
Blood pressure: 90/70
Bimanual vaginal examination: slightly enlarged uterus with swelling and tenderness in the right fornix and dark, bloodstained discharge.

When asked, Clare could report pain in the tips of her shoulder blades. This referred pain is sometimes experienced by women who have ectopic pregnancy. Diagnosis may also be made by raised plasma βhCG levels and ultrasound as well as urinary pregnancy testing (Wasley 1988).

Clare was admitted to the gynaecology ward of the local hospital and prepared for theatre.

Treatment for ectopic pregnancy

If a patient is suspected to have ectopic pregnancy, she is always taken to theatre for laparoscopic investigation. All or part of the affected uterine tube is removed (total or partial salpingectomy) and any remaining part of the tube is surgically reconstructed.

A major problem associated with this type of operation is that it is always undertaken as an emergency so that, although it is known that future fertility may be impaired between 30 to 60 per cent, there is little opportunity for doctors or nurses to discuss this with the patient. It is known, however, that the egg is chemically attracted to the fimbriae once it has been released into the pelvic cavity, and that it may sometimes be released from the right ovary yet enter the left uterine tube. To discourage migration and ensure that eggs enter the undamaged uterine tube, some surgeons recommend removing the ovary on the affected side. This means that there will be no delay as future eggs move towards the uterus.

The operation is performed through an incision made transversely just above the symphysis pubis called *Pfannenstiel incision* (see Fig. 5.4). Wounds in this position heal well and achieve a good cosmetic result. Closure is usually with silk sutures or clips.

Several studies have been undertaken to document the effect on future fertility, but numbers remain too small for statistical analysis (Editorial: *BMJ* 1976).

Whatever the future of her fertility, the chance of survival for the woman is excellent as soon as bleeding is stopped, and recovery is rapid.

Pre-operative nursing care

In this emergency situation, minimal preparation is made for theatre, even if the uterine tube has not ruptured, because it may still do so. The length of time between conception and rupture is variable, although it is not usually more than about six weeks after Day One of the last menstrual period. The progesterone only pill

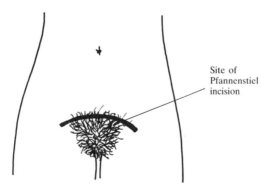

Site of
Pfannenstiel
incision

Figure 5.4 Site of Pfannenstiel incision.

increases risk of ectopic pregnancy (see Chapter 2) and the irregular bleeding associated with it means that estimation of the last menses may be difficult.

The nurse responsible for pre-operative care must confirm the following:

- The patient is wearing only a theatre gown;
- Dentures, prostheses, cosmetics and all jewellery except a wedding ring have been removed;
- Details on the identity band are correct;
- Urinalysis has been performed;
- The doctor has obtained a sample of blood for haemoglobin estimation and grouping and that at least two units of blood have been cross-matched;
- The stomach is empty (at least four hours since the last meal) to prevent aspiration and inhalation of gastric contents;
- The upper part of the suprapubic hair is shaved, since the incision will be made in this region.

Emotional reaction to ectopic pregnancy

Before she goes to theatre, the patient will be required to sign a consent form and this will involve an explanation of the operation, usually from the doctor. However, someone who has just been admitted to hospital in an emergency, feeling anxious and in pain, may be unable to remember, or even to absorb all the information given. Under these circumstances, it is essential that the nurse responsible for the patient's care should be available when she has recovered from the effects of surgery and anaesthesia to explain what has happened and the possible implications for her fertility.

Since routine, planned surgery is known to generate anxiety both before and after the operation (Wilson-Barnett 1979), it is reasonable to assume that in an emergency the degree of stress experienced will probably be greater. Many studies by nurses and psychologists have demonstrated the effectiveness of psychological preparation before surgery (Ridgeway and Mathews 1982) and at least two studies by British nurses have indicated that providing information can reduce the incidence of post-operative complications (Hayward 1975, Boore 1978). However, most research concerning ectopic pregnancy has been conducted by doctors and focuses on epidemiology and future prospects for fertility. Although little nursing research has taken place, it is likely that the patient will feel distressed due to the following conditions:

- The trauma of emergency admission;
- Loss of pregnancy;
- Altered self concept;
- Possible effects on future fertility.

(Cowen 1986)

Because data have not been gathered systematically to document reaction to ectopic pregnancy, there is little indication of the extent to which the individual will experience grief or loss. However, Oakley *et al.* (1984), writing about miscarriage in general, express a belief that ectopic pregnancy may be particularly difficult to accept because it is invisible and the woman may scarcely have realised that a pregnancy occurred at all. Chapter 4 contains guidelines for the nurse counselling couples who are grieving about spontaneous abortion, and these may also be helpful in a situation where ectopic pregnancy has occurred.

Post-operative nursing care

■   The model by Roper *et al.* (1985) was chosen for Clare during her post-operative recovery because it is based on an Activities of Living (AL) Model, and Clare's ALs were so severely disrupted that she was entirely dependent on the nursing and medical staff (see Care Plan 5.1 on page 112). The revised model described by Roper *et al.* lists twelve ALs which are affected by many different influencing factors (physical, psychological, cultural and socio-economic). Change in response to these alters not only throughout the life span of the individual but also over much shorter periods of time, including a period of illness or dependence. The use of this model could be criticised as it was applied to Clare, because its contribution towards planning psychological care is somewhat limited, although the ALs listed include communication. However, it was possible for Clare's nurse to adapt the model so that Clare and her husband were given the opportunity to express their feelings about the pregnancy and their future plans. Care Plan 5.2 (on page 120) illustrates the continuing care needed after the immediate post-operative phase. Women do not usually stay in hospital for more than five or six days.

Incidence and aetiology of ectopic pregnancy

There is much well-documented evidence to suggest that the incidence of ectopic pregnancy is increasing (Beral 1975, Chaukin 1982). Westrom *et al.* (1981) reported the number of ectopic pregnancies in a general practice over a twenty year period for all women between 15 and 39 years of age. The rate was estimated at one per 1,000 conceptions at the beginning of the study, but increased gradually as the research progressed. Risk increased with age, being greatest for women in their late twenties and thirties. Risk factors included the following:

- Inflammation of the pelvic organs;
- Scarring from previous surgery;
- Use of the progesterone-only pill;
- Use of an IUCD;
- Developmental abnormalities of the uterine tubes;
- Previous ectopic pregnancy.

Care plan 5.1 (Roper, Logan and Tierney: Activities of Living model)

Name: Clare Parry

Treatment/condition: Salpingectomy for ectopic pregnancy. Post-operative care

Assessment and care plan:

Activity of Living	Date & Time of Assessment	Assessment	Problems	Goal	Nursing Intervention	Evaluation
Maintaining a safe environment	20.02.89 10 pm	Returned to ward from theatre. Vital signs: Pulse –70 beats/minute BP: –110/70 Vaginal loss: slight, dark. Skin warm, well perfused. See also 'Breathing'	(1) Shock and haemorrhage (potential) (2) Postural hypotension on first getting out of bed (potential)	(1) Monitor vital signs (pulse, BP, respiratory rate) to detect any change in condition early (2) Prevent postural hypotension	(1) Monitor vital signs and vaginal loss at half hourly intervals until within normal limits, then four hourly (Normal limits: pulse 60–80 beats/minute BP 110/70–130/80 respiratory rate 14–20 breaths/minute) (2) Assist Clare to sitting position. Ensure she does not feel dizzy prior to standing	20.02.89 10.30 pm Condition stable 12.30 pm Condition stable 21.02.89 2.30 am Four hourly observations: condition stable 21.02.89 Out of bed for half an hour BP 110/70 Not dizzy or faint
Communication	20.02.89 10 pm	Drowsy, but coherent	None			
Breathing	20.02.89 10 pm	Respiratory rate: 16 per minute	Post-operative chest infection	Clare will not develop post-	(1) Position with pillows so that	22.02.89 Respiratory rate: 16 per

Activity of living	Date/time	Assessment	Problem	Goal	Nursing intervention	Evaluation
		Deep and regular. Pale but not cyanosed. Skin warm and well perfused	(potential)	operative chest infection	Clare can expand her chest fully and secretions do not pool	minute. Deep and regular. Clare has learned to support the wound when coughing. She has no evidence of chest infection
					(2) Encourage deep breathing exercises taught by physiotherapist. Encourage Clare to cough and expectorate, holding the wound to support it	
					(3) Monitor respiratory rate and depth four hourly. (Normal range 14–20 breaths/minute)	
					(4) Observe colour, consistency and amount of sputum	
Eating and drinking	20.02.89 10 pm	Two units of blood transfused in theatre. Intravenous fluids in progress (1 litre of dextrose/saline to be administered over 8 hours). Fasting after anaesthetic. Says her mouth is dry and complains of nausea	(1) Dry mouth (actual) (2) Nausea (actual) (3) Fasting (actual) (4) Anorexia due to nausea (potential)	(1) Clare's mouth will feel moist and comfortable (2) She will not feel nauseated (3) She will not fast longer than necessary (4) She will not become anorexic	(1) Offer mouthwashes two hourly, help clean teeth. Observe condition of oral mucosa (2) Give 10 mg metochlorpromapide intramuscularly for nausea and monitor effectiveness (3) The doctor or experienced nurse will use stethoscope to listen for bowel	21.02.89 12 am Clare no longer feels nauseated. She has drunk 50 ml of water and is no longer thirsty. Intravenous fluids may be discontinued 22.02.89 2 pm Clare is tolerating fluids and diet

Activity of Living	Date & Time of Assessment	Assessment	Problems	Goal	Nursing Intervention	Evaluation
					sounds. Offer sips of water progressing to free fluids when they become apparent, then a light diet if tolerated. Discontinue intravenous fluids on the advice of medical staff	
Elimination	20.02.89 10 pm	Bladder emptied via catheter before surgery (300 ml). Has not passed urine since return to wards. Bowels last opened yesterday	(1) Urinary tract infection due to catheterisation (potential) (2) Urinary retention due to handling of bladder (potential) (3) Constipation due to lack of mobility (potential)	(1) Will pass urine within 12 hours of surgery (2) Will not develop urinary tract infection (3) Will not become constipated	(1) Monitor urinary output. Record on fluid balance chart (2) Offer commode, not bedpans (3) As soon as Clare is tolerating fluids ensure that she drinks at least two litres daily (4) Monitor urine for signs of infection (colour, odour, complaints of dysuria, send clean catch specimen for bacteriological examination) (5) As soon as Clare is	21.02.89 12 am Clare is tolerating oral fluids (see eating and drinking). She has passed 600 mls of urine 22.02.89 12 am Clare is tolerating a normal diet. Her bowels have opened. She has no evidence of urinary tract infection

eating offer a diet containing fibre
(6) Give aperients as prescribed if Clare does not open her bowels within three days

Activity	Date	Assessment	Problem	Goal	Nursing action	Evaluation
Personal cleansing and dressing	20.02.89 10 pm	Wearing hospital gown. State of hygiene good. Vaginal discharge: small amounts of old, dark blood	Movement restricted by IVI – will need help to wash etc. (actual). Vaginal discharge (actual)	Help Clare with personal hygiene until intravenous fluids are discontinued. Minimise discomfort/ inconvenience of vaginal discharge	Offer help with washing, combing hair, cleaning teeth. Until IV fluids are discontinued Perform vulval toilet and provide sanitary towels two hourly	21.02.89 12 am Clare may attend to her own hygiene needs. Says she is pleased about this – dislikes accepting help from nurses. Vaginal discharge: minimal
Controlling body temperature	20.02.89 10 pm	Oral temperature: 37.5°C Skin feels warm	(1) Mild pyrexia (actual) (2) Could later develop wound infection (potential). (See maintaining safe environment and elimination)	Clare's temperature will return to normal limits within 48 hours of surgery	(1) Monitor temperature four hourly. Report changes to medical staff (2) Nurse with one blanket (3) Observe all possible sites for infection (see breathing and elimination)	21.02.89 9 am Clare's temperature is 37.2°C. Her skin feels warm. She does not complain of feeling hot 22.02.89 12 am Temperature: 36.9°C
Mobilising	20.02.89 10 pm	In bed with intravenous infusion. Says	Reduced mobility due to: (a) IVI (actual)	(1) Early ambulation to prevent all	(1) Help Clare out of bed and encourage her to walk around	20.02.89 11.30 pm Omnopon 15 mg intra-

Activity of Living	Date & Time of Assessment	Assessment	Problems	Goal	Nursing Intervention	Evaluation
		the wound site hurts	(b) wound pain (actual) Problems arising from reduced mobility: (a) Inflamed pressure areas (potential) (b) Deep venous thrombosis (potential) (c) Constipation (potential – see elimination) (d) Urinary stasis (potential – see elimination)	hazards of bedrest identified (2) Pain control to permit early ambulation	bed. Encourage her to sit in a chair for short periods (2) Encourage leg exercises taught by physiotherapist to avoid deep venous thrombosis (3) Give analgesia as prescribed: omnopon 15 mg intramuscularly (three doses prescribed), then control pain with mild analgesia (paracetamol) especially before physiotherapy	muscularly has successfully controlled wound pain

21.02.89
Clare has been out of bed for 15 minutes

22.02.89
Clare is able to walk short distances without discomfort. Her pressure areas are not inflamed. She has no evidence of deep venous thrombosis

24.02.89
Clare is now able to move around the ward without pain, but is concerned about coping with household tasks when she returns home, especially lifting her daughter. A new assessment, goals etc. now need to be completed in preparation for discharge |

Activity of living	Date	Assessment	Problem	Goal	Nursing action	Evaluation
Working and playing	20.02.89 7.30 pm on admission	Clare is married with one child, aged 3 years. She does not work outside the home at present. Formerly she was a lecturer in higher education 21.02.89 post-operatively. Clare's husband always helps with housework. She is not on close terms with other families nearby. Her parents and brother do not live in the same town. She normally leads a fairly sedentary life	Clare will return home within 5–6 days to run her home and look after her daughter aged 3. She has no nearby family to help (actual)	Clare and her husband will begin to plan ahead for Clare's extended recovery at home	Clare and her husband will be told the probable length of admission, and that when she goes home she will need help with household tasks for at least three weeks. Although the wound will by then be sealed, healing will still not be complete for several months. Heavy lifting should be avoided for at least two months	24.02.89 Clare and her husband have discussed how they will cope when she first goes home. He will take two weeks annual leave, then Clare's mother will stay for a few days
Expressing sexuality	20.02.89 11 pm	Clare is drowsy but obviously distressed. She did not realise she was pregnant. She does not know	(1) Loss of pregnancy, guilt (actual) (2) Effect on body image (potential)	Clare will voice her feelings to her nurse and her husband, and they will not be afraid to show their emotions	(1) Allow Clare to express her fears and emotions (2) Give information about the possible effect of surgery on future fertility	23.02.89 Clare has discussed how she feels. She and her husband have decided to use a barrier method of contraception until they are ready to decide

Activity of Living	Date & Time of Assessment	Assessment	Problems	Goal	Nursing Intervention	Evaluation
		whether she would have been happy or not, but is upset for her husband who would have liked another baby			(3) Give information about suitable forms of contraception	whether they want to establish another pregnancy
Sleeping and resting	20.02.89 10 pm	At first drowsy from anaesthetic. Reassessment 21.02.89 Says she normally sleeps from 11 pm to 6 am. Sometimes she wakes and has difficulty sleeping again. Does not wish to have night sedation	(1) Often sleeps poorly (actual) (2) Normal sleep pattern may be disrupted in hospital (potential)	Clare's normal sleep pattern will be disrupted as little as possible	(1) Clare is not disturbed between 11 pm and 6 am, but knows she may call the nurse if unable to sleep (2) Control wound pain/discomfort	24.02.89 Clare says she is able to sleep fairly well in hospital providing that wound discomfort is relieved

21.02.89 2 pm	Clare is now awake and recovered from the anaesthetic. She is relieved that the operation is over. She has heard of ectopic pregnancy and perceives it as a life-threatening condition	Fear for mortality – ectopic pregnancy is a 'life-threatening' condition	Clare will discuss her fears	Spend time with Clare and allow her to discuss her fears. Give her full explanations of her condition	24.02.89 Clare has discussed how she feels. She demonstrates an appreciation that ectopic pregnancy can be a life-threatening condition, but its outcome, as in her own case, is usually favourable as far as the woman's general health is concerned
Dying					

The Model by Roper *et al.* (1985) was used to plan care for Clare Parry because ectopic pregnancy is a potentially life-threatening condition which severely disrupts most or all of the activities of daily living. Looking critically at the care plan it is possible to see that, although physical problems can be identified quite well within the framework of the model, the care required in this emergency situation is likely to change very rapidly. From your own experience of the care of critically ill patients do you think that it would be realistic to prepare a care plan and adapt it as rapidly as the need seems here? Could a standard care plan have any use in this situation? What would be the implications for psychological care of the individual patient and her family if a standard format was used? Roper's Model can be used to help plan care for discharge and to identify areas where patient-teaching is required (see 'Working and playing' and 'Expressing sexuality') but as Care Plan 5.2 shows, a new plan may have to be devised for the later stages of recovery.

Care plan 5.2 (Roper, Logan and Tierney: Activities of Living model)

Name: Clare Parry

Treatment/condition: Rehabilitation following salpingectomy for ectopic pregnancy

Activity of Living	Date of Assessment	Assessment	Problems	Goal	Nursing Intervention	Evaluation
Maintaining a safe environment	23.02.89	Ambulant. Vital signs stable and within normal limits. Vaginal loss minimal. Discomfort in suture line, no oozing. Apyrexial	(1) Discomfort in suture line (actual) (2) Reluctant to move due to discomfort (potential)	Prevent discomfort in suture line	(a) Examine wound for evidence of infection/ haematoma. Monitor temperature four hourly (b) Encourage Clare to shower (not bath) – to prevent secondary infection of wound/cross infection (c) Offer mild analgesia (paracetamol) four hourly and monitor effectiveness – to reduce discomfort and encourage ambulation (d) Explain to Clare the importance of walking and moving to avoid hazards of bedrest. Reassure her that sutures will	23.02.89 No evidence of infection/haematoma. Wound looks clean and dry. Non-adherent dressing applied. Apyrexial. Analgesia given four hourly. Clare reports that for much of the time she is pain free. She understands that she must not stay in bed 25.02.89 Sutures removed. Wound appears clean and dry

	Date	Assessment	Problem	Goal	Nursing intervention	Evaluation
					be removed on the fifth post operative day (e) Apply non-adherent dressing – to promote tissue repair, prevent infection and irritation by clothing	
Elimination	23.02.89	Fluid balance chart in progress. Urine tends to be concentrated. No dysuria or frequency. Bowels not opened since surgery. Usual pattern – daily	(1) Urinary tract infection (potential) (2) Constipation (actual)	(1) Clare will not develop a urinary tract infection (2) Clare will no longer be constipated	(1) Encourage Clare to drink at least two litres of clear fluids daily. Monitor output (2) Give two glycerine suppositories and monitor effectiveness. Advise Clare to eat a fibre-rich diet, pointing out suitable items on menu	23.02.89 Importance of taking adequate oral fluids emphasised. Suppositories given. Bowels opened once. Dietary advice given 25.02.89 No urinary tract infection. No constipation
Expressing sexuality	23.02.89	Not sure whether she wants to become pregnant again. Has asked for contraceptive advice	Requires a highly reliable form of contraception (POP and IUCD unsuitable as they alter tubal motility and may increase risk of another ectopic pregnancy)	Clare will be aware of options open to her and know where to obtain a suitable form of contraception	Provide verbal and written information about contraception. Make an appointment for Clare at the family planning clinic	Clare feels that a barrier method of contraception would be most suitable until she and her husband decide whether to establish another pregnancy. Has discussed this with her husband. Appointment at the family planning clinic has been arranged

Inflammation often damages the delicate fimbriae, so they are occluded. Alternately, the entire tube may become attached to another pelvic organ by adhesions. Peristaltic action may be reduced, slowing the passage of the egg so that it is still inside the tube after the time of normal implantation. In Westrom's study, ectopic pregnancy was seven times more likely to occur during phases of acute inflammation.

Both the progesterone-only pill and the IUCD exert part of their contraceptive action by altering tubal mobility, so their relationship to ectopic pregnancy is not surprising.

References

Beral, V. (1975) 'An epidemiological study of recent trends in ectopic pregnancy', *British Journal of Obstetrics* 82, pp. 775–82.

Boore, J. (1978) *Prescription for Recovery*, London: Royal College of Nursing.

Chaukin, W. (1982) 'The rise in ectopic pregnancy – exploration of possible reasons', *International Journal of Gynaecology and Obstetrics* 20, pp. 341–50.

Cowen, S. (1986) 'Ectopic pregnancy care', In: Webb, C. (ed.) *Using Nursing Models: Women's Health*, Sevenoaks: Hodder and Stoughton, pp. 127–39.

Editorial: (1976) 'Tubal pregnancy and surgery', *British Medical Journal* 1, pp. 607–8.

Hayward, J. (1975) *Information – Prescription against Pain*, London: Royal College of Nursing.

HMSO (1979) *Report on Confidential Enquiries into Maternal Deaths in England and Wales 1973–1975*, London: HMSO, p. 98.

Lucas, C. and Hassim, A.M. (1970) 'Place of culdocentesis in the diagnosis of ectopic pregnancy', *British Medical Journal* 1, pp. 200–2.

Macafee, C.A.J. (1984) 'Ectopic pregnancy', In: Chamberlain, G. (ed.) *Contemporary Gynaecology*, London: Butterworths, pp. 57–61.

Nash, T.G. (1974) 'Extra-uterine pregnancy', *Nursing Times* 70 (42), pp. 1623–4.

Oakley, A. *et al.* (1984) 'Miscarriage', London: Fontana.

Patel, Y.A. (1985) 'Ectopic pregnancies: five years hospital experience', *The Practitioner* 229, pp. 269–71.

Ridgeway, V. and Mathews, A. (1982) 'Psychological preparation for surgery: a comparison of methods', *British Journal of Clinical Psychology* 21, pp. 271–80.

Roper, N., Logan, W.W. and Tierney, A.J. (1985) *The Elements of Nursing*, 2nd ed., Edinburgh: Churchill Livingstone.

Wasley, G. (1988) 'Urinary pregnancy testing', *Nursing Times* 84 (36), pp. 42–3.

Westrom, L. *et al.* (1981) 'Incidence, trends and risks of ectopic pregnancy in a population of women', *British Medical Journal* 1, pp. 15–18.

Wilson-Barnett, J. (1979) *Stress in Hospital*, Edinburgh: Churchill Livingstone.

6   Inflammation and Infection

Vaginal discharge

Vaginal discharge may originate from the vagina, the cervix or higher up the genital tract. It is a symptom, not a disease, and may indicate the presence of infection, menstrual disorder or a tumour (benign or malignant). Although discharge frequently reflects a minor problem, easily corrected, it can be extremely worrying and embarrassing to the woman who may endure it for some time before seeking help.

Some women worry about the normal secretion produced by the cervical glands. This is particularly noticeable in the fertile phase of the menstrual cycle. Women taking hormone replacement therapy may also notice increased vaginal discharge.

■   Stella Bastion was aware of a slight, persistent discharge which sometimes stained her clothes, but ignored it until she noticed it becoming profuse and bloodstained, particularly after intercourse. She mentioned the discharge to the nurse at the Family Planning Clinic when she called for a repeat prescription of contraceptive pills. The nurse asked about the colour and consistency of the discharge and its relationship to intercourse. Stella could not remember when it had first become noticeable, but reported that the discharge was not associated with itching, soreness or odour, and that intercourse was painless. She had not taken any drugs other than the pill and had no reason to believe she might be pregnant. The nurse suggested that Stella should see the doctor, explaining that vaginal discharge, though common, can have many different causes and should be thoroughly investigated. The doctor performed a general and pelvic examination and sent a specimen for culture and sensitivity testing.

Speculum examination revealed that Stella had a cervical erosion which had become infected.

Cervical erosion

Before puberty, the cervical canal and surface of the cervix projecting into the vagina are covered with a delicate layer of columnar epithelium (see Fig. 6.1). At puberty,

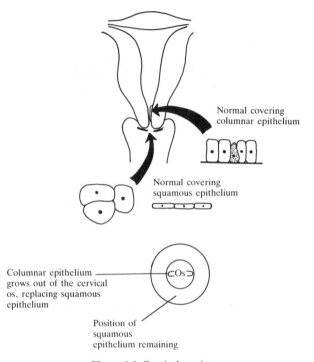

Normal covering
columnar epithelium

Normal covering
squamous epithelium

Columnar epithelium
grows out of the cervical
os, replacing squamous
epithelium

Position of
squamous
epithelium remaining

Figure 6.1 Cervical erosion.

columnar epithelium surrounding the cervical os is usually replaced with squamous
epithelium. This is tougher and more able to resist trauma and infection. Columnar
cells still line the os and provide cervical secretion.

Cervical erosion is a common condition in which the squamous epithelium again
becomes overgrown by columnar cells. This frequently happens when normal hormonal balance is disrupted by pregnancy, or the pill. Occasionally, for some reason
not apparent, the cervix does not become completely re-epithelialised at puberty.

A cervical erosion looks raw and feels velvety to the doctor performing the
examination, but is painless although the columnar cells are more likely to become
injured or infected.

■   Stella was upset because she had heard that cervical erosion is often followed
by malignant changes. She was reassured that there is no basis for this
common misconception (Goldacre 1978). Cervical erosion often disappears
spontaneously if the woman discontinues the pill.

Treatment of cervical erosion
Mild cervicitis is treated by *cryotherapy*, a treatment usually performed in the Outpatient Department since it is quick and painless. The cryoprobe is cooled to extremely

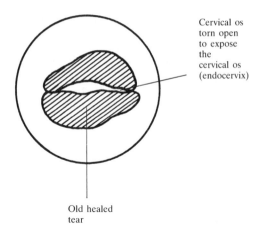

Cervical os
torn open
to expose
the
cervical os
(endocervix)

Old healed
tear

Figure 6.2 Cervical ectropion.

low temperature (−50°C), then applied to the damaged area. Tissue adheres to the cold metal and separates when the cryoprobe is removed. Women must be warned that they will experience watery discharge for about two weeks and should not use tampons during this time or have intercourse to avoid introducing infection to the raw area. They should return to the doctor if the discharge becomes offensive or blood-stained. The raw area gradually becomes re-epithelialised.

More extensive lesions must be treated with *diathermy* and a general anaesthetic will probably be necessary. The discharge is likely to be more offensive than following cryotherapy and takes longer to resolve because trauma is greater.

Trachelorrhaphy
Trachelorrhaphy is excision of a badly torn or infected area on the cervix. Fortunately, with improved obstetric practice it is now seldom necessary. When the cervix is badly torn after delivery the condition is called *ectropion* (see Fig. 6.2).

Vulvitis

Vulvitis may occur for a number of reasons, some trivial, some reflecting serious underlying pathology (see Table 6.1). Not all women seek help, some older women in particular may not appreciate that something could be seriously wrong.

Hypertrophic dystrophy (leucoplakia)

The descriptive term *leucoplakia* ('white patches'), is a condition which tends to occur more often in older women. Atypical cells arising from the dermis increase the rate of mitosis, giving rise to white patches surrounded by areas of inflammation, soreness or irritation. Similar lesions can be caused by other dermatological conditions or even

Table 6.1 Inflammation of the vulva: possible causes and nursing intervention

Cause	Nursing intervention
Nylon underwear, close-fitting jeans	Advise about hygiene and the need to wear loose clothing made of natural fibres when the environment is hot
Allergic dermatitis which may be due to washing powder, scented soap, etc	Try to establish cause. Advise to wash clothes in mild soap and rinse thoroughly
Psychological; over zealous personal hygiene, douching, use of vaginal deodorants	Discussion of personal hygiene and what constitutes reasonable cleanliness. Exploration of anxieties and phobias. May need psychiatric referral in extreme cases
Vaginal discharge	Take high vaginal swab for micro-organisms. Test urine for glucose
Foreign objects inserted into vagina, e.g. tampons, contraceptive sponge	Gentle speculum examination with good light source. Report signs of vaginal discharge and send swabs to laboratory
Infestation	Look for signs of scabies, pediculosis pubis (crab lice)

Systemic disease can give rise to vaginal discharge, the most common being diabetes mellitus, or the vulval area may be affected by conditions found on the rest of the skin, e.g. psoriasis, rashes due to a number of causes. Medical advice should be sought

haemorrhoids. Histology is therefore essential and, if the lesions are localised, they can be excised.

Hypertrophic dystrophy is thought to be a pre-cancerous condition. Some gynaecologists believe that 50 per cent of all cases of carcinoma of the vulva follow hypertrophic dystrophy.

Other inflammatory conditions of the vulva (vulval dystrophies)

Lichen planus

This is a chronic disease of unknown aetiology. The woman complains of pruritus (itching) more frequently than soreness or discharge. Small red-brown patches appear on the labia and histology reveals characteristic inflammatory changes. Lesions can be treated effectively with topically applied steroid creams.

Scleroderma (*Lichen sclerosus et atrophicus*)

The lesions are round or irregular indurated white areas with a characteristic red-brown border. Aetiology is unknown. Initially, the woman may be unaware of them, but they tend to leave scars as they heal, sometimes altering the size and shape of the introitus. Sometimes they cause irritation or hypertrophic changes, so biopsy is necessary.

Bartholin's cyst

Bartholin's glands, which lubricate the vulva, lie behind the vestibule. They are covered with skin and muscle and normally cannot be palpated. They are alveolar (racemose) glands, lined with cuboid epithelium, and their secretion travels down a duct about 2 cm long to reach the vaginal orifice, lateral to the hymen (see Fig. 6.3). Sometimes the duct can become blocked, giving rise to a painless swelling which becomes palpable. Infection may supervene, and an acute painful abscess will result. Treatment involves opening the abscess to facilitate drainage. The walls of the abscess are sutured to the surrounding skin to leave a large orifice. This procedure, called *marsupialisation* (from the Greek *marsipos*, a bag) is performed in the hope that a new duct will form as healing occurs, so the gland can be conserved. The wound is kept open for the first 24–48 hours with a loose ribbon gauze pack inserted gently to avoid further trauma to the wound edges. When the nurse removes the pack she must remember that this is a highly sensitive area, well-supplied with nerve endings. Great care will therefore be necessary. The woman will benefit if given an analgesic before the procedure, allowing enough time for it to take full effect.

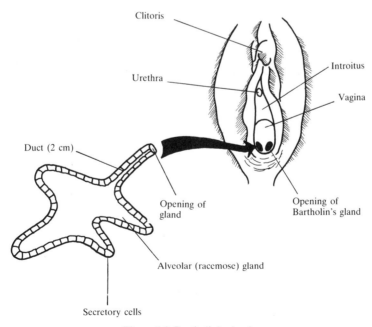

Figure 6.3 Bartholin's gland.

Recurrent Bartholinitis may eventually have to be treated by excising the gland. Since the area is highly vascular, a haematoma may form post-operatively. Removal of both glands is always avoided if possible, because vaginal moistening will be diminished.

Like many other infections of the genital tract, Bartholinitis may be caused by a wide range of organisms, including the bacteria responsible for gonorrhoea. Most women know about sexually transmitted infections and may secretly fear they are infected when they notice a vaginal discharge.

Special clinics (genitourinary medicine clinics)

Women may visit their GP because they are worried about infection or inflammation of the genital tract, or they may go to a special clinic. Some may be reluctant to seek help at a clinic specialising in the treatment of sexually transmitted disease (STD), but the service is usually quick and efficient and absolute confidentiality is assured. In many cases, diagnosis can be established the first time the woman attends. Therefore treatment can be provided immediately.

If a woman goes to her GP specimens must be sent to a laboratory at a neighbouring hospital, delaying diagnosis and treatment. Most bacteria and viruses causing sexually transmitted infections are fragile, and will not survive long outside the tissues. Delay therefore adds to the risk of false negative diagnosis.

Many special clinics do not operate an official appointment system, to provide an efficient service for people who might otherwise have to ask employers for time away from work. However, waiting can be protracted, especially in the lunch hour and evening. Some clinics are open at weekends when they are likely to be busy.

In the days before the National Health Service, treatment for sexually transmitted infections was provided free of charge at specially organised clinics. These became attached to particular hospitals when the NHS was established, but were often geographically separated because of their origins, or resited unobtrusively in the basement. Potential clients were often faced with the embarrassment of having to ask exactly where they should go. Today, many clinics have been re-allocated in more pleasant surroundings, helping to dispel some of the old stigma. Many people who are afraid they may have an infection prove on examination to be infection free. Others require check-ups because they have had sex with someone other than their usual partner or request pyschosexual counselling. Not all conditions treated are necessarily sexually transmitted and staff have many opportunities to provide health education. If an infection is diagnosed however, clients must return to ensure that treatment has been successful. Nurses can do much to support women at a stressful time when diagnostic procedures may prove uncomfortable or embarrassing.

Follow-up visits are important to ensure that treatment has been effective; women will not be encouraged to return if they dislike the atmosphere of the clinic or sense disapproval. This is particularly likely to upset women who have caught infections from a regular partner.

■ When Lisa Small noticed that she had developed vaginal discharge, it seemed that recently everything had gone wrong. She already suspected that her boy-friend had slept with someone else. Initially Lisa's discharge was white and irritant, but after a few days it became copious and offensive. She was terrified she might have 'VD'. Her friend encouraged her to go to the nearby STD clinic. At first Lisa was appalled, but Carole pointed out that as Lisa was reluctant to go to her own GP, she had little choice.

At first Lisa thought she would go to a clinic in a neighbouring town in case she saw anyone she knew locally. However, she became worried about lo-cating another clinic and establishing when it was open. She had seen infor-mation leaflets in the family planning clinic, but was reluctant to take one. Lisa spent a sleepless night, worse because she felt itchy and sore, but decided to go to the clinic next morning.

On arrival at the clinic, Lisa was greeted by a clerk who asked whether she had attended previously before recording her name, age and address. She noticed that her personal details were written inside a folder with only a number stamped on the cover and she was given a card with her number written on it, although the nurse addressed her by name. Lisa was told that the doctor would ask about her general medical, gynaecological and sexual history, before obtaining a specimen of discharge to find if she had any infec-tion. This would involve a speculum examination to obtain material from the cervix and vagina, as well as a cervical smear. A specimen would be taken from the urethra, and this would probably be the most unpleasant part of the examination, since it is such a sensitive area. As well as entering the urinary tract, some infectious agents may gain access to the rectal mucosa, possibly because they drain downwards in discharge or contaminated menstrual blood. It would therefore be necessary to obtain a swab from the rectum. This would involve inserting a proctoscope to open the anal sphincters to ensure that an adequate specimen could be obtained. Although uncomfortable, this part of the examination would soon be over.

The nurse explained that she would help to collect the specimens. The results would probably be available within half an hour, since they would be examined in the clinic. She asked whether Lisa was aware of any drug allergies, particularly to antibiotics, or if there was any possibility she could be pregnant, since this might affect any treatment prescribed. Lisa did not think she could be pregnant because she was taking the pill. In more doubtful cases, a preg-nancy test can be performed in the clinic.

The nurse obtained a specimen of blood to be sent to the laboratory and tested Lisa's urine for albumin and glucose. Diabetics are especially prone to infection because of their disordered metabolism and elevated blood sugar levels. They often develop vaginal infections, particularly *Candida*. This might be the first sign of diabetes.

After Lisa had spoken to the doctor, the nurse returned to help prepare her for the physical examination. Women usually find this embarrassing since the doctor will need a good light (probably an anglepoise lamp) to visualise the genital area, with the woman in the lithotomy position (see page 9). This position is otherwise used mainly in theatre, when the woman is anaesthetised.

Diagnostic procedures and specimen handling

During examination, material is obtained from the vagina, cervix, urethra and rectum, smeared onto microscope slides and examined immediately (see Table 6.2). Part of each specimen is inoculated onto culture media (see Fig. 6.4) and placed in an incubator. All slides and cultures must be prepared with a scrupulous, non-touch technique in order to maintain asepsis and prevent contamination of the environment. This will avoid the growth of extraneous micro-organisms. Cultures are collected from the clinic at the end of the day so that bacteria can be grown and identified in the laboratory. This helps to confirm the findings made straight away, in the clinic. Sensitivity to antibiotics can only be tested when bacteria are grown in culture. This is very important in view of the increasing reports of antibiotic resistance among bacteria, including *Neisseria gonorrhoea*. The blood of all clients is obtained to test for syphilis in the laboratory.

As all specimens obtained in the STD clinic contain potentially infectious material, they must be handled carefully to avoid contamination and spillage, and marked with 'Biohazard' or 'Danger of Infection' labels, before transport to the laboratory in plastic bags. Particular care must be taken when blood is handled because at least two viruses – hepatitis B and human immunodeficiency virus (HIV) are parenterally transmitted. Although historically the carriage rate of both has apparently been highest in homosexual and bisexual men, *anybody* can become infected, and all nurses and

Table 6.2 Gram staining

Most bacteria can be classified as *Gram positive* or *Gram negative* according to uptake of microscope dyes. This has practical importance for identification and treatment since the two groups tend to be susceptible to different antibiotics.

Procedure
1. The microscope slide, with a thin film of the specimen spread over it, is passed through the hot flame of a bunsen burner to 'fix' (kill) the organisms
2. The film is covered with gentian violet (also known as crystal violet) dye to stain all the bacteria. This stain is rinsed away quickly to prevent over-colouration
3. The film is covered with iodine, which helps the gentian violet to stain more intensely ('fixes' the stain), then rinsed away
4. The slide is rinsed with alcohol (usually ethanol, but can be acetone or mixtures) to decolorise the Gram negative bacteria
5. The film is covered with a red counterstain such as Safranin, which stains the Gram negative bacteria. After a final rinse and drying, the Gram positive bacteria can be identified because they retain the gentian violet

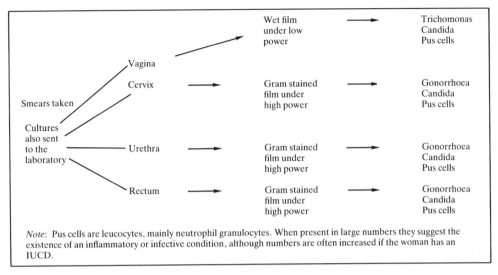

Figure 6.4 Examination of specimens in the clinic.

doctors must adopt sensible precautions to protect themselves. Well-fitting latex gloves should be worn when handling specimens or performing venepuncture. Needles and syringes should be placed, immediately, without separation into a special 'Sharps' box. If blood and other body fluids are spilt, they should be mopped up at once using disposable wipes, by someone wearing latex gloves and a plastic apron. The area must be disinfected by an agent know to destroy hepatitis B and HIV. Compared to most other viruses, neither of these is particularly robust, and both are destroyed by hypochlorite disinfectants (bleaches) (Spire *et al.* 1984). In hospital, hypochlorite granules may be used. In the hospital or home, a freshly prepared solution of household bleach, diluted one part bleach to ten parts water, is effective against HIV. Protection of staff is very important when dealing with potentially infected patients and clients, but it is essential for nurses to appreciate that most infection control precautions depend on knowledge of microbiological principles and if these are understood and properly applied, transmission of infection should be preventable without the need for exaggerated precautions likely to be distressing for the client. Bacteria and viruses responsible for sexually transmitted conditions are not infectious in the same way as those causing colds or influenza. This is why they depend on intimate contact between one person and another to spread. No harm can result from ordinary social contact with infected people, and avoiding touch adds to their distress by making them feel 'unclean'.

■   Microscope examinations showed that Lisa had an infection caused by *Trichomonas vaginalis*.

Trichomoniasis

Trichomonas vaginalis is a highly motile flagellate protozoan (see Fig. 6.5) which causes an offensive, frothy, yellow-green discharge. Speculum examination of a woman who has a severe infection will reveal inflamed, oedematous vaginal walls and cervix. The vulva, perineum and insides of the thighs may become sore. The organisms are transmitted from one partner to the other during sexual intercourse but, although they are readily demonstrable in the vagina of an infected woman, they are difficult to isolate from men. This has caused some authorities to suggest that *Trichomonas* may sometimes also be transmitted by a non-sexual route, possibly on fomites such as towels, or in swimming pools (Catterall and Nichol 1969). Women as well as men sometimes remain asymptomatic, probably acting as carriers, so both partners need treatment even if diagnosis is made in only one of them. This needs emphasising to clients; unless *Trichomonas* is adequately treated in *both*, protozoa may be passed back from one to the other.

■   Lisa was relieved to learn that, although an infection had been found, it could be cured effectively by a course of tablets. The drug of choice is metronidazole (Flagyl). Lisa wanted to know whether she had caught the infection from her boyfriend. The nurse explained this was possible, particularly as some women appear to carry *Trichomonas* for a long time before developing symptoms, but that sexual transmission is possibly not the only route, and Lisa could have become infected by some other means.

Most people who attend an STD clinic receive treatment as out-patients, unsupervised, so before they leave the nurse must ensure they know exactly what to do. When metronidazole is prescribed the following points need emphasis:

- One tablet (200 mg) should be taken three times a day, after meals.
- Tablets should be taken at regular intervals throughout the day and the entire course should be completed. The level of drug in the blood could otherwise fall too low to destroy the infection.
- Alcohol should be avoided until all tablets have been taken (there have been reports of fits and confusional states following the ingestion of alcohol and metronidazole).
- Clients should return to the clinic one week later to ensure that treatment has been successful. Occasionally people taking metronidazole have experienced skin rashes, headaches, and gastrointestinal upsets. If side effects are encountered, clients should return earlier.
- Intercourse should be avoided until a check-up has shown treatment to be effective. Infection might otherwise be passed on to someone else or the woman might become re-infected, especially if the vaginal mucosa is not fully healed.

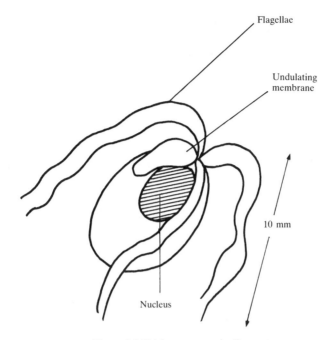

Flagellae

Undulating
membrane

10 mm

Nucleus

Figure 6.5 Trichomonas vaginalis.

The incidence of trichomoniasis appears to be declining, possibly because metronidazole is now widely used in dentistry, and bowel surgery.

Contact tracing

The aim of contact tracing is to ensure that all potentially infected people are examined and treated as speedily as possible to prevent spread. This is one of the main reasons for identifying and treating infection during the first visit to the clinic. If gonorrhoea or syphilis is diagnosed, it is essential for all partners to be followed up. STD clinics employ one or more contact tracers who will, if necessary, correspond with or personally visit individuals and persuade them to be examined.

The success of contact tracing depends on clients providing full, truthful accounts of all their partners but, with casual encounters, names and addresses may genuinely not be known. It is usually possible to obtain a description however and, over the years, clinics tend to build up 'dossiers'.

The difficulty of establishing the possible source of infection is one of the main reasons for the introduction of the term 'sexually transmitted disease'. The term 'venereal disease' with all its stigma is considered rather old-fashioned today. It implies that infection is spread exclusively by the sexual route. Three infections are classified as venereal: gonorrhoea, syphilis and chancroid (soft sore) mainly a tropical disease, seldom seen in Britain. Even for these, spread may occur via a non-sexual route. However, the term 'venereal' has medico-legal implications. Among adults these infections are mainly spread sexually; if a man or woman catches gonorrhoea or syphilis from his or her partner the most reasonable explanation is infidelity, which may be used as grounds for divorce.

People with non-venereal sexually transmitted infections are not routinely followed up, partly through economic considerations, and also because these conditions, though distressing, do not have the devastating long term effects of gonorrhoea or syphilis.

Contact tracing is generally undertaken by specially trained members of staff (often former nurses or social workers) away from the clinical areas. Clients will be most co-operative if they feel goodwill towards the clinic and, as this will reflect on the way they have been treated, nurses can do much to promote the success of contact tracing. They can also encourage clients to attend follow-up appointments, comply with drug regimens and avoid intercourse until they are infection-free.

Prevalence of sexually transmitted diseases

Gonorrhoea and syphilis are *notifiable* diseases, i.e. doctors have a legal responsibility to report the number of new cases to the Medical Officer of Environmental Health as part of public health measures in helping to identify and control communicable disease. The Public Health Laboratory Service (PHLS) collates figures and sends a weekly report of outbreaks of all types of communicable disease to medical microbiologists and relevant clinical staff every week. Annual reports are made of the incidence of gonorrhoea and syphilis. Although reporting other sexually transmitted conditions is not a legal requirement, staff at PHLS welcome reports.

Careful monitoring has shown that sexually transmitted diseases remain among the most commonly diagnosed infectious conditions in this country. In 1986 the number of new cases rose to 647,000, an increase of 7 per cent over 1985, and more than 10 per cent since 1976 (DHSS 1988). The greatest increase was seen among female attenders, who now account for 46 per cent of all conditions seen in STD clinics. This increase may be due in part to improved diagnostic techniques and willingness to attend clinics but other factors almost certainly play a part (Adler 1986). Attitudes towards sexual behaviour are more liberal and more effective methods of contraception have removed fears of unwanted pregnancy. Older barrier methods offered some protection against infection but oral contraceptives and the IUCD do not. Today, people travel more often for business as well as pleasure and, with the weakening of family ties, are more likely to live and work far from home, where loneliness may act a spur to sexual experimentation. The number of new cases of gonorrhoea and syphilis have traditionally been regarded as an index of promiscuity but in 1986 these accounted for only 7 per cent of new conditions seen as compared to 16 per cent in 1976. Decrease was greatest for males, perhaps reflecting a change in sexual behaviour among homosexuals in response to the health education message concerning HIV in the mid 1980s. Increases in the numbers of sexually transmitted infections reported are mainly owing to non-specific genital infections and warts.

Discovery that she has such a condition is likely to shock a woman. Nurses who work in STD clinics see people at their most vulnerable and may have to provide sympathetic help in the face of recrimination, bitterness and resentment. Anger may be directed at the nurse by a client so distressed that she does not know how to express her feelings. Nurses who work in clinics must consider their own attitudes towards aggression and have opportunity to develop skills for helping to defuse a stressful situation.

Other sexually transmitted diseases

Candidiasis (thrush)

Candida albicans is a fungus related to the yeasts. It reproduces mainly by a vegetative process called budding and can survive under adverse conditions by forming spores (see Fig. 6.6). *Candida* can be demonstrated by Gram staining vaginal, cervical and urethral smears. It may infect men although it is more readily detectable in women.

Candida is not necessarily a sexually transmitted infection but, if it is isolated from the vagina, it is usually also present in the genital tract of the woman's partner. In men, *Candida* is usually asymptomatic, although it may occasionally cause balanitis. It

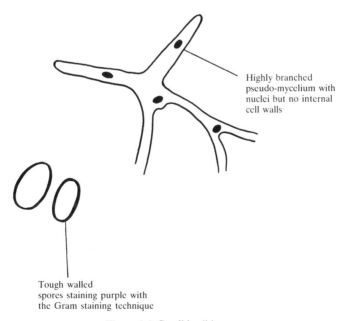

Highly branched pseudo-mycelium with nuclei but no internal cell walls

Tough walled spores staining purple with the Gram staining technique

Figure 6.6 Candida albicans.

may also inhabit the mouth or lower bowel, often developing in response to antibiotic treatment which inadvertently destroys part of the normal gut flora, allowing *Candida* to grow unchecked. Upsets of the normal, vaginal pH (4.5) may also suppress the usual bacteria and promote candidiasis. The woman then complains of 'thrush', recognisable as a thick, irritant discharge with a characteristic yeasty odour. This often happens when normal hormone balance is disrupted by pregnancy or the contraceptive pill. Existing infection may allow *Candida* to develop.

Candidiasis can be treated with a topical fungicidal agent such as nystatin or clotrimazole (Canesten). There are claims that clotrimazole is more effective.

Women may be given clotrimazole cream and pessaries. The nurse must explain how to use them:

- The cream, which is soothing, may be applied to the vulval area whenever necessary.
- The pessaries must be inserted as high as possible into the vagina using the applicator provided. This is best done at night after going to bed as they can easily be dislodged. As they liquefy the pessaries may stain clothing, so most women prefer to wear a sanitary pad.
- Completion of the course of treatment and follow-up are essential, as with any other infection.

Clotrimazole can be purchased without prescription, although self-medication is unwise.

Some women (particularly diabetics or those taking the pill) may find *Candida* a recurrent problem. The vaginal walls become inflamed and extremely painful. If the characteristic white patches are removed with a swab, a raw bleeding area will be exposed. In these cases a course of nystatin tablets may be prescribed.

Various self-help remedies have also been found effective, and women will probably be grateful if nurses can tell them about these. Cotton underwear is cooler and more comfortable than nylon. It can be boiled to prevent re-infection. Soap has a drying effect on the skin, and can increase soreness. Some women prefer to use warm water and baby oil. Patting rather than rubbing dry may help. Live yoghurt contains *Lactobacilli* similar (but not identical) to those normally found in the adult female vagina. Local applications may be soothing.

Incidence of candidiasis has increased by 63 per cent since 1976.

Genital herpes

There are two types of herpes simplex virus. Type 1 causes cold sores which usually develop around the lips. Type 2 causes blisters similar in appearance, which develop primarily on the genitals, although it is now recognised that cross-infection from one area to another can occur. The herpes virus normally enters the body via the mucous membranes or a skin lesion. There is usually some prodromal discomfort before symptoms appear. The lesion is a characteristic raised vesicle developing into a fluid-filled a pustule containing highly infectious virus particles. As the pustule heals, a scar forms and the lesion ceases to be infectious. Lesions can develop on the cervix, labia or vulva. They are extremely painful, especially during micturition. Secondary infection is common.

Women experiencing primary infection develop a systemic illness similar to influenza (pyrexia, headache, general malaise), but occasionally symptoms are more severe. There may be severe headaches, back pain, and enlarged lymph nodes in the groin. Diagnosis is confirmed by clinical examination and identifying virus particles from the exudate under the electron microscope.

Improved diagnostic facilities and publicity have increased the number of cases of genital herpes reported in recent years Between 1985 and 1986, the number of new cases declined for the first time, although in the past ten years incidence overall has trebled. The decline we are now beginning to see may be due to a resurgence of interest in barrier methods of contraception.

After the primary infection has resolved, both men and women continue as carriers of the now dormant virus. They usually experience repeated episodes of inflammation when they are again infectious.

Genital herpes is a worrying infection on several counts:

- The lesions are extremely painful. Urinary retention may occur in severe cases. Ice packs or topically applied anaesthetic ointment may be helpful.
- There is no reliable cure. Acyclovir, an anti-viral agent, can help alleviate symptoms (orally, intravenously or topically applied) but to be fully effective treatment must begin in the prodromal stages, before lesions appear. Acyclovir seems more effective during primary than secondary attacks.
- The virus can infect the eyes, so clients and nurses must wear plastic disposable gloves when topical preparations are applied, to avoid disseminating virus particles on the fingers.
- If a baby is born during a primary attack, infection can be transmitted during passage down the birth canal, causing encephalitis, which can be fatal. Caesarean section is justified.
- There appears to be a link between herpes simplex Type 2 and cervical cancer, since women who have encountered the virus appear to be particularly prone to this malignancy. Many doctors recommend two year cervical smears after herpes infection (see Chapter 12). The possible relationship has been described in the lay literature. Nurses must therefore be aware that women may have fears they feel unable to voice.
- Vaccine is not yet available because there are technical difficulties involved with developing immunisation against viruses, although clinical trials are in progress (Mims 1987).

On the positive side, nurses can explain to women that between attacks they are not infectious.

Victims may be grateful to hear about a self help group called the Herpes Association, c/o Spare Rib Ltd., 27 Clerkenwell Close, London EC1.

Genital warts (*Condylomata acuminata*)

Genital warts are caused by a papilloma virus which has come under suspicion as a possible causative agent of cervical cancer (Deitch and Smith 1983). Virus particles have been demonstrated inside the cells of genital warts but do not appear very different to viruses causing warts in other parts of the skin.

Most genital warts appear to be sexually transmitted; 70 per cent of partners are also affected, but incubation seems to extend over several months. Warts develop mainly in moist areas, usually the vagina, vulva and on the cervix, either singly or in clusters. Size is variable. The largest can measure 10 cm. Incidence has increased over the past ten years and now accounts for 10–14 per cent of all new cases seen in Special Clinics.

Warts look unsightly and cause discomfort because they catch on clothing. They develop most rapidly when hygiene is poor, so the importance of careful washing and drying must be emphasised. Growth is also rapid during pregnancy. Treatment demands patience. Warts can be painted with a solution of 20 per cent podophyllin or trichloro-acetic acid but, as these preparations burn the skin, great care must be taken to prevent contact with any other area. They must be re-applied on a regular basis and care must be taken to ensure that the woman knows exactly when to wash them off. In severe cases cryotherapy may be necessary.

Non-specific genital infection

In the past clients sometimes complained of vaginal discharge but repeated microscopy failed to show any causative agent. This condition was referred to as non-specific urethritis owing to the symptoms which developed in the male partner. Today, the greater magnification possible with the electron microscope will often indicate presence of an organism called *Chlamydia trachomatis* which microbiologists classify in a group intermediate between bacteria and viruses. *Chlamydia* is similar to bacteria in its sensitivity to antibiotics but, like viruses, can multiply only inside host cells. Various other members of the group have been identified and are known to cause diseases as diverse as psittacosis (spread from birds to man) and trachoma, a major cause of blindness in the Third World.

Chlamydia trachomatis can cause severe urethritis in men, although asymptomatic carriage is also possible. In women it infects the cervix, occasionally giving rise to vaginal discharge, but silent infection can occur and may be extremely damaging. Infection spreads upwards from the cervix, giving rise to pelvic inflammatory disease, sometimes resulting in infertility (Wilson 1985). Chlamydial infections can be treated effectively with tetracyclines, doxycycline or sulphonamides given to both partners. Today the infection is regarded as having the same damaging side effects to women as gonorrhoea (see page 141).

The incidence of NSGU is rising, and it is now the most commonly recorded STD, accounting for about a quarter of all new cases diagnosed. Although it is still more common in males, incidence is rising faster in females.

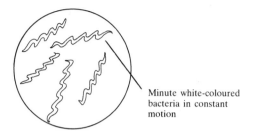

Minute white-coloured
bacteria in constant
motion

Figure 6.7 Treponema pallidum.

Syphilis

The causative organism of syphilis is *Treponema pallidum*, a minute, highly motile spirochaete with a characteristic appearance when visualised by the special technique of dark ground microscopy (see Fig. 6.7). Nowadays this chronic and extremely damaging infection occurs more commonly in homosexuals, but women sometimes become infected.

Syphilis is spread almost exclusively by the sexual route in adults (occasionally spread from lesions on the hands or lips have been reported).

Two other diseases, yaws and pinta, are caused by spirochaetes, but are less damaging because they do not attack the nervous system. Both diseases are widespread in undeveloped parts of the world, but non-sexual transmission is possible although immigrants who have yaws are often treated in STD clinics in this country.

Treponema pallidum enters the body via the mucous membrane of the genital area or mouth, reaches the subcutaneous tissues and eventually gives rise to the lesion of primary syphilis, called the *chancre*. The incubation period is extended (9–90 days) but, on average, the chancre normally appears five or six weeks after exposure to infection, though not always at the exact site of penetration. Chancres are often disregarded because they are painless and may be invisible inside the vagina or on the cervix. Textbooks describe a typical 'punched out' lesion with a well-defined edge, but there may be considerable variation. Lymph nodes in the groin become enlarged but this also is painless.

The secondary stage develops about two months later. Again, it may be overlooked because symptoms of headache, sore throat, pyrexia and general malaise can be so easily mistaken for influenza. The typical copper-coloured skin rash does not always appear, or may be dismissed because it is non-irritant. During the appearance of the rash, the individual is highly infectious and the surfaces of the papules teem with treponemes. It is during this phase of the disease that wart-like lesions called *condylomata lata* may appear in damp areas (mucous membranes, axillae). Their irregular outline and covering of grey-white slough has earned the name of 'snail-track' ulcers. When the slough separates, the underlying lesion looks dull and red.

The lesions of primary and secondary syphilis heal without treatment and the disease enters its latent phase, although in the early years the individual remains infectious. Tertiary syphilis may not manifest itself until twenty or more years later. The typical lesion this time is the gumma, an ulcer with an asymetrical shape tending to heal from the centre rather than the outside. Gummata can appear anywhere on the skin and can be highly destructive, eroding deep underlying tissues including bone. Typical sites include the lower part of the leg (just below the knee), buttocks, face, inside of the mouth and on the tongue.

Quaternary syphilis may involve the cardiovascular or nervous system, with far-reaching, sometimes fatal, effects. Cardiovascular complications occur when the aortic wall is invaded by treponemes, resulting in aortic aneurism or aortic incompetence. Approximately 10 per cent of those untreated develop neurosyphilis. This may take the form of tabes dorsalis, a condition in which the lower part of the spinal cord degenerates. Since the passage of nervous impulses between the brain and lower limbs becomes disrupted, there may be pain and a loss of control, accompanied by a sensation of walking on 'cotton wool' because the individual can no longer feel his/her feet. Urinary and faecal incontinence may develop.

General paralysis of the insane, one of the most feared complications of advanced syphilis, is manifested by gradually increasing lack of memory, poor concentration and slow but subtle personality changes which ultimately culminate in dementia.

Another particularly worrying aspect is the possibility of congenital spread from mother to baby across the placenta. This may result in spontaneous abortion or the birth of a baby with the typical stigmata of congenital syphilis. Fortunately this happens very rarely today because all pregnant women have their blood tested for syphilis during the first trimester. If they are infected, treatment with penicillin will be effective since it can cross the placental barrier, providing it is given before fetal damage has occurred.

Although material gently scraped from a primary or secondary lesion may reveal spirochaetes, syphilis is usually diagnosed by one of several possible blood tests also used to monitor the effectiveness of treatment (see Table 6.3). The infection is usually treated by a course of penicillin (or equivalent antibiotic if the individual is allergic) but, as it is usually given on an outpatient basis, the woman must know exactly what she should do to comply with treatment. The information the nurse can give is itemised below:

- A course of penicillin injections will normally clear the infection completely. Once completely eradicated, syphilis will leave *no* lasting damage. Relapse is rare with modern therapy, but it can occur if treatment starts late or if dosage of the antibiotic is inadequate.
- To be effective, injections must be given intramuscularly (procaine penicillin 6,000,000 units) every day so that a constant level of drug circulates in the bloodstream.
- The course will last between 10 and 14 days, depending on the clinic. Over weekends, staff will make arrangements for injections to be given (in the accident and emergency department or by ward staff).
- Injections can be extremely painful, and this may be a reason for default, so their vital importance must be emphasised.

Table 6.3 Blood tests used to detect syphilis

1. *Wasserman Reaction (WR)*
   A standard complement-fixation test that has now been superseded by more modern tests which are easier to perform

2. *Venereal disease research laboratory test (VDRL)*
   A flocculation test which is used routinely to confirm diagnosis and to monitor the course of the disease since it quantifies the amount of treponemal antibodies in the bloodstream. Valuable for screening

3. *Fluorescent treponemal antibody test (FTA)*
   A test that has the advantage of giving a positive result earlier in the course of the disease than any other test yet developed. Not normally used for screening as it is expensive

4. *Treponemal immobilisation test*
   Technically difficult to perform but sometimes necessary if there is doubt over the diagnosis since it is highly specific. Not suitable for routine screening

5. *Treponemal pallidum haemagglutination test (TPHA)*
   A very sensitive test which can sometimes remain positive for considerable periods of time despite completion of an otherwise apparently successful course of treatment. Not suitable for routine screening

- Between four and twelve hours after the first injection, clients may experience headache, pyrexia, joint pain, rigors and oedema around the lesions. This is the Jarisch Herxheimer reaction, which occurs most frequently when treatment is commenced in the early stages of disease. Various theories have been postulated, but the cause remains obscure. Though frightening, it is not harmful.

Since treatment takes place over several days and follow-up, including blood tests, will be required over a prolonged period, nurses have the opportunity to get to know clients well. Contact tracing is vital and clients should not have intercourse for a considerable period of time; the duration recommended is likely to vary from one clinic to another.

Gonorrhoea

The delicate Gram-negative diplococcus *Neisseria gonorrhoeae* which causes gonorrhoea (see Fig. 6.8) cannot survive long outside the body, so spread among adults depends on the sexual route. The squamous epithelium of the adult vagina is resistant to infection: tissues most likely to become infected are the more delicate cells of the urethra, Bartholin's glands and columnar cells of the cervix. The incubation period is up to ten days. In men a painful, purulent urethral discharge develops, prompting them to seek medical help quickly. In women, infection is often silent; estimates of latent infection vary between 50 and 70 per cent. The bacteria can travel upwards, infecting the uterine tubes and causing inflammation, scarring and infertility. This condition is referred to as *pelvic inflammatory disease*. It can be caused by other micro-organisms, including *Chlamydia*.

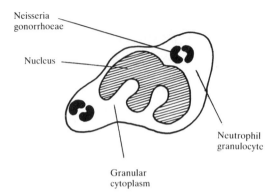

Figure 6.8 Neisseria gonorrhoeae.

Inflammation of the uterine tubes (salpingitis) can present either as an acute or chronic infection, responsible for prolonged pelvic discomfort and general malaise. If the woman does succeed in becoming pregnant, the baby's eyes may become infected as it travels down the birth canal, causing ophthalmia neonatorum. This condition, characterised by purulent discharge, may cause blindness unless treated promptly with antibiotics. It is a notifiable disease.

Occasionally young girls become infected with gonorrhea before puberty. Bacteria invade the vaginal and vulval mucosa because the cells are too delicate to withstand infection. Some cases occur through child abuse, but it is thought that, among this age group, infection might possibly be spread on fomites such as damp towels.

Gonorrhoea is an extremely damaging infection associated with serious long-term health problems. However, these are preventable providing the woman receives treatment promptly. Infection is revealed by Gram staining and treatment is effective with a single large oral dose of ampicillin (2–3 gms) combined with probenecid, a drug which prevents rapid excretion of the antibiotic via the kidneys. It is therefore possible to maintain sufficiently high levels of antibiotic in the blood to destroy infection. If culture and sensitivity testing indicates penicillin resistance, or if the client is allergic to it, tetracycline, vibramycin or spectinomycin may be given. Follow-up with repeated diagnostic tests and contact tracing are vital. Clients should not have intercourse until repeat tests are negative, because many antibiotic-resistant strains are known to exist especially overseas where the drugs may be purchased without prescription. Unfortunately, many women do not realise they have been exposed to infection until late in the course of the disease.

Acute pelvic inflammatory disease

■   Sarah Brewer had experienced pelvic discomfort for some time. One afternoon the pain became so severe that came home early to rest in bed. During the evening she felt much worse, and her flatmate called the GP. After

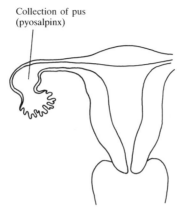

Collection of pus
(pyosalpinx)

Figure 6.9 Pyosalpinx.

examining Sarah, he decided that she should go to hospital straight away. Severe pelvic pain can be due to acute pelvic inflammatory disease, ectopic pregnancy or appendicitis. The outcome of any of these can be serious if diagnosis and treatment are delayed. Pelvic inflammatory disease was suspected because on vaginal examination, the fornices looked inflamed and felt tender. Sarah was told she had an infection, which would best be treated by antibiotics and rest in bed to help the inflammation subside and minimise damage to the delicate uterine tubes. A sample of blood was sent to the laboratory. When there is acute infection, leucocyte count is raised (mainly because more neutrophils are released into the blood) and the erythrocyte sedimentation rate is elevated. Infection may cause pus to collect in the uterine tubes forming an abscess called a pyosalpinx (see Fig. 6.9). Antibiotics will not help the abscess to resolve because the drug cannot penetrate to the bacteria deep inside it, so surgical drainage is necessary via the laparoscope. However, Sarah was relieved to hear that her condition was not sufficiently serious to warrant laparoscopy.

In cases of pelvic inflammatory disease it is often impossible to identify the causative organism. For this reason it is usual to give several drugs together to achieve as broad a spectrum as possible. Cephradrine may be given to destroy aerobic bacteria and metronidazole for anaerobes. Once the infection has begun to resolve, intravenous administration may be discontinued and the drugs may be given by some other route (intramuscularly, orally, or rectally).

■   Sarah was given some analgesia and once this had begun to work, she was allowed to sleep. The next morning her nursing needs were assessed and a nursing care plan drawn up to help meet them (see Care Plan 6.1 on page 146).

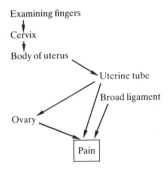

Figure 6.10 Cervical excitation.

Rehabilitation and advice on discharge
Before she left hospital, Sarah was given the following advice:

- Initially she should continue to rest as much as she had in hospital, gradually returning to normal levels of activity over the next week or so. Comments made by women who have undergone gynaecological treatment suggest a need for realistic advice before discharge, tailored to meet the needs of the individual, rather than a standard package of general information (Gould and Wilson-Barnett 1985). Discussion with Sarah revealed that her work as a physical education teacher was strenuous. She was encouraged to postpone return to work until after the Summer vacation, which was shortly to begin.
- Sarah was reminded to keep to a sensible diet and take plenty of fluids.
- She was instructed to complete the course of antibiotics, taking the tablets at regular intervals throughout the day before meals to ensure complete absorption.
- Sarah was advised not to have intercourse until the course of antibiotics had been completed. Her usual method of contraception was discussed. The intrauterine contraceptive device is not suitable for women who have had pelvic inflammatory disease, as it may lead to further inflammation.

Women who have had pelvic inflammatory disease have an increased risk of ectopic pregnancy (see Chapter 5) and infertility (see Chapter 8) because of permanent scarring to the uterine tubes. It is not possible to predict the extent of the damage, and the amount of information given to the individual must be gauged carefully. Sarah was not yet ready to settle down with one partner or think about starting a family. However, it was explained that should she ever develop pelvic pain again, she must seek treatment urgently, and should mention that she had had a pelvic infection if she ever required gynaecological treatment of any kind.

Aquired immune deficiency syndrome

The human immunodeficiency virus (HIV) causes a spectrum of diseases. In order of increasing severity these are:

- Persistent generalised lymphadenopathy (PGL)
- AIDS related complex (ARC)
- Aquired immune deficiency syndrome (AIDS)

There is evidence that, as with all infectious agents, exposure to the pathogen does not necessarily mean that the individual will develop overt disease (Adler 1986). Although the incubation period is a long one, sometimes up to several years, there is at present no available blood test for HIV itself, only for the antibody which the body produces after exposure to the virus. A positive antibody test indicates that the body has been exposed to HIV and has responded to it (*seroconversion*). Evidence presently available suggests that not all those who seroconvert will necessarily progress to chronic infection, although they are assumed to be infectious.

HIV has worrying features:

- The viruses attack cells of the immune system (T helper cells, macrophages) and prevent initiation of the immune response necessary to protect the body against a range of infectious agents which in health are not harmful. The individual becomes highly susceptible to fungal, protozoal and some virus and bacterial diseases. The clinical picture and course of the illness are largely dependent on the particular opportunistic infections to which the individual falls victim (OHE Briefing January 1988).
- Susceptibility to certain types of malignancy is increased (Kaposi's sarcoma, anorectal cancer, non-Hodgkin's lymphoma).
- HIV attacks cells of the nervous system giving rise to various neurological manifestations. Personality change and dementia may occur (Carne 1987).
- The course of the disease is difficult to predict and, as the factors which trigger active virus replication within host cells have yet to be identified, it is not possible to determine those individuals in whom HIV will remain latent and those in whom it will cause disease.
- Seroconversion may take up to three months, so the blood test for antibodies is of limited value, because they take so long to develop and because exposure to HIV could still occur after the test has been performed.
- It is believed that infection persists for life and the individual remains infectious to others.
- Although life can be extended (OHE Briefing January 1988) by medical advances and skilled nursing care, AIDS itself is inevitably fatal. At present there is much speculation about the number of people with PGL and ARC who will go on to develop the full syndrome (Pinching 1987).
- Although most pathogens spread sexually and parenterally are generally not highly virulent and although HIV is readily destroyed by heat and disinfectants,

Care plan 6.1 (Roper, Logan and Tierney: Activities of Living model)

Name: Sarah Brewer

Treatment/condition: Pelvic inflammatory disease

Assessment and care plan:

Activity of Living	Date & Time of Assessment	Assessment	Problems	Goal	Nursing Intervention	Evaluation
Maintaining a safe environment	10.07.89 9 am	*Vital signs:* Temperature – 38.8°C Pulse – 100 beats/minute BP – 120/80 *Vaginal loss:* nil. Has acute abdominal pain	(1) Pyrexia (actual – see 'Controlling body temperature') (2) Pain (actual – see 'Rest and sleep') (3) Infection – permanent damage to uterine tubes (actual)	Reduce further damage by: (a) bedrest (b) giving intravenous antibiotics as prescribed	(1) Provide help/ perform ALs as necessary while Sarah is in bed (2) Give intravenous antibiotics as prescribed	15.07.89 Temperature and pulse within normal limits. Signs of pelvic infection subsiding. Sarah is now taking oral antibiotics and may begin to mobilise gradually. Her pain has diminished
Communication	10.07.89 9 am	Sarah is fearful and reluctant to talk to the nurse at first. She has been told about the probable nature of her infection by the doctor and has	(1) Refusal to talk to nurses (actual) (2) Transfers anger to boyfriend (actual)	Give Sarah the opportunity to participate in her own care, and to discuss her feelings of distress with someone of her choice when she feels able	Explain to Sarah that she will be in hospital for some days, and that her privacy will be respected, but that her nurse is available to discuss feelings and help plan care, and that Sarah has a right to say what she feels her	15.07.89 Over a period of several days Sarah has become more communicative and has helped in the planning of her own care, although she is still withdrawn at times

nursing needs are

	Date	Assessment	Problem	Goal	Nursing action	Evaluation
		expressed anger towards an old boyfriend whom she no longer sees				
Breathing	10.07.89 9 am	Respiratory rate: 22 breaths/minute, regular. Skin warm and pink. No cyanosis	Elevated respiratory rate due to pyrexia and heightened metabolic rate (actual)	Sarah's respiratory rate will return within normal limits (14–20/minute) as the infection resolves	Monitor respiratory rate four hourly. Report changes to medical staff	12.07.89 Respiratory rate now 18 breaths/minute, monitored four hourly
Eating and drinking	10.07.89 9 am	Complaining of thirst. Last had a drink at 7 pm. Has not eaten since breakfast, but says she is not hungry. Does not have to starve for theatre. Intravenous fluids in progress	(1) Thirst due to pyrexia (actual) (2) Anorexia (potential – more protein and calories are needed during pyrexia) (3) Sore, dry mouth (actual)	(1) Prevent dehydration (2) Provide an acceptable, highly nutritious diet (3) Provide mouthcare	(1) Encourage Sarah to drink at least two litres of clear fluids daily and explain why this is important (2) Monitor fluid balance. Observe colour and specific gravity of urine (indicates concentration) (3) Care of intravenous infusion (4) Mouth care. Encourage Sarah to clean her teeth after every meal with a soft toothbrush. Teeth should be cleaned *before* breakfast and	11.07.89 9 pm Sarah has drunk two litres of fluid since admission and no longer feels thirsty. Her mouth is clean and moist. She says she feels hungry. 12.07.89 9 pm Sarah is drinking two litres of fluid per 24 hours. Her IVI has been discontinued. She is not in negative fluid balance. She is eating most of the food provided

Activity of Living	Date & Time of Assessment	Assessment	Problems	Goal	Nursing Intervention	Evaluation
					before settling for the night (5) Offer small, attractive meals frequently, high in calories and protein	
Eliminating	10.07.89 9 am	Sarah has passed 500 ml of urine since she arrived on the ward. Bowels last opened yesterday. Dislikes using a bedpan	(1) Dislikes using bedpan (actual) (2) Constipation while confined to bed (potential)	(1) Give privacy when using commode/bedpan to avoid embarrassment (2) Avoid constipation. Ensure high fluid intake (see eating and drinking)	(1) Reassure Sarah that the curtains will be drawn when she uses a bedpan, and the nurse will ask before she enters (2a) Offer fibre-rich diet and explain its importance (2b) Take Sarah to the WC if she wishes to open her bowels (2c) Give aperients as prescribed	10.07.89 9 pm Sarah has passed 1,500 ml urine 12.07.89 Sarah is not in negative fluid balance. She has tolerated her high fibre diet (see eating and drinking). She has opened her bowels twice
Personal cleansing and dressing	10.07.89 9 am	Hot and sweaty. Hygiene otherwise good. Says she would like a bath	(1) Hot and sweaty (actual) (2) Cannot bath because she is confined to bed (actual) (3) Movements restricted by IVI (actual)	Sarah will feel cool and comfortable	Help Sarah to wash and put on a clean night-dress. Help comb hair and clean teeth as required	10.07.89 2 pm Sarah says she feels more comfortable 12.07.89 2 pm Sarah is now able to attend to her own hygiene needs as the IVI has been discontinued

	Date	Assessment	Problem	Goal	Nursing action	Evaluation
Controlling body temperature	10.07.89 9 am	Oral temperature: 38.8°C Says she feels hot and sweaty. Looks hot and uncomfortable	Pyrexia (actual)	To reduce temperature to less than 37.5°C within 48 hours	(a) Monitor temperature four hourly, report changes to medical staff (b) Supply fresh bedclothes as required. Avoid use of more than one blanket (c) Provide fan (d) Assist with hygiene needs as frequently as desired (e) Tepid sponge if temperature above 38.5°C persists, ensuring that temperature does not fall too rapidly (f) Give intravenous antibiotics as prescribed. Monitor effectiveness (g) Give soluble aspirin as prescribed until temperature is below 37.5°C.	10.07.89 12 am Temperature 37.5°C Sarah says she feels cooler 11.07.89 9 am Temperature now 37°C. Aspirin discontinued
Mobilising	10.07.89 9 am	Knows that she will be confined to bed until the infection resolves. Movement further restricted by:	(1) Sore, inflamed pressure areas (potential) (2) Constipation (potential – see 'Elimination'	Avoid hazards of bedrest	(1a) Advise Sarah to alter her position at least every hour and explain the reason for this (1b) Monitor condition of skin twice daily (2) See 'Elimination'	12.07.89 Sarah's pressure areas are intact. She has no evidence of deep venous thrombosis

Activity of Living	Date & Time of Assessment	Assessment	Problems	Goal	Nursing Intervention	Evaluation
		– Pain – Intravenous infusion	nation') (3) Deep venous thrombosis (potential)		(3) Teach leg exercises. Observe calves for pain and signs of inflammation	
Working and playing	10.07.89 9 am	Sarah teaches physical education at a local school. For recreation she plays tennis, badminton and squash. She reads but dislikes sewing and knitting. She regards herself as 'an energetic person'	Boredom (potential)	Sarah will come to terms with the temporary enforced inactivity of bedrest	Spend time talking to Sarah. Introduce her to other patients. Help her to find ways of passing the time	12.10.89 Sarah spends her days talking, reading and resting. She says she feels miserable at being in bed, especially as she begins to feel better. Her frustration is evident, but she continues to feel more tired than expected
Expressing sexuality	10.07.89	Nature of the infection has been explained by the doctor. Sarah says she feels 'dirty' and 'embarrassed'. She has no boyfriend at present	Damaged self esteem because she realises that her infection may have been sexually transmitted (actual)	Sarah will feel able to discuss her feelings. Tactful health education will be provided	Give Sarah the opportunity to discuss her feelings. Provide further information about pelvic inflammatory disease	15.07.89 Sarah and her nurse have talked about pelvic inflammatory disease and its implications. She realises that a 'sexually transmitted disease' is not necessarily a 'venereal' one. She feels very angry with her previous boyfriend

		Assessment	Problems	Goals	Nursing actions	Evaluation
						whom she continues to regard as the source of her infection. She is more 'angry' than 'hurt'
Sleeping and resting	10.07.89 9 am	Sarah has had a sleepless night because she was hot and in pain. Normally she sleeps well (11 pm–6.30 am) Her active day helps her to rest	(1) Pain (actual) (2) Pyrexia (actual – see temperature control) (3) Difficulty resting due to lack of exercise (potential)	Sarah's pain will be controlled and she will be given opportunities to sleep and rest, pointing out the need for this as part of continuing recovery at home	(1) Give aspirin four hourly as prescribed and monitor effectiveness (2) Help to make more comfortable in bed (3) Avoid disturbing between 11 pm and 6.30 am	10.07.89 12 am Sarah's pain has diminished 11.07.89 9 am Sarah said she slept quite well and has only mild pelvic discomfort Her parents know of her admission and she will stay with them when she leaves hospital. She still feels tired

The model chosen to plan care for Sarah was the one developed by Roper et al. (1985) to illustrate how problems can be identified for a patient confined to bed during the acute stages of an illness, when most or all activities of living are likely to be seriously disrupted. Physical problems have been readily identified, and using this approach it has also been possible to deliver psychological care, even though Roper's model has sometimes been criticised for failing in this respect. When Sarah leaves hospital her usual lifestyle will require modification until she is completely well, and she will require some health education. Her needs are outlined in the text.

Having read this section you could write a care plan using Roper's model to help plan the care Sarah will need before she leaves hospital. Would another model perhaps be more appropriate here? You might, in addition, read the section on Orem's model (1985) on page 86 and use this instead.

figures released by the Communicable Disease Surveillance Centre in England and Wales, and equivalent bodies in the USA and other countries, suggest that numbers of infected people are increasing. In the absence of any national or large scale screening programme the number of seroconverted (therefore infectious) people in the community is impossible to estimate.

In the USA and Britain, HIV disease emerged as a condition affecting the homosexual population chiefly, although in Africa women are infected as often as men. Epidemiological patterns are changing now, however, and women in Britain should receive health education and HIV for the following reasons:

- HIV can be transmitted during normal heterosexual intercourse, so women *are* vulnerable even though epidemiologists agree that at the present time females are still more likely to become infected via the parenteral route through intravenous drug abuse (OHE Briefing January 1988) or transfusion with contaminated blood. They will also be at risk however from sexual contact with intravenous drug abusers and from men who have had sex in African countries.
- HIV can be transmitted from an infected mother to her child *in utero*, at parturition, and possibly via breast milk.
- Pregnancy in a seropositive but otherwise asymptomatic woman is thought to be a co-factor in the development of fully expressed AIDS. A woman receiving antenatal care has a right to receive this information and to be screened *at her request, with her informed consent* providing she has received appropriate counselling. HIV seropositive status is adequate grounds for legal termination of pregnancy. The ethical issue of routine screening, both for the woman's own sake and to estimate the epidemiological behaviour of the disease, is hotly debated at present by doctors, nurses and the public.
- Some latent viral infections may act as co-factors in the development of AIDS. Those presently under suspicion include cytomegalovirus, herpes simplex and the varicella-zoster virus (chicken pox, shingles), which affect women as often as men.
- As with any sexually transmitted infection, the more partners the greater the risk of infection.

Although the possibility of developing AIDS may seem remote for most women, it must be remembered that new facts about the virus are emerging all the time and numbers of people infected are increasing at an epidemic rate; neurological symptoms have only recently been documented, for example. There may be other sinister manifestations of HIV and unsuspected modes of transmission which could increase risks for women in the future.

References

Adler, M. (1986) *ABC of Sexually Transmitted Diseases* Articles from the British Medical Journal, London: British Medical Association.

Adler, M. (1987) 'Acquired immune deficiency syndrome', *British Medical Journal* 1, pp. 1145–7.

Carne, C.A. (1987) 'ABC of AIDS: neurological manifestations', *British Medical Journal* 294, pp. 1339–401.

Catterall, R.D. and Nichol, C. (1969) 'Transmission of Trichomonas', *British Medical Journal* 1, pp. 765–6.

Deitch, K.V. and Smith, J.E. (1983) 'Cervical dysplasia and condylomata acuminata in young women', *Journal of Obstetric, Gynaecological and Neonatal Nursing* 12 (3), pp. 155–8.

DHSS (1988) *New Cases seen at NHS Genitourinary Medicine Clinics in England 1976–1986*, Statistical Bulletin July 2nd, London: HMSO.

Goldacre, M.J. *et al.* (1978) 'Epidemiological and clinical significance of cervical erosion in women attending a Family Planning Clinic', *British Medical Journal* 285, pp. 748–50.

Gould, D.J. and Wilson-Barnett, J. (1985) 'A comparison of recovery following hysterectomy and major cardiac surgery', *Journal of Advanced Nursing* 10, pp. 315–23.

Mims, C.A. (1987) *The Pathogenesis of Infectious Disease*, London: Academic Press.

Office of Health Economics (1988) *HIV and AIDS in the UK*, London: Whitehall.

Pinching, A.J. (1987) *Evidence to the Social Services Committee Enquiry into Problems Associated with AIDS*, London: HMSO. Volume 1.

Pratt, R. (1988) *A Strategy for Nursing Care*, 2nd ed., London: Edward Arnold.

Roper, N., Logan, W.W. and Tierney, A.J. (1985) *The Elements of Nursing*, 2nd ed., Edinburgh: Churchill Livingstone.

Spire, B. *et al.* (1984) 'Inactivation of lymphadenopathy-associated virus by chemical disinfectants', *Lancet* 2, pp. 899–900.

Wilson, H. (1985) 'Chlamydia trachomatis and infertility', *New Zealand Nursing Journal* 77 (13), pp. 24–6.

7   Menstruation and its Disorders

Nurses need to understand normal functioning before they can discuss the treatment of menstrual problems or help patients/clients to judge the likely time of ovulation in order to achieve or avoid conception. This chapter will explain the physiology of the menstrual cycle and its normal variations, then give an account of menstrual disorders. The female reproductive cycle is under endocrine control, so discussion will open with a description of the ovaries and their hormones.

The ovaries and their hormones

The paired ovaries are small, almond-shaped organs lying in the pelvic cavity (see Fig. 7.1). They have two functions:

- To produce eggs (*ova*);
- To secrete the female sex hormones, *oestrogen* and *progesterone*.

Both of these hormones belong to the group of chemicals called *steroids*. Despite their similar chemical structure, their effects on the body are quite different. Oestrogen is released in large quantities throughout the reproductive years and is responsible for the female secondary sexual characteristics. Progesterone, produced in smaller quantities, prepares the uterus to receive a fertilised egg each month, and plays an important role in pregnancy and lactation.

Sex steroids are secreted in minimal quantities (if at all) before puberty and their levels decline dramatically after the menopause (see Chapter 9). However, the adrenal cortex produces oestrogens from puberty onwards, and this continues after the menopause. Both ovaries and adrenal cortex secrete very small quantities of male hormones known collectively as *androgens*. In animals, androgens are considered responsible for the female sex drive (*libido*) and are thought to be associated with aggressive behaviour. It is not known whether this is true in humans. Androgens are mentioned here because some drugs used to alleviate menstrual disorders behave like androgens. Treatment may occasionally result in weight gain and virilisation.

The menstrual cycle

Release of oestrogen and progesterone from the ovary is controlled by two further hormones, follicle stimulating hormone (FSH) and lutenising hormone (LH) from the

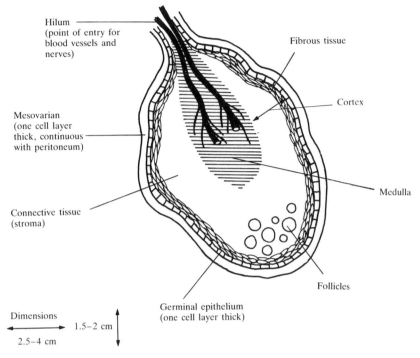

Hilum
(point of entry for
blood vessels and
nerves)

Fibrous tissue

Cortex

Mesovarian
(one cell layer
thick, continuous
with peritoneum)

Medulla

Connective tissue
(stroma)

Follicles

Germinal epithelium
(one cell layer thick)

Dimensions

1.5–2 cm

2.5–4 cm

Figure 7.1 Structure of the ovary.

anterior pituitary gland at the base of the brain. Collectively, FSH and LH are referred to as *gonadotrophins*. Plasma concentrations at different stages of the menstrual cycle are shown in Fig. 7.2. Release of ovarian hormones also occurs cyclically and levels fluctuate throughout the month under the influence of the gonadotrophins. (Rate of release of oestrogen from the adrenal cortex does not vary.)

The menstrual cycle is a complex series of events summarised below:

1. Approximately every twenty-eight days plasma concentrations of gonadotrophins (mainly FSH from the anterior pituitary) increase. When they reach the ovary they stimulate the development of several follicles, each containing an egg. This is the follicular stage of development, lasting up to the time when one of the eggs is released (ovulation). As the follicles grow, they release oestrogen into the bloodstream.

2. On Day Fourteen of the 'average' cycle, one (occasionally two) of the follicles will release an egg which enters a uterine tube via the pelvic cavity (see Fig. 7.3). The egg travels down the uterine tube towards the uterus.

3. The cells of the follicle left behind after ovulation persist as a structure called the *corpus luteum*, which secretes both oestrogen and progesterone. Progesterone prepares the uterus to receive a fertilised egg. It causes the endometrium (uterine lining) to become thicker, with extra blood vessels and coiled glands which secrete

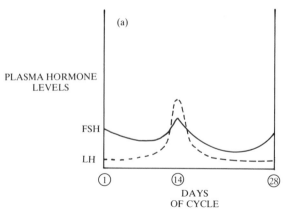

(a) Gonadotrophin release during a 28 day menstrual cycle.

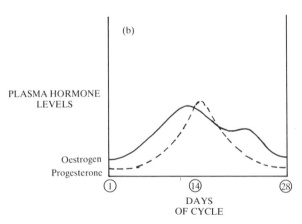

(b) Release of the ovarian hormones during a 28 day menstrual cycle.

Figure 7.2 Release of gonadotrophins, oestrogen and progesterone throughout the menstrual cycle.

glycogen, helping to nourish the fertilised egg. This is the secretory phase of the cycle, which begins as soon as ovulation has occurred. It ends with the onset of menstruation. From Fig. 7.2 the levels of gonadotrophins are seen to reach a peak just before ovulation (28–40 hours).
4. As the secretory phase draws to a close, the release of gonadotrophins declines. During the last few days of the cycle, the corpus luteum begins to degenerate unless the egg has been fertilised. The failing cells of the corpus luteum cease to produce oestrogen and progesterone. Menstruation begins as the endometrium sloughs away from the uterine walls and is lost via the vagina. Menstruation is the third and final stage of the cycle.

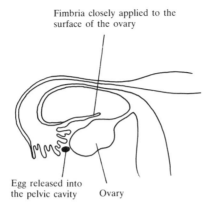

Figure 7.3 Relationship of the ovary to the uterine tube.

The 'average' menstrual cycle, shown in Fig. 7.4, lasts twenty-eight days. Bleeding, which is variable in amount, continues for about five days. The first day of menstruation is always regarded by convention as Day One of the cycle and for the mythical 'average' cycle, ovulation will occur on Day Fourteen.

Control of the sex steroids

Gonadotrophins control release of oestrogen and progesterone by a negative feed-back mechanism (see Fig. 7.5). There is an inverse relationship between the levels of ovarian hormones in the bloodstream and gonadotrophins. At the beginning of the cycle, when menstruation is ceasing, oestrogen levels are low. This prompts the

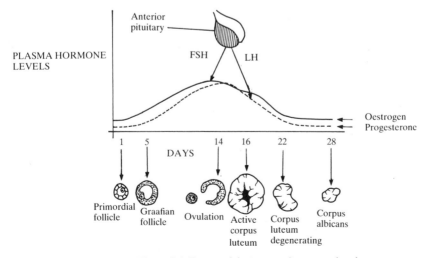

Figure 7.4 Events of the 'average' menstrual cycle.

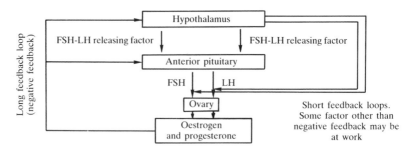

Figure 7.5 Negative feedback control of the ovarian hormones.

anterior pituitary to release FSH which stimulates follicular development. As the follicles mature, the amount of circulating oestrogen increases. This progressively inhibits FSH secretion, but initiates release of LH. The sudden release of LH just before Day Fourteen of the 'average' cycle is called *the LH surge*. It prompts ovulation to occur soon afterwards. Women with fertility problems sometimes fail to ovulate because of a low LH surge (see Chapter 8). Both LH and FSH are needed to stimulate ovulation, however. Experiments have shown that LH, in the absence of FSH, is ineffective.

   Once ovulation has occurred, the corpus luteum continues to release large quantities of oestrogen and progesterone, inhibiting secretion of FSH and LH. Unless pregnancy occurs, the life span of the corpus luteum is limited to about fourteen days. When it degenerates the production of oestrogen and progesterone ceases. Withdrawal of sex steroids results in menstruation, but inhibition of FSH is lifted as their levels decline. As the beginning of the next cycle is initiated, FSH levels begin to increase again.

Control of FSH and LH

Release of gonadotrophins is controlled by a hormone called *FSH-LH releasing factor* from the hypothalamus, a small but vital control area of tissue positioned immediately above the pituitary gland (see Fig. 7.6). FSH-LH releasing factor travels to the anterior pituitary via a capillary network (*hypothalamic-hypophyseal portal system*) stimulating some of its cells to release FSH and LH. The existence of releasing factor was not suspected until the late 1950s. Physiologists have yet to determine full details of the control system. It is evident that negative feedback is not entirely responsible for all aspects of control. Some researchers believe there must be an inhibitory factor to prevent release of LH until just before ovulation although they have been unable to isolate it.

Other control systems

Although precise control mechanisms for releasing factor and gonadotrophins have not been elucidated, it is apparent that there is some influence from the higher centres of the brain, particularly those affecting emotion (see Fig. 7.7). It is common knowl-

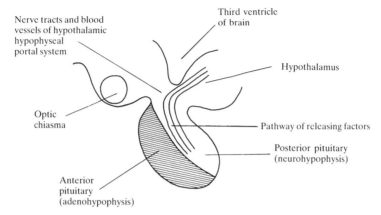

Figure 7.6 Anatomical relationship of the hypothalamus and pituitary gland.

edge that unsettling events (starting a new job, leaving home) can delay or speed up the arrival of a period.

The hypothalamus controls many vital physiological functions (including thirst, appetite, temperature) and co-ordinates nervous connections from all over the brain, including centres which influence emotion. Even when a woman normally experiences regular menses, excitements or upsets may interfere.

Animal experiments have demonstrated that environmental changes, particularly hours of daylight, may influence reproductive cycles. There is some evidence that environmental factors play a role (though of minor importance) in women, the brain acting as a co-ordinator sorting out and relaying information to the endocrine system via the hypothalamus.

Some mammals (for example, domestic cats) ovulate only *after* copulation. This is controlled by a reflex mechanism. There is little evidence for reflex ovulation in women, although the timing of ovulation might possibly be modified by tactile stimuli.

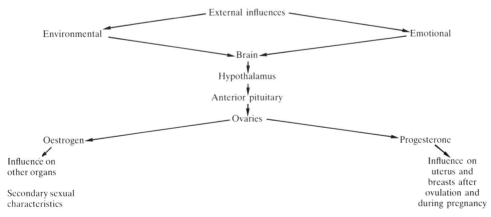

Figure 7.7 Pathways of information flow between the brain and reproductive organs.

Normal variations of the menstrual cycle

For some women the menstrual cycle may always be erratic, while for others it may be regular, but rather long. When the cycle is extended, it is the follicular phase, the time before ovulation, that is protracted. Once the LH surge has been initiated and ovulation has occurred, the remaining secretory phase will always be of the same fixed length. This is an important practical point for nurses to remember when helping patients/clients to identify the time of ovulation in order to achieve or avoid conception.

Although cycles as long as forty-five days or as short as twenty days are considered normal, gynaecology books, including those written with lay readership in mind, tend to emphasise the 'average' cycle, and women may be concerned about the timing of their periods, especially if they are trying to avoid or become pregnant.

Natural methods of family planning

Natural family planning methods are discussed in this chapter because success depends on teaching women to recognise the signs of ovulation. Intercourse can then be avoided when conception is possible. Several methods exist, but all demand very high levels of commitment, and are best taught to both partners since co-operation and mutual agreement about the need for periodic abstinence are vital. However, for many couples natural methods of family planning are the only acceptable forms of contraception, due to cultural or religious beliefs or a desire to avoid invasive procedures and drugs. Teaching is best undertaken on an individual basis by an experienced counsellor, who may often be a lay person. Some couples learn techniques from self-help manuals, but then lack the support which seems to be the key to success. Self-instruction may also encourage couples to develop their own 'rules' and these may account for the high levels of failure reported. Torrance and Milligan (1986) provide evidence to show that 19 per cent of women (aged 15–44) relying on periodic abstinence became pregnant during the first year. However, these estimations may be biased, since only women using natural methods incorrectly become known to the medical and nursing services.

Research is helping to define the fertile period more precisely. To practise natural methods, couples need to know the following:

- Exactly when ovulation occurs;
- How long the egg remains viable;
- How long sperms remain able to fertilise eggs.

Viability of eggs and sperms

Eggs are believed to remain viable for 24–48 hours, but recent research described by Torrance and Milligan (1986) suggests that sperm are able to survive in the female genital tract considerably longer. Cervical mucus from women trying to become pregnant by artificial insemination contained motile sperm up to 120 hours (five days) after deposition. Further experiments demonstrated that *in vitro* these sperms could still penetrate and fertilise eggs. Any couple practising natural methods must be warned about the protracted survival of sperm. There is also a danger that fertilisation of 'old' eggs and sperms may give rise to embryos with genetic abnormalities (Johnson and Everitt, 1984). This may result either in spontaneous abortion or the birth of a handicapped child.

Recognising the time of ovulation

For many years the success of the 'safe period' was doomed by attempts to apply animal physiology to humans.

Human females (and their close relatives, the great apes) are unique in having a menstrual cycle. All other female mammals have an oestrus cycle, bleeding when they are fertile. Victorian women mistakenly advised to restrict intercourse to the middle of the cycle experienced some disappointment with this method. Nevertheless it received Vatican approval in 1853, its high failure rate no doubt accounting for the term 'Vatican Roulette' by which it became known. The source of error did not become apparent until the 1930s.

As with many other important scientific advances, female reproductive mechanisms were discovered by two researchers working independently: Knaus in Austria and Ogino in Japan. Their work, published in 1929, involved recovery of human eggs from menstrual flow and suggested that the fertile period occurred mid-cycle.

Following the work of Knaus and Ogino, women learned how to calculate their fertile period using the calendar method. This is seldom used today because it is inefficient and restrictive. Women were advised to record the lengths of their cycles to establish a pattern for at least six months before relying on the method. For those whose cycles were irregular, the potential fertile period could be considerable and failures possibly occurred due to the unrealistic length of abstinence.

Today, there are three methods of natural family planning:

- The temperature method;
- The Billings method;
- The muco-thermic method (a combination of the other two).

The temperature (thermic) method
This is based on the ability of progesterone, released after ovulation, to cause a slight rise in basal metabolism (see Fig. 8.4, page 201). This may be transient or sustained throughout the secretory phase. A slight dip in temperature immediately prior to ovulation also occurs in 10–15 per cent of women. Temperature must be taken at the same time every morning and recorded on a chart, so that a pattern emerges. The main difficulty lies with human error. Temperature rise is very small ($0.2–0.5°C$) and may not be easy to detect even if the couple are highly motivated and able to keep accurate records. The situation has improved since the availability of electronic thermometers, but couples must still be warned about other conditions, such as infection, which may obscure results.

The Billings method (mucus method, Australian method)
This method, first developed by an Australian team (Billings and Westland 1980) is based on hormonally controlled changes in the cervical mucus, causing its consistency and appearance to alter at different stages throughout the cycle. It has attracted considerable attention in recent years and seems to be more accurate than the temperature method because the changes are more easily observed.

In the early part of the follicular phase, cervical mucus forms a thick plug occluding the cervical os, which sperms are unable to penetrate. As the amount of oestrogen released by the follicles increases, the cervical mucus becomes more abundant (cervical cascade) and changes in character. Around the time of ovulation it becomes profuse, clear, slippery and bears a striking resemblance to egg white. The *Spinnbarkeit phenomenon* can now be demonstrated: a drop of mucus suspended between two microscope slides (or the fingers) can be stretched into a thread reaching 15 cm at the time of ovulation (see Fig. 7.8). A drop of mucus allowed to dry shows a typical pattern called 'ferning'. During this time, sperm can easily penetrate the mucus but, once the egg is no longer viable, the hostile plug again develops to occlude the os.

Over 90 per cent of women can be taught to recognise these changes (Torrance and Milligan 1986). Billings and Westland (1980), describing the method, argue that it has been used successfully in some societies for many years. These authors are careful, however, to point out its limitations. It is suitable only for couples in a stable relationship as a very high level of commitment is required. The woman must record her observations on a special chart for at least a month before relying on it to ensure that she can recognise her fertile period. Complete abstinence is necessary throughout this time because spermicides, hormones and even the natural lubricant secretions released during intercourse, may obscure the pattern. Complete reliance on the method is advocated without additional precautions for the same reason.

The muco-thermic method is a combination of the Billings and temperature methods and is safer, since it provides a double check for the estimated time of ovulation.

Changes in the vaginal epithelium also occur at ovulation (see Chapter 8). They can only be observed under the microscope and have no value for couples trying to avoid pregnancy, but can be used to help confirm ovulation during fertility investigations.

Predicting ovulation by modern methods
More objective methods of detecting ovulation are now becoming available. These provide much greater precision in determining the fertile period. Most rely on detecting the 'peak' levels of oestradiol in the plasma just before ovulation or identification of the LH surge. A number of rapid and reliable hormone assay techniques have been developed suitable for laboratory tests, and reagent strips for LH and oestradiol metabolites in urine are now available for use in the home. Ultrasonography can trace the development of the enlarging follicle in women hoping to undergo *in vitro* fertilisation (IVF).

Members of the general public committed to 'natural' lifestyles or undergoing fertility investigations need to know about these new developments and to have a sound understanding of the events of the menstrual cycle.

Understanding of the menstrual cycle is crucial for nurses working with gynaecology patients/clients, so a more detailed account is given below.

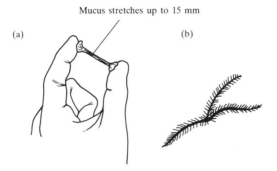

Figure 7.8 (a) Spinnbarkeit formation; (b) ferning of dry mucus on a microscope slide.

The menstrual cycle: a more detailed account

The follicles containing the eggs are called *primordial follicles*. During development and when they enlarge and change appearance, they are referred to as *Graffian* follicles after the biologist who first described them (see Fig. 7.9).

During the follicular phase of the cycle, the increasing levels of FSH stimulate the follicle to enlarge and a layer of cells called *granulosa cells* develops around it. Ovarian tissue gives rise to thick-walled cells called *theca cells* which lie outside the granulosa cells and enclose them. Oestrogen and later progesterone are released mainly from the theca cells. As the follicle develops, both theca and granulosa cells begin to secrete a thick fluid containing high concentrations of oestrogen. Plasma levels of oestrogen also increase. As follicular fluid accumulates, a space called *the antrum* develops inside the follicle, pushing the egg towards one end. The size of the Graffian follicle increases steadily and, as the time of ovulation approaches, it moves to the edge of the ovary, coming to lie just beneath the surface. By the time of ovulation, the follicle is about 1.5 mm in diameter and would be visible to the naked eye if the ovaries were examined via the laparoscope.

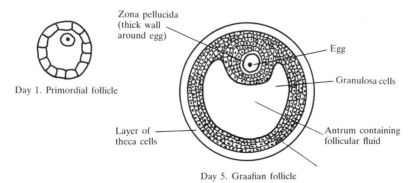

Figure 7.9 Structure and development of the Graafian follicle.

Just before ovulation, a protrusion called the *stigma* develops on the outer wall of the follicle and swells rapidly. Within approximately thirty minutes follicular fluid begins to ooze out via the stigma, which opens suddenly, allowing the fluid to escape and carry the egg into the pelvic cavity.

The escaping fluid may cause local irritation, and a small amount of bleeding may occur from the ovary, resulting in a transient pain called *mittleschmertz* (middle pain), experienced by approximately 25 per cent of women.

Nature is profligate. Together the ovaries contain about 400,000 eggs, although many degenerate without maturing: throughout the reproductive years, only about 400 will be released.

Every month approximately twenty follicles are stimulated to develop by FSH, but, after Day Five or Six of the cycle, one (or occasionally two) follicle begins to grow faster than all the others, which then die. This phenomenon is called *atresia*. Despite many theories, the mechanism is obscure.

Once the egg has been released, the theca cells undergo rapid physical and chemical change called *lutenisation*. They enlarge and become yellow due to the deposition of fatty substances which give rise to steroid hormones. By Day Twenty-two of the typical cycle, the corpus luteum may be as large as 1.5 mm in diameter and is still secreting oestrogen and progesterone. From this point onwards, it begins to degenerate (unless pregnancy has occurred) and its secretory function is gradually lost. As the fatty components disappear, the cells change from yellow to white and the structure is now called the *corpus albicans*. Over the next few weeks, it will gradually be replaced by scar tissue, giving the surface of the ovary a characteristic pitted appearance.

Cyclical changes in the uterus

Although nurses must be able to explain all aspects of the menstrual cycle to patients and clients in terms they can understand, they will probably be asked most often about the process of menstruation itself, because bleeding is the visible, obvious indicator of cyclical change. Endometrial changes occur in three phases (see Fig. 7.10):

- The stage of proliferation corresponding to the follicular phase of the cycle;
- The secretory stage following ovulation;
- Menstruation.

The proliferative phase
The proliferative phase commences on approximately Day Five of the 'average' cycle, coinciding with the end of menstruation. At this time, the endometrium lining the uterus persists as a thin layer, and the remaining epithelial cells which have not been shed lie deep inside the endometrial glands. Release of oestrogen before ovulation causes the epithelial cells to divide rapidly and by Day Seven the uterine cavity is again completely covered by an epithelial layer. This increases steadily in thickness as ovulation approaches. The endometrial glands and blood vessels become more numerous. At ovulation, the endometrium is 2–3 mm thick.

The secretory phase
Throughout the secretory phase following ovulation, oestrogen continues to promote endometrial development, while progesterone from the corpus luteum prepares it

to receive a fertilised egg. Blood supply is stimulated to increase further, and the endometrial glands, now highly coiled, secrete glycogen. By the time the egg would implant, if it had been fertilised, the endometrium is about 5 mm thick. If implantation does not occur, the corpus luteum degenerates, the supply of oestrogen and progesterone ceases abruptly and the endometrium is shed.

Menstruation
During the twenty-four hours immediately preceding menstruation, the blood vessels supplying the endometrium constrict so the blood supply to the cells lying over them is reduced suddenly. These cells die, and blood begins to seep into the endometrium, resulting in the formation of small haemorrhagic areas. The endometrium gradually sloughs away from the uterine wall and the egg is carried with it.

Menstruation: nursing assessment

Women often worry about the amount and appearance of menstrual flow. Typical loss consists of 35 ml of blood and 35 ml of serous fluid every month, but this varies not only between one individual and another, but from one cycle to the next and between days of the same period. The question: 'Are your periods normal?' is not therefore likely to yield much useful information. When a nurse is assessing a client it may be more helpful to ask more specific questions about:

- The length of the last period;
- Whether the flow was heavier or lighter than usual;
- The appearance of vaginal loss, including colour and presence or absence of clots;
- The number of sanitary towels or tampons used (this can only give an approximation of loss because some women change more often than others, and the absorbency of different brands can vary. More accurate assessment, if necessary, can be made with pre-weighed towels);
- Whether there has been pain or discomfort, when it occurred, and whether it was unusual;
- Odour, if the woman has recently had an induced or spontaneous abortion, or if there is any reason to suspect infection;
- Any other symptoms associated with menstruation (depression, tearfulness, sore, swollen breasts or abdomen, headaches).

Some women lose more blood on the first day of their period while for others bleeding begins slowly and is heaviest on the second or third day. Although bleeding is chiefly arterial (75 per cent), the vessels concerned are very small. Even when loss is heavy, women can be reassured that haemorrhaging will never occur when they menstruate. It may be helpful to point out that flow will generally be greatest when standing (sitting or lying causes blood to pool in the vagina) and that only a small quantity of blood is sufficient to colour a large quantity of water red (in the WC).

Blood mixed with fluid secretions looks pale and bright. Heavy flow is often darker and may contain clots. The uterus releases an anticoagulant called *fibrinolysin* which delays clotting until blood has escaped through the cervical os. Sometimes fragments

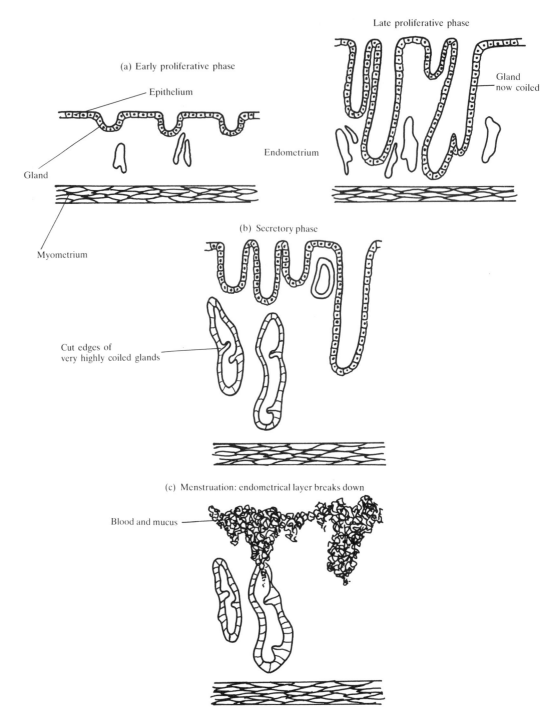

Figure 7.10 The endometrial cycle.

of endometrial tissue escape and this again is normal.

The uterus contracts at the onset of menstruation, helping to expel blood. The agents responsible are a group of chemicals called prostaglandins. One of their most important general properties is to cause smooth muscle, including myometrium, to contract. Contractions are frequently painful, explaining why the onset of menstruation is often accompanied by pelvic discomfort.

Most women experience menstrual discomfort at one time or another, but occasionally periods become so heavy or painful that everyday life is disrupted. The rest of this chapter is concerned with menstrual problems.

Dysmenorrhoea

Dysmenorrhoea is pain experienced during menstruation. *Primary dysmenorrhoea* is diagnosed in the absence of demonstrable pelvic pathology, *secondary dysmenorrhoea* when there is evidence of pelvic pathology or the woman has an IUCD. Aetiology, medical treatment and nursing approach differ.

Primary dysmenorrhoea

Primary dysmenorrhoea most often occurs in nulliparous young women once ovulatory cycles are established. It may come as a shock to girls who have experienced a few anovulatory, painless cycles. Usual complaint is of low backache and colicky pain in the pelvic area which may continue down the thighs or into the vulva. Distribution is quite distinct from pain caused by secondary dysmenorrhoea (see Fig. 7.11).

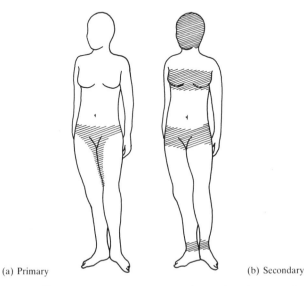

(a) Primary   (b) Secondary

Figure 7.11 Sites of discomfort in primary and secondary dysmenorrhoea.

Primary dysmenorrhoea is due to excess prostaglandin (F2). Elevated levels have been detected in the endometrium and menstrual flow of girls reporting severe menstrual pain. Locally, prostaglandins induce the myometrium to contract. Ischaemia results. Prostaglandin also enters the systemic circulation and may cause nausea, vomiting, diarrhoea or faintness. The reason for elevated levels of prostaglandin is not known.

Primary dysmenorrhoea is most effectively treated by drugs which inhibit or reduce prostaglandin synthesis. These include aspirin (which can be purchased over the counter), mefenamic acid (Ponstan), distalgesic and indomethacin, all of which require prescription. Beta receptor stimulators such as salbutamol also inhibit prostaglandin release but are seldom used in clinical practice because the dose required for effective treatment has too many side effects on the cardiovascular system.

At one time girls complaining of severe period pains might be admitted to hospital for D and C, but this treatment is now seldom used because of the risk of incompetent cervix (see Chapter 4). Women taking the pill often find that their periods become less painful because they no longer ovulate.

The prevalence of primary dysmenorrhoea in the general population is difficult to establish. Most women suffer some discomfort at one time or another but, even when pain is sufficiently disabling to disrupt normal activities, help may not be sought. A survey of women aged 15–50 registered in one general practice indicated that 14 per cent regularly experienced pains, with peak prevalence occurring between the ages of 15 and 20 (Richards 1979).

Although dysmenorrhoea is temporary, it can be severe, resulting in loss of work, school and recreational opportunities. Traditional beliefs prevalent throughout the nineteenth century that women's lives are inevitably dominated by their uteri and ovaries (English and Ehrenreich 1973) are now waning, yet menstrual pain is still frequently regarded as such an everyday occurrence that it has attracted little research attention (Roberts 1984).

In view of the relationship between stress and disease, several nurse researchers have explored possible links between dysmenorrhoea, life events and social support. Jordan and Meckler (1982), conducting a survey of 156 student nurses, found dysmenorrhoea to occur most often among those who had had recent life changes, but the pain was unaffected by available social support. Brown and Woods (1984) using the same questionnaire, observed that, in a sample of women aged between 18 and 35 years, pain appeared to be problematic for women with negative attitudes towards menstruation. Such attitudes may have been generated by the experience of pain itself, but the authors do not comment on this.

■   Julie Astor's painful periods resulted in loss of time at school, so she asked the school nurse if the pill might help. Although there may sometimes be very good medical or social reasons for prescribing the pill to young girls, it is not necessarily the treatment of first choice because the hormones it contains alter normal endocrine function. In particular, oestrogen may fuse the epiphyses of the long bones prematurely, possibly preventing the girl from attaining her full height. The school nurse, taking a sympathetic approach, recommended a number of other strategies for symptomatic relief. She emphasised that dysmenorrhoea is a common problem which troubles many girls and suggested aspirin and rest with a local source of heat when pain became severe. Julie could do various other things to help herself such as eating a high fibre diet to prevent constipation and taking regular exercise to improve circulation generally – which would help relieve ischaemia to the pelvic area.

Secondary dysmenorrhoea

Secondary dysmenorrhoea is not usually experienced until the woman reaches her mid twenties. It is a dragging rather than a colicky pain, occurring in the pelvic area, back and breasts, sometimes accompanied by headaches. It may result from pelvic pathology such as fibroids or endometriosis, described later in this chapter. Medical intervention is necessary to diagnose and treat the underlying cause, so women in this age group should always be advised to seek help. In the meantime rest, local warmth and mild analgesia can be recommended.

Membranous dysmenorrhoea

This is a rare condition. The entire endometrium is shed as a 'cast', accompanied by severe abdominal pain. Flow then reduces and the pain subsides. Membranous dysmenorrhoea can be relieved by hormone therapy or hysterectomy in an older woman whose family is complete.

Premenstrual tension syndrome (PMS)

The cyclical appearance of a cluster of symptoms before menstruation was first described by the American gynaecologist Frank in the 1940s. Much subsequent work has been conducted in Britain by Dalton (1969, 1971), a GP whose extensive descriptions of individual case studies showed that women complained of a wide range of physical and emotional symptoms during the twelve days or so preceding menstruation (see Table 7.1).

PMS has attracted considerable research attention and is said to affect up to 50 per cent of women at some time in their lives (Sutherland and Stewart 1965). There is no doubt that it has considerable impact on family life. Brown (1986) found that in a sample of eight-three women there were reports of seventy-four different, recurring symptoms, though anxiety and irritability were mentioned most often. Partners offered various supportive and coping strategies. Anger was also a common reaction, particularly in couples in the lower socioeconomic groups.

Average age of presentation is 35 years, but symptoms can appear at puberty (Beard 1984). A retrospective study, conducted among 630 women attending a PMS clinic, indicated that symptoms usually develop for the first time after childbirth (Brush 1985). Women taking combined oral contraceptives do not generally suffer from

PMS, but often develop it when they discontinue. Relationship between PMS and the progesterone-only pill has not yet been investigated.

Aetiology of PMS
Numerous theories have been suggested but none convincingly explain all the symptoms of PMS:

- *Diminished levels of progesterone.* Researchers at St. Thomas's Hospital in London found that progesterone levels were depressed throughout the secretory phase of the cycle in 30 per cent of women experiencing PMS. Some women have been helped by injections of natural progesterone (it cannot be taken orally) or oral progestogens such as Duphaston, but the benefits of hormone treatment for the remaining 70 per cent whose progesterone levels were apparently normal is questionable ('Talking Point' – British Medical Journal 1979).
- *Elevated prolactin levels.* Prolactin is a hormone released from the anterior pituitary which stimulates lactation. Secretion is usually suppressed by a hormone inhibitor, but levels are sometimes elevated in women who have PMS. Secretion can be suppressed by a drug called bromocriptine, although numerous side effects have been reported (nausea, faintness, lassitude, hypotension).
- *Diminished aldosterone levels.* Some women with PMS have depressed levels of aldosterone, a mineralocorticoid hormone released from the adrenal cortex which helps to control water and electrolyte balance. Deficiency may account for fluid retention which is common with PMS. However, not *all* women investigated for PMS have depressed aldosterone levels.

Treatment of PMS
Overall it appears that PMS is an endocrine problem of multiple and complex aetiology, with different women experiencing subtly different forms of endocrine upset. It therefore seems unlikely that a single treatment regime will prove 100 per cent effective for all. This is an important point for nurses to remember if they are asked for advice because popular treatments for PMS are often discussed in women's magazines and many of the drugs recommended can be obtained without prescription.

Pyridoxine (vitamin B6) was found by the research team at St Thomas's Hospital to help relieve headache, depression and oedema, but may cause peripheral neuropathy if taken in excessive doses. It seems to exert its effects by relieving vitamin deficiency associated with lack of *tryptophan*, and sometimes also helps to alleviate depression associated with oral contraceptives. Tryptophan is an amino acid usually included in a normal diet. One of its functions is to act as a neurotransmitter in the brain. Reduced levels of neurotransmitter can result in depression. Pyridoxine can be replaced by taking vitamin B-complex tablets regularly, but why individuals should become deficient when eating an apparently healthy diet remains obscure. It has been argued that the female is not well adapted to the regular demands of menstruation occurring in Western society where family size is small and the period of lactation relatively short. Frequent menstruation might somehow disrupt pyridoxine metabolism. According to

Table 7.1 Main features of the premenstrual tension syndrome (documented by Dalton and others)

Fluid retention	Weight gain (up to 3 kg)
	Painful, heavy breasts
	Abdominal distension
	Feeling bloated
Pain	Headache
	Backache
	Muscle stiffness
	Fatigue
Autonomic reactions	Dizziness/faintness
	Nausea
	Vomiting
	Sweating
	Hot flushes
Mood changes	Tension
	Irritability
	Crying
	Depression
Loss of concentration	Forgetfulness
	Clumsiness
	Indecision
	Insomnia
Other	Chest pain
	Palpitations
	Numbness
	Tingling sensations

a second hypothesis, pyridoxine may operate as a prolactin inhibitor by counteracting the effects of another neurotransmitter, *dopamine*, which has also been implicated in mood disturbance.

Prostaglandin El is necessary to help maintain normal endocrine balance and, if deficient, may contribute to PMS. The body converts a chemical called *gammalinoleic acid* (GLA) to prostaglandin El. GLA is a constituent of many vegetables usually included in a healthy diet but is destroyed in products like polyunsaturated margarines exposed to heat during production. A deficiency state may therefore result. GLA is finding popularity as a self-help treatment for PMS, marketed as Efamol, extracted from the seed of the evening primrose. It is obtainable from health shops without prescription.

Women who seek medical advice may be given diuretics to help reduce the uncomfortable effects of fluid retention. Tranquillisers may sometimes also be prescribed. However, many women regard PMS as a disagreeable problem which does not merit medical intervention because it is part of everyday life, yet may still welcome advice or helpful suggestions from a nurse. Much can be done to encourage self-help:

- The woman can be told about vitamin B supplements and Efamol, although she should not expect them necessarily to prevent all her symptoms.
- She can be advised about a diet containing adequate vitamins and polyunsaturated fat, and to avoid constipation. Reducing salt (sodium chloride) intake may help alleviate fluid retention.
- Exercise can be beneficial because it encourages relaxation and sleep and promotes the release of locally acting hormones called *endorphins* which reduce the sensation of pain. A particular task (bread-making, polishing), as well as providing rhythmic exercise, may help to remove tension and direct aggressive feelings away from other people.
- Massage helps relieve stress. Aches or pains may be alleviated by local heat, rest or aspirin.
- Some women find relief in crying and should be reassured that this is normal, not a sign of weakness.
- Discussion with other people (partners, friends, members of a self-help group), not necessarily at a time when PMS is actually being experienced, can help. Self-awareness will enable women to understand their own behaviour and perhaps explain to their partners that it is not wilful. They will benefit if the nurse shows them how to report symptoms and moods on a menstrual chart (see Table 7.2). Stress can then sometimes be avoided at a vulnerable time and women will realise that they are not alone in their mood swings.

Psychiatric problems and PMS
The menstrual cycle is reported to exert a powerful influence on women's behaviour (Friedman 1984). Early work by Dalton revealed countless examples of women who performed less efficiently at home and work just before and during their periods. Further research indicated that women were more likely to make suicide attempts (Mandell and Mandell 1967), and more likely to commit a criminal offence (Jacob and Charles 1970, Dalton 1980), at this time. PMS has twice been accepted as a mental disease under the 1957 Homicide Act and at least two charges of murder have been commuted to manslaughter for reasons of diminished responsibility (*Lancet* 1981). However, early research has been criticised because of its poor design and lack of control subjects. Women have always been aware that they were being asked about PMS and this may have encouraged them to interpret moods in relation to menstruation which may have been coincidental. Women have also been asked about PMS *after* they have committed offences or been admitted to psychiatric hospitals – prospective studies involving reports of PMS and later examination of behaviour do not appear to have been attempted. This situation is criticised by Roberts and Garling (1981) who point out that, if women are willing to accept menstrual problems as explanations for ill health, this may go against them when applying for jobs or responsible positions in society.

   Research by nurses has indicated that PMS may be due to negative attitudes acquired during socialisation (Woods *et al.* 1985). PMS is a tiresome problem encountered by large numbers of women but there is little evidence that menstrual distress alone will drive an otherwise normal individual to desperate behaviour; psychiatric referral is necessary for only a small number of women (Sampson 1984).

Table 7.2 PMS diary

Name		Month	

Record how you feel each day according to the five point scale below under the column headed 'Problems'. In the column headed 'Symptoms noted' describe how you feel. Circle each day you menstruate.

1. No symptoms
2. Some symptoms beginning/just noticeable
3. Moderate symptoms, but under control
4. Symptoms not really under control, but bearable/coping is possible
5. Symptoms not controlled at all/not coping at all

Day of cycle	Problems	Symptoms noted
1		
2		
3		
4		
5		
6		
7		
8		
9		
10		
11		
12		
13		
14		
15		
16		
17		
18		

Table 7.2 (cont.)

Day of cycle	Problems	Symptoms noted
19		
20		
21		
22		
23		
24		
25		
26		
27		
28		

Amenorrhoea

Amenorrhoea (absence of menstrual periods) may be primary, when periods pre-viously occurred, or secondary, when established menstruation ceases. The most common explanation for secondary amenorrhoea is pregnancy. The causes, investi-gations and treatment for amenorrhoea are discussed in Chapters 8 and 14.

Vaginal bleeding

The remainder of this chapter is concerned with abnormal vaginal bleeding for which women should be encouraged to seek medical advice; heavy bleeding (*menorrhagia*) and intermenstrual bleeding (*metrorrhagia*). Bleeding may be due to benign condi-tions or malignancy; problems faced by women who have malignant conditions are discussed in Chapter 12. Additionally, there are non-gynaecological reasons for menorrhagia, such as thyrotoxicosis or clotting disorders, but these are rare.

Menorrhagia

Non-malignant causes of vaginal bleeding are shown in Fig. 7.12. The most common reason is probably uterine fibroids.

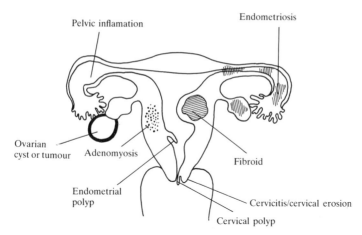

Figure 7.12 Non-malignant causes of vaginal bleeding.

■   Susan Harris had a D and C because her periods were heavy, prolonged and
painful (see Chapter 1). Vaginal examination showed her uterus to be
enlarged, and examination under anaesthetic suggested the presence of a
single large fibroid.
    Susan was 42 and had two teenage children. She was not, therefore, sur-
prised when the gynaecologist mentioned the possibility of hysterectomy.
Several of her friends had had this operation for the same reason.

Fibroids (leiomyomata)

Fibroids are found in 15–20 per cent of women aged 35 years or more. They are
benign tumours of connective tissue usually described according to location (Fig.
7.13). Fibroids may be no larger than millet seeds or many centimetres in diameter.
Small ones may be asymptomatic and treatment will not therefore be required. Larger
fibroids, which may be single or multiple, cause menorrhagia by increasing the surface
area of the uterine cavity so that a greater expanse of endometrium is shed at menstruation. Pelvic congestion may occur further increasing loss. Large fibroids may
press on the bowel (causing constipation) or on the bladder (causing urinary frequency
or retention) but seldom become malignant, although they may necrose or calcify.
Growth is stimulated by oestrogen: after the menopause fibroids regress.

Treatment
If fibroids are asymptomatic no treatment is required, but when they interfere with
health they must be removed, either individually (*myomectomy*) or by hysterectomy.

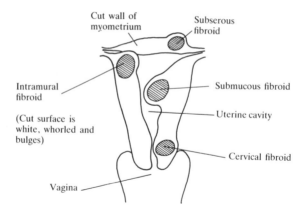

Figure 7.13 Fibroids.

Myomectomy

Myomectomy is only possible when there are a few large fibroids which the surgeon can dissect out of the myometrium, an operation often technically difficult to perform. Sometimes women request myomectomy because they are hoping to become pregnant. Unfortunately, fibroids tend to recur and pregnancy is unlikely because they act as foreign bodies, interfering with implantation. Blood loss can be considerable with this operation and a haematoma may form. Suturing weakens the uterine wall.

Types of hysterectomy

Total abdominal hysterectomy

In total abdominal hysterectomy, the body of the uterus and cervix are removed (see Fig. 7.14) leaving the ovaries and uterine tubes. Ovarian conservation is important for pre-menopausal women because the sudden withdrawal of oestrogen can lead to unpleasant side effects (see Chapter 9). Normally the ovaries are removed only if there is evidence of disease. An attempt is made to retain some ovarian tissue wherever possible because it will still be able to secrete hormones. Removing the cervix takes away the risk of later developing carcinoma at this site: cervical carcinoma is not an uncommon malignancy (see Chapter 12).

Subtotal hysterectomy

Subtotal hysterectomy is seldom performed today, unless the operation is technically so difficult that the cervix cannot be removed. The nurse must ensure that the woman knows she must continue to have regular smear tests.

Wertheim's hysterectomy

Wertheim's hysterectomy is a radical procedure performed when there is evidence of advanced malignancy of the genital tract. It involves the removal of the uterus, ovaries, uterine tubes, surrounding connective tissue and lymph ducts (*parametrium*), and the upper part of the vagina. Clearly women must be told about this and receive

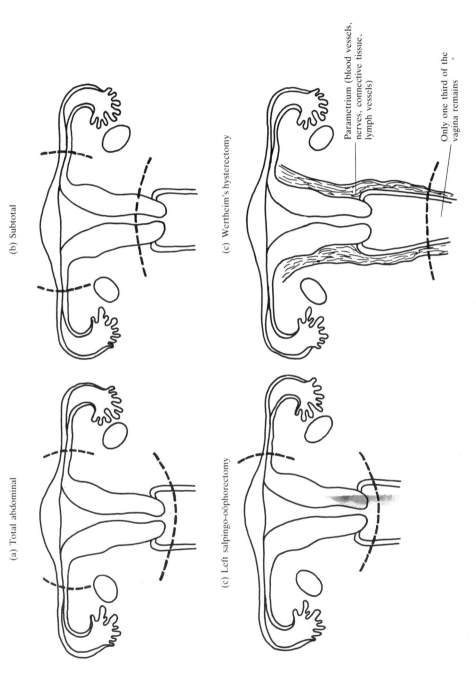

(a) Total abdominal

(b) Subtotal

(c) Left salpingo-oöphorectomy

(c) Wertheim's hysterectomy

Parametrium (blood vessels, nerves, connective tissue, lymph vessels)

Only one third of the vagina remains

Figure 7.14 Types of hysterectomy.

counselling as part of their preparation for surgery; as well as ceasing to menstruate and being unable to have any more children, sexual activity will be restricted.

Vaginal hysterectomy
Vaginal hysterectomy involves removal of the body of the uterus via the vagina, leaving the ovaries intact. It is most often performed for older women who have some degree of uterine prolapse, and may accompany a repair operation (*colporrhaphy*). The care of women undergoing vaginal hysterectomy is discussed in Chapter 10.

Pre-operative nursing care: total abdominal hysterectomy

■   Susan Harris was admitted one day before surgery to help her become accustomed to the ward and staff. She also needed to have a number of pre-operative investigations (see Care Plan 1.1, page 13).

Webb (1986) believes that, as women undergoing routine gynaecological surgery share many common needs pre-operatively, a standard care plan is appropriate. However, patients' home circumstances and needs for information are likely to vary, so these must be taken into consideration when after-care is planned. There is evidence that patients can be taught about routine events in hospital (what to expect in the recovery room and during early post-operative recovery) in groups as well as individually (Lindeman and Van Aernam 1971). However, opportunity must be given for individual questions, dealt with in private if necessary.

■   Orem's Model (1985) was used to plan Susan's care in preparation for discharge and the first few weeks at home (see Care Plan 7.1 on page 180).

Recovery from hysterectomy: research studies
Until the 1980s, gynaecological nursing attracted little attention as a subject for research (Hockey and Mcleod Clark 1979). Large numbers of women underwent hysterectomy every year, but little was known of their emotional reactions to surgery or recovery. Studies by doctors suggested that mortality and major physical problems were rare (Cole 1977), while psychologists reported increased incidence of psychiatric problems, decreased self-esteem and regret concerning loss of menstruation and fertility. However, many of these studies reflected the views of the researcher rather than a true representation of the data. Samples were generally small and studies were often conducted retrospectively; women who had had psychiatric problems for years were interviewed and problems then related to surgery, when no direct relationship could be demonstrated (see Gould 1986). The findings of these methodologically unsound studies did not agree with the findings of a research team in Oxford (Gath 1980) who, by interviewing and assessing the psychological status of women before as well as after

Care plan 7.1 (Orem's Self Care model)

Name: Susan Harris

Treatment/condition: Total abdominal hysterectomy

Universal Self Care Requisites	Therapeutic Self Care Requisites	Self Care Agency	Self Care Deficits	Nursing Systems	Nursing Agency	Future
Maintain sufficient intake of oxygen	At risk of post-anaesthetic respiratory infection	Breathing unassisted. Tissues appear oxygenated. Understands rationale for breathing exercises four hourly and is able to perform them	None at present	Supportive	Continue encouraging breathing exercises. Monitor temperature for early signs of infection	Self caring
Maintain sufficient intake of fluid	At risk of urinary tract infection. Therefore should maintain fluid intake of two litres daily while in hospital	Understands rationale for increased fluid intake. Able to drink fluids independently now IV fluids discontinued. Understands purpose of fluid balance chart and will maintain own record. Unable to supply self with fluids due to decreased mobility	Needs to be supplied with fluids of choice frequently	Partially compensatory	Supply fluids of choice at frequent intervals (hourly). Monitor Susan's record keeping of fluid balance. Obtain midstream specimen of urine for routine bacteriological culture and sensitivity	Self caring
Maintain sufficient intake of food	Increased demands of nutrients for healing –	Concerned about weight gain due to	None at present	Supportive/ educative	Dietary consultation to	Weight maintenance

Universal Self Care Requisites	Therapeutic Self Care Requisites	Self Care Agency	Self Care Deficits	Nursing Systems	Nursing Agency	Future
	well balanced diet with vitamin C and protein. At risk of temporary constipation related to post-operative opiate analgesia – include increased fibre in diet. At risk of post-operative weight gain	reduced exercise. While in hospital will receive appropriate diet. *Discharge planning*: Unassessed knowledge for appropriate decision-making about diet. Shopping and food preparation may be hampered due to decreased energy and mobility. Unassessed support of family about need for weight maintenance. Daughter will stay for two weeks following discharge	*On discharge*: Daughter will need to know about diet		include both Susan and her daughter	will be a continuous demand and will have to be monitored by Susan
Provision of care associated with elimination	At risk of urinary tract infection. At risk of temporary constipation related to post-operative opiate analgesia and decreased mobility. Expected vaginal discharge, for at least 2–3 weeks	*Bowels*: usual pattern is once daily in the morning. Understands expected constipation and rationale for increased fibre and increased activity. *Vaginal discharge*: Understands that vaginal discharge is expected for 2–3 weeks and action to be taken if discharge becomes profuse or changes to bright red. Currently using two pads/day	None at present	Supportive	Monitor bowel pattern. Monitor vaginal discharge	Self caring

Maintain balance between rest and activity	Expected temporary fatigue related to major surgical procedure. Abdominal muscles compromised for 2–3 months while incision healing	Understands temporary fatigue but concerned about usual housework: 'Can't stand to see dust and cobwebs.' Usual activities involving abdominal muscles will be altered: – driving – working – cleaning and lifting. Daughter will stay for two weeks following discharge	*In hospital*: none *Discharge planning*: Modified activity	Supportive/ educative	Explore with Susan the alterations provoked by compromised abdominal muscles, i.e. household tasks, driving. Encourage Susan and her daughter to set order for priority for activities and explore other available resources	Self caring
Maintain balance between solitude and social interaction	Alteration in usual activities related to temporary fatigue and decreased mobility	*Hospital*: self caring *Discharge planning*: Possible decrease in social contact related to not being able to drive for six weeks. Will be home alone when daughter leaves after two weeks. Says she is worried about spending all day alone	Potential loneliness with dimished resources to cope	Supportive	Explore with Susan and daughter setting up social contact with friends for when daughter leaves. Find alternatives for the six week limitation on driving	Self caring

Universal Self Care Requisites	Therapeutic Self Care Requisites	Self Care Agency	Self Care Deficits	Nursing Systems	Nursing Agency	Future
Prevention of hazards to life, well being and functioning	Healing of abdominal muscles will take 2–3 months. Heavy lifting (more than a full kettle) should be avoided, as well as prolonged periods of standing	Understands temporary limitations but in discussions is concerned about knowing when to begin resuming normal activities	Knowledge deficit regarding return to usual activities	Supportive/educative	Discuss gradual return to activities which should be determined by her progress and how she feels, emphasising her role as judge of her own progress	Self caring
Promote normality	Alteration in body structure, while not visible, may have impact on self concept particularly gender identity. Loss of body part will result in grieving. Temporary physical constraints on sexual functioning related to healing tissues and vaginal discharge	Susan is concerned that the discomforts of early convalescence will continue and affect sexual activity. Views loss of childbearing capacity as normal. Susan says she enjoyed having and raising her children, but is looking forward to enjoying her grandchildren and time with her husband	Temporary alteration in usual sexual functioning	Supportive/educative	Provide time to express feelings and concerns about temporary restriction in sexual functioning. Explore alternative ways of expressing affection if this issue is of concern	Good

Recovery from hysterectomy has been the subject of several nursing research studies. Findings suggest that women are likely to have particular concern about this operation and its effects, and benefit if warned about possible problems during short and longer term recovery in advance. Most seem keen to participate in their own care, so Orem's model (1985) seems particularly suitable for planning care. However, Orem's model is not used as frequently in this country as the model by Roper et al. (1985). Try Roper's approach (see page 111) to planning care for Susan, either writing a whole care plan, or just a few of the problems reported, putting them into the activities of living framework employed by Roper. How do you think these two approaches compare?

surgery, found that women undergoing hysterectomy were no more depressed or neurotic than others in the general population, and that the operation reduced the incidence of psychiatric symptomatalogy by improving health.

In the early 1980s, nurses became increasingly concerned about women's longer term recovery following routine hysterectomy, and a number of studies have now been completed in the USA (see Kuczynski 1982, Cosper and Fuller 1979) and in this country, where the DHSS funded a four month follow-up study of women who had hysterectomy with ovarian conservation for non-malignant lesions (see Webb and Wilson-Barnett 1983a and b, Webb 1983), and a further follow-up eleven months later (see Gould 1986, Gould and Wilson-Barnett 1985).

There was very little evidence of clinical depression in these studies, but responses to questions about physical recovery were far less encouraging. Table 7.3 reveals the range of physical problems occurring during the eleven months, while Table 7.4 indicates those which appeared for the first time late in recovery, long after women would have attended their routine six-week follow-up appointment. Nearly half the women interviewed could be considered to have had a serious complication, and nearly half had experienced at least three post-operative problems. However, most were discharged within fourteen days of surgery and, apart from the follow-up visit to the Outpatient Department six weeks later, had little contact with medical or nursing staff although over half had seen their GP at least once during the eleven month period. In thirty-three cases, this was in relation to gynaecological problems, and thirteen required another referral to the gynaecologist (see Table 7.5).

At the time of the hospital interview, thirty women worked full-time outside the home, and thirty-two worked part-time. Jobs were mainly of a clerical nature, and women took an average of 9.6 weeks to return. In the sample as a whole few women abandoned any activity whether associated with work or leisure completely, and in the

Table 7.3 Symptoms experienced during the eleven month recovery period

Change of appetite	21.1%
Weight increase	27.6%
Weight decrease	14.4%
Urinary problems	28.2%
Bowel problems	23.5%
Sleep disturbance	22.3%
Vaginal bleeding/discharge	17.6%
Wound problems	28.2%
General aches and pains	37.6%
Fatigue	58.8%
Vertigo	31.7%

Note: Reproduced by kind permission of *Nursing Times* where this table first appeared on 4 June 1986, 82 (23) pp. 43–5.

Table 7.4 Symptoms developing late
in the post-operative period (after
four months)

	Number
Appetite change	4
Urinary	8
Bowel problems	3
Sleeping problems	9
Vaginal loss	7
Wound problems	7
Fatigue	5
Vertigo	14
Vasomotor disturbance	2
Depression	9

Note: Reproduced by kind permission of *Nursing Times* where this table first appeared on 4 June 1986, 82 (23) pp. 43–5.

four cases where this happened, hysterectomy was never blamed. Five women found new leisure activities and four worked for the first time after the operation. These women attributed their ability to the beneficial effects of surgery.

Very few factors seemed to predict poor recovery, although older women generally fared least well, and those who had experienced more life events throughout the eleven months reported more physical symptoms, which were generally of a more serious nature.

Table 7.5 Gynaecological referral

Reasons	*No.*
Post coital bleeding	2
Problems with colporrhapy (performed at the same time as hysterectomy)	4
Failure to heal	2
Vaginal adhesions	1
Senile vaginitis	1
Pelvic pain	1
Abscess formation	1
Extrauterine endometriosis	1
TOTAL	13

Note: Reproduced by kind permission of *Nursing Times* where this table first appeared on 4 June 1986, 82 (23) pp. 43–5.

Another major cause for concern was the lack of preparation received for discharge and continuing recovery at home: twenty-one women said they could remember no information at all, a further thirty-seven said they had been given general advice ('don't lift heavy weights' – 'amount unspecified' – 'have sex or drive a car for six weeks') and only sixteen could remember information of a specific nature. Information when provided came from a number of sources, mainly the ward sister or consultant. When asked about advice that would have been helpful, women would like to have been told about:

- Exactly what to expect during recovery;
- Possible side effects;
- Length of time necessary before feeling completely well;
- Exactly when different activities could safely be resumed.

In the early stages of this research study, ward nurses often expressed surprise that women's recovery from hysterectomy should be considered a topic worthy of investigation in view of its 'routine' nature and apparent lack of problems. Careful documentation of events after discharge suggested that many problems did in fact exist, and that women would have worried less if they had been forewarned. To the individuals themselves and their families there was nothing 'routine' about hysterectomy.

Endometriosis

Endometriosis is proliferation of endometrial tissue outside the uterine cavity. If it is confined to the myometrium it is called *adenomyosis* (internal endometriosis), but it is often found at sites outside the uterus, including the ovaries, uterine tubes and surface of the bowel. Lesions are usually restricted to the pelvic area, although there have been reports of endometrial tissue from distant sites, including the lungs.

Aetiology is obscure, but a number of theories have been suggested:

- Retrograde flow of menstrual blood up the uterine tubes, carrying endometrial cells into the pelvic cavity.
- Lymphatic or blood-born spread carrying endometrial tissue to distant sites.
- Embryological migration of cells destined to become endometrium from the uterus to other pelvic sites.
- Transfer on surgical instruments during pelvic operations. Endometrial tissue has been recovered from scars, where it is particularly likely to cause problems.

Spread probably occurs in several different ways depending on the site affected. Symptoms develop every month under the influence of oestrogen. The extraneous endometrium undergoes the same cyclical changes that would occur if it was normally situated but the blood, unable to escape, forms cysts (often called 'chocolate cysts' because the blood becomes dark and viscous as fluid is absorbed). Areas of fibrosis and adhesions form around the cyst and may cause pain.

Women complain of *worse* pain before menstruation; symptoms vary according to the site of lesions, but dyspareunia is common. Endometriosis occurs most often among women who have delayed having a family. It may therefore be detected during fertility investigations. Such women often have problems conceiving but, if pregnancy does occur, the pain and discomfort associated every month with endometriosis often disappears spontaneously when periods return.

Endometriosis may be treated by hysterectomy, although this may not eliminate all extrauterine lesions. Women may also be given the drug danazol (see page 187). Problems disappear after the menopause when oestrogen levels fall.

Dysfunctional uterine bleeding

Sometimes women complain of heavy periods or intermenstrual bleeding for which hysterectomy is performed, yet no organic lesions are demonstrated and there is no evidence of systemic disease. Twenty-eight per cent of women in Gould's sample (1986) fell into this category. At one time it was felt that these women, who had no demonstrable pelvic pathology, were having unnecessary surgery, helping to confirm a popular view that too many hysterectomies are performed. However, this type of bleeding, called dysfunctional uterine bleeding, is associated with characteristic histological changes in the endometrium and is thought to be caused by imbalance of oestrogen to progesterone throughout the luteal phase of the cycle. It appears that the corpus luteum either persists for too long, resulting in over-secretion of progesterone, or degenerates too quickly, resulting in under-secretion. Other cases may be due to excessive levels of endometrial prostaglandins.

Treatment
Occasionally symptoms disappear without treatment, but for many women everyday activities remain so disrupted that intervention is necessary. Many women are happy to undergo hysterectomy but others prefer drug therapy to help alleviate symptoms. The following drugs are commonly used:

- Antifibrinolytic agents (e.g. aminocaproic acid) given orally during menstruation to prevent excess bleeding by inducing coagulation. Another drug, ethamsylate, reduces capillary fragility, but effectiveness is doubtful.
- Oestrogen and progesterone given as the combined pill relieve dysfunctional uterine bleeding very effectively by correcting hormonal imbalance. However, many women affected are approaching the menopause, when long term therapy with sex steroids is generally avoided (see Chapter 2).
- Prostaglandin inhibitors (e.g. aspirin, mefenamic acid, indomethacin) prevent the vasodilatory effects of prostaglandin E2 and have beneficial analgesic effects, but taken long term may damage the gastric mucosa.
- Danazol reduces blood loss effectively although bleeding is likely to recur as soon as the woman stops taking it. Danazol is a synthetic sex steroid chemically related to testosterone. It works by inhibiting gonadotrophin release from the pituitary and opposes the effects of oestrogen. Danazol is said to have little virilising effect at a dosage of 400 mg daily, but higher doses may be necessary to relieve symptoms and a number of side effects may then be experienced. These include amenorrhoea, weight gain, hot flushes, loss of libido, hirsuitism, and voice changes caused by thickening of the vocal cords.

These changes are reversible and not experienced by all women. Others may experience mild symptoms which they find tolerable. However, given the potentially androgenic effects of danazol, it is not surprising that many women prefer surgery. The masculising effect of the drug may further damage feminine self-esteem at a time when a woman may already feel unattractive because she is continually bleeding. Those people who criticise women for their readiness to accept surgery as a drastic and invasive form of treatment, and gynaecologists for their readiness to perform it, would do well to remember this.

There are some women for whom danazol is definitely *not* suitable. It impairs glucose tolerance and opposes the effects of insulin and is unsuitable for women who have diabetes mellitus. Those who are overweight may develop Type 2 (adult onset) diabetes.

Resources

A book that can be recommended to clients:

Breitkoff, L. and Bakoulis, G. (1988) *Coping with Endometriosis*, Wellingborough: Grapevine Press.

Associations

National Association for Premenstrual Tension Syndrome
P.O. Box TN13 3PS
Sevenoaks, Kent.

References

Beard, M. (1984) *Understanding Premenstrual Tension*, London: Pan.
Billings, A. and Westland, A. (1980) *Natural Family Planning*, London: Allen Lane.
Brown, A. (1986) 'Personal and family impact of premenstrual symptoms', *Journal of Obstetric, Gynaecological and Neonatal Nursing* 15 (1), pp. 31–7.
Brown, M.A. and Woods, N.F. (1984) 'Correlates of dysmenorrhoea: a challenge to past stereotypes', *Journal of Obstetric, Gynaecological and Neonatal Nursing* 13 (4), pp. 259–66.
Brush, M.G. (1985) 'The premenstrual syndrome before and after pregnancy', *Maternal and Child Health* 10 (1), pp. 19–20.
Cole, P. (1977) 'Elective hysterectomy', *American Journal of Obstetrics and Gynaecology* 129, pp. 117–23.
Cosper, B. and Fuller, S. (1979) 'Characteristics of post-operative recovery following hysterectomy', *Journal of Obstetrics, Gynaecological and Neonatal Nursing* 7 (3), pp. 4–11.
Dalton, K. (1969) *The Menstrual Cycle*, London: Pelican.
Dalton, K. (1971) *The Menstrual Cycle*, 2nd ed. New York: Pantheon.
Dalton, K. (1980) 'Cyclical criminal acts in premenstrual syndrome', *Lancet* 2, pp. 1070–1.
Dumas, R.R. and Leonard, C. (1963) 'The effect of nursing on the incidence of post-operative vomiting', *Nursing Research* 1, pp. 12–15.
English, D. and Ehrenreich, B. (1973) *Complaints and Disorders*, New York: The Feminist Press.

Frank, R.T. (1961) 'The hormonal causes of premenstrual tension', *Archives of Neurology and Psychiatry* 26 (5), pp. 1053–7.

Friedman, R.C. (1984) 'Behaviour and the menstrual cycle', New York: Marcel Dekker.

Gath, D.M. (1980) 'Psychiatric aspects of hysterectomy' In: Robins, L. *et al.* (eds.) *The Social Consequences of Psychiatric Illness*, New York: Brunner-Mazel, pp. 33–45.

Gould, D.J. (1986) 'Hidden problems after a hysterectomy', *Nursing Times* 82 (23), pp. 43–6.

Gould, D.J. and Wilson-Barnett, J. (1985) 'A comparison of recovery following hysterectomy and major cardiac surgery', *Journal of Advanced Nursing* 10, pp. 315–23.

Hockey, L. and McLeod Clark, J. (1979) *Research for Nursing: A Guide for the Enquiring Nurse*, London: HM and M Publishers.

Jacob, T.J. and Charles, E. (1970) 'Correlation of psychiatric symptomatology and the menstrual cycle in an outpatient population', *American Journal of Psychiatry* 126 (10), pp. 1504–8.

Johnson, M. and Everitt, B. (1984) *Essential Reproduction*, Oxford: Blackwell Scientific.

Jordan, J. and Meckler, J.R. (1982) 'The relationship between life events, social supports and dysmenorrhoea', *Research in Nursing and Health* 5, pp. 73–9.

Kuczynski, J. (1982) 'After the hysterectomy', *Nursing Mirror* 155 (6), pp. 42–6.

Lancet (1981) 'Premenstrual syndrome: a disease of the mind?', *Lancet* 2, pp. 1238–40.

Lindeman, C.A. and Van Aernam, B. (1971) 'Effects of structured and unstructured pre-operative teaching', *Nursing Research* 20, pp. 319–32.

Mandell, A.J. and Mandell, M.P. (1967) 'Suicide and the menstrual cycle', *Journal of American Medical Association* 200, pp. 792–3.

Orem, D. (1985) *Nursing – Concepts of Practice*, New York: McGraw-Hill.

Richards, D.H. (1979) 'A general practice view of functional disorders associated with menstruation', *Research Clinical Forums* 1, pp. 39–45.

Roberts, D.W.T. (1984) 'Dysmenorrhoea' In: Chamberlain, G. (ed.) *Contemporary Gynaecology*, London: Butterworths, pp. 1–4.

Roberts, S. and Garling, J. (1981) 'The menstrual myth revisited', *Nursing Forum* 20 (3), pp. 267–72.

Sampson, G.A. (1984) 'The role of the psychiatrist in the treatment of premenstrual syndrome', *Maternal and Child Health* 9 (3), pp. 96–101.

Sutherland, H. and Stewart, I. (1965) 'A critical analysis of the premenstrual syndrome', *Lancet* 1, pp. 1180–3.

'Talking point: Premenstrual tension syndrome' *British Medical Journal* (1979) 286, pp. 212–13.

Torrance, C. and Milligan, S. (1986) 'How safe is the safe period?', *Nursing Times* 82 (26), pp. 37–8.

Webb, C. (1983) 'Hysterectomy – dispelling the myths', *Nursing Times* 79 (47), pp. 52–4; 79 (48), pp. 44–6.

Webb, C. (1986) 'Care plan for a woman having an abdominal hysterectomy, based on Roy's Adaptation Model' In: Webb, C. (ed.) *Using Nursing Models: Women's Health*, Sevenoaks: Hodder and Stoughton, pp. 140–53.

Webb, C. and Wilson-Barnett, J. (1983a) 'Self concept, support and hysterectomy', *International Journal of Nursing Studies* 20 (2), pp. 97–107.

Webb, C. and Wilson-Barnett, J. (1983b) 'Hysterectomy: a study in coping with recovery', *Journal of Advanced Nursing* 8, pp. 311–19.

Woods, N.F. *et al.* (1985) 'Major life events, daily stressors and premenstrual symptoms', *Nursing Research* 34, pp. 263–7.

Woods, N.F. (1985) 'Relationship of socialisation and stress to perimenstrual symptoms, disability and menstrual disorders', *Nursing Research* 34, pp. 145–9.

8   Subfertility

'Subfertility' is defined as failure to conceive after a couple have had unprotected intercourse for twelve months or longer. Couples may think their situation is unique: all around there are people with children and, in the media, family life is portrayed as ideal. However, subfertility is more common than most people imagine, although until recently few statistical records were available.

Incidence

The first major study to document incidence, causes, treatment and outcome of subfertility was conducted by Hull *et al.* (1985) in a health district in the South of England. Hull's team established that in a population of 7,000, 708 couples were referred to a specialist clinic, an incidence of one in six couples of childbearing age.

■   Christine and Kevin Meadows, both aged 28, had not taken contraceptive precautions for over a year. Christine was not unduly upset for the first few months when her period arrived but, as time went by, her growing surprise turned to dismay. She began to feel jealous of other women with children, and to feel resentful towards her sister who had two children. Christine eventually decided to take action because of an incident at a party to which she and Kevin had been invited. The conversation turned towards children and Christine was asked whether she had a family. She heard herself explaining rather coldly that she had a career which she did not want to interrupt just yet. Another guest, some years older than Christine, assured her that she would soon change her mind once a baby arrived. In the discussion which followed, Christine heard someone else commenting upon a friend's childless marriage and the emptiness of a home without children for which elegant possessions and expensive foreign holidays could never compensate. She told Kevin she wanted to leave and cried all the way home. Christine was now frightened that she and Kevin might be unable to have a baby of their own. Kevin became very quiet. He had had the same idea.

Childlessness, Stigma and Society Norms

■   Like many other people confronted by possible infertility, Christine and Kevin at first denied that anything might be wrong, from themselves and from each other, yet secretly both were anxious. Christine felt resentful of other women who apparently became pregnant without difficulty and frustrated when she thought of all the years of carefully practised contraception. Kevin was concerned that he might somehow be 'to blame' for their failure and felt guilty. Neither Christine nor Kevin had analysed *why* they wanted a baby, but both were sure it was right for them to start a family together.

Oakely (1979), asking 60 women pregnant for the first time why they wanted a baby, found their responses varied and vague, yet their desire to have children was strong. McCormick (1980) points out that individuals who are unable to conceive may feel as though they have lost control over an important part of their lives, especially if they have apparently controlled fertility successfully by contraception. Childlessness may generate keen disappointment, sufficient to result in psychological disorder. In some cultures and religions, infertility is regarded as no less than a disaster. Even for those whose religious or cultural beliefs do not reflect this ideology, knowledge that they are unable to procreate may take away their raison d'être.

Health care professionals have long been aware of the anguish of people unable to conceive. Newill (1974) argues that everybody in this predicament deserves sympathy and medical help but fertility treatment is specialised and expensive at a time when health care resources are scarce. Some people would argue that in a heavily populated country in a planet overcrowded to the extent that many go hungry, resources are misdirected if used to generate more lives. Because so many unplanned pregnancies and abortions occur, it has been suggested that finance should be directed towards improving contraception rather than fertility. However, research into the mechanism of conception is likely to provide information which will be of value in both spheres. The Declaration of Human Rights (1948) states that it is the right of every individual to have children and, as Newill points out, the childless can scarcely be expected to live without procreation because of the contraceptive failures or irresponsibilities of others.

Acknowledging the problem

In approximately one third of cases, subfertility occurs because the woman has some problem and, in another third, problems are associated with the man. In the remaining third, fertility problems are contributed by both partners. For example, the man may have a low sperm count and the woman's periods may be infrequent. This explains why people who have had children with previous partners may experience later difficulties. Thus there are two types of subfertility:

- *Primary infertility* when the woman has never become pregnant;
- *Secondary infertility* when the woman has conceived at least once.

Most normal healthy couples conceive within twelve months of unprotected intercourse but there are no hard and fast rules for commencing fertility investigations. Most doctors agree that tests should begin after a year but, if a problem is anticipated from the outset (previous pelvic inflammatory disease, anovulatory cycles) or if the woman is reaching the age when fertility is naturally declining, investigations may begin earlier. The number of tests that GPs are willing to perform are variable, as is the provision of fertility services across the country. Although the approach taken will depend on the individuals concerned, it is likely that investigations and treatment will be more thorough if the couple are referred to a specialist centre with experienced staff and good laboratory services.

One of the first investigations is to check that ovulation is regular. Most women experience occasional anovulatory cycles, and regular cyclical bleeds are possible in the complete absence of ovulation. The only real proof of ovulation is pregnancy, but a certain amount of presumptive evidence can be obtained to suggest that it is occurring.

One of the least invasive methods is regular temperature recording to detect the slight transient fall, then rise, in basal body temperature just before ovulation (see Chapter 7).

The fertility clinic

■ Eventually Christine and Kevin went to their GP, who referred them to a fertility clinic. They were greeted by the nurse specialist who would co-ordinate all the tests and treatments they would undergo. She explained that, although the cause of subfertility can sometimes be detected quite quickly, this is not always the case. Sometimes investigations and treatment take months or years. Christine and Kevin would probably need several appointments. Some tests and treatments have to take place at particular times in the woman's menstrual cycle. This may lead to unavoidable delays or inconvenience even in a big clinic with good laboratory facilities.

All the time the nurse was observing Christine and Kevin carefully. Fertility investigations place an enormous strain on a relationship, especially in view of uncomfortable and embarrassing procedures which may have to be repeated, and the need to have intercourse at specified times in relation to these. To withstand emotional trauma, the relationship must be stable and the couple must be genuinely motivated towards having a baby. However, cursory and inadequate assessment of the couple's relationship and psychological status are among the main grievances of women experiencing fertility investigations (Pfeffer and Woolett 1983). Couples need plenty of opportunity to talk to staff before they can be expected to express their feelings openly, and may need time to come to terms with their reactions towards attendance. By requesting fertility investigations they have acknowledged to themselves, to each other and to outsiders that they are finding it difficult to achieve what for most people is taken for granted. Before they sought help, they could pretend that this problem did not exist. They need time to alter self-concept and feelings towards each other.

The nurse showed them the nursing assessment form, but suggested they should discuss their reactions to the tests later. She explained her role and described what would happen during this first visit, emphasising that the tests and treatments performed, and their order, depend on the problems experienced by the particular couple. Variations also depend on the doctor and specialist centre concerned. It is important for couples to be given this information so they do not compare their own experiences inappropriately with others'. Nevertheless, people who are undergoing fertility treatments can benefit enormously from the support of others in the same position (Christianson 1986). Several groups have been set up nationally (see page 220) and some clinics have established their own. The nurse drew attention to the addresses of these organisations.

Experts agree that people undergoing fertility investigations benefit from participation and should be regarded as active partners rather than passive participants in care (Winston 1986). They need to be informed sympathetically but realistically about progress. Nurses working in this field play a major role supporting clients, providing continuity of care sometimes over long periods of time, counselling and teaching. Women may be admitted to hospital for some investigations, but length of stay is usually short and, as they are in good health, they do not normally require much physical nursing care. They rely heavily on developing a good relationship with nurses in the clinic. The RCN established a Fertility Nurses' Interest Group in 1987, which allows nurses with a special interest in this topic to update knowledge and keep abreast of research findings and improve quality of care.

Medical examination

For both partners, investigations begin with a medical examination. This provides an opportunity for both partners to discuss any worries privately with the doctor. Even in the closest relationships there may be incidents, often occurring before the partners met, which one may prefer not to disclose to the other. Women may have had a previous pregnancy terminated or one of the partners may have had a sexually transmitted infection which could affect fertility.

The male

- The man is asked about previous illness, infections and current health. Sexually transmitted infections (gonorrhoea, non-specific urethritis) can reduce fertility by scarring the male urethra. Mumps after puberty may cause orchitis.

- Sperm production is continuous and can be affected by a range of factors, including previous surgery such as orchidopexy. A temperature slightly below normal body temperature is most conducive to spermatogenesis; this may be why the testes hang outside the main abdominal cavity where the temperature is about 2°C lower. Men who have had undescended testicles may have low sperm counts. A *varicocele* (collection of veins similar to varicose veins in the testis) may increase temperature and reduce spermatogenesis. Varicoceles may be surgically repaired and sperm production then improves.
- It is important to obtain details of occupation. Exposure to heat (in a boiler house or foundry) and to some chemicals may reduce spermatogenesis (Elkington 1986).
- Social habits – alcohol consumption, cigarette smoking and sometimes very strenuous exercise – can depress sperm count temporarily.
- Some drugs reduce fertility (for example, sulphasalazine used to treat ulcerative colitis; this is reversible when the drug is no longer taken).
- The man must be asked about the regularity and timing of coitus. He must achieve orgasm to ensure release of semen. In the study by Hull *et al.* (1985) six per cent of cases of subfertility were related to problems with coitus.
- During physical examination, development of the male secondary sexual characteristics is noted. Normal development implies normal testosterone secretion. Absence of secondary sexual characteristics might indicate a genetic defect such as *Klinefelter's Syndrome* (see Chapter 14).
- The male genitals are examined in case there is any previously undetected abnormality. The vasa deferentia are palpated to ensure both are intact. Congenital damage or occlusion are rare causes of infertility, but have been reported.

The female

- The woman is asked about her present health, any drugs she may be taking and her past medical history, particularly infections. Gonorrhoea and chlamydial infections may damage the uterine tubes. Scarring and adhesions can also result from previous inflammatory conditions such as appendicitis. Mumps after puberty may cause oöphoritis. Recent evidence suggests that high caffeine intake may possibly affect ability to conceive (Wilcox *et al.* 1988).
- Enquiries will be made about previous obstetric history. Infection damaging the pelvic organs can follow childbirth, spontaneous or induced abortion.
- Menstrual history must be recorded. This may indicate that the woman in not ovulating. A very long or irregular cycle may mean that it is difficult to time intercourse so that it occurs at the most fertile time. Many people believe, mistakenly, that ovulation takes place exactly in the middle of the cycle, but the

egg leaves the ovary 13–14 days before Day One of the *next* cycle. For women whose cycles are longer or shorter than 28 days this will not be precisely midway between one period and the next. Irregular or very light periods may suggest anovulatory cycles.

- The woman will have a general medical examination to check development of the female secondary sexual characteristics, verifying production of adequate oestrogen, and a pelvic examination to detect any gynaecological problems (fibroids, endometriosis, or rarely, gross physical abnormalities such as congenital absence of the uterus).

There is a theory that anxiety may interfere with conception, especially when the couple become distressed at failure to establish pregnancy (Edelmann and Connolly 1986). The truth of this is difficult to establish. In many cases no good reason can be found to explain subfertility although, as diagnostic techniques improve, this number is diminishing. Nevertheless, 25 per cent of the couples in Hull's sample (1985) fell into this category. Most people have heard stories of couples who abandoned fertility treatment to adopt a child only to conceive a short while later. The number of cases in which this has happened has never been documented. There are instances of women who became pregnant after years of trying when they either gave up work or took a job, and there have been cases where young girls, under great stress and worried about the possibility of unplanned pregnancy, have conceived. Evidence is mixed. There are nervous connections between the hypothalamus and higher centres of the brain which presumably allow information to be relayed between the two, and it is known that animals exposed to stress often fail to breed. But human beings differ from other animals, and these analogies are not likely to be of much help or comfort to clients.

■   The doctor could find no immediate reason to suggest why Christine and Kevin were failing to conceive except that some of Christine's cycles might be anovulatory because her periods were rather light. He arranged some preliminary investigations. These included a skull X-ray for Christine and tests to check whether she was ovulating. Kevin was to have semen analysis. The nurse arranged these, explaining why they were important and what each would involve.

Subfertility: some causes

Hyperprolactinaemia

Prolactin is a hormone released from the anterior pituitary, entering the bloodstream in intermittent pulses. Release increases tenfold during pregnancy, when prolactin prepares the breasts for lactation. For many years it has been known that women who secrete excessive amounts of prolactin when they are *not* pregnant have difficulty conceiving. Periods may stop altogether, or become scanty, and a milky secretion may escape from the nipples (*galactorrhoea*).

Prolactin secretion can increase without pregnancy in a number of pathological conditions:

- *Small pituitary tumours*. These are adenomas (tumours of glandular tissue), nearly always benign and less than 10 cm in diameter.
- *Accompanying hypothyroidism* due to interference with secretion of hormone releasing factors from the hypothalamus.
- As a side effect of some drugs (methyldopa, metoclopramide, cimetidine, some sedatives and tranquillisers).

Elevated prolactin levels prevent the ovaries responding to FSH and LH. They probably also have a direct effect on the hypothalamus, preventing secretion of gonadotrophin releasing factor. High levels of prolactin during lactation have a natural contraceptive effect. The occasional pregnancies which sometimes result may occur because of the intermittent manner in which prolactin is secreted. Contraceptive effect may be temporarily altered as circulating levels fluctuate.

The main reason for hyperprolactinaemia in young, asymptomatic women is a benign pituitary adenoma, easily detected by skull X-ray (see Fig. 8.1). It has been suggested that hyperprolactinaemia is one of the most common causes of female subfertility (Laycock and Wise 1982). X-rays are worth performing early in the sequence of investigations because they are both easy to carry out and non-invasive.

Figure 8.1 shows that nerve fibres carrying information from the eyes to the brain run close to the *sella turcica*, the bony cavity in the skull occupied by the pituitary. Any tumour of the pituitary will act as a space-occupying lesion, and may interfere

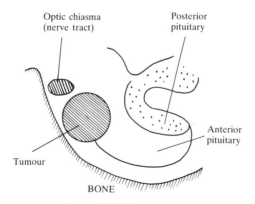

Figure 8.1 Pituitary adenoma.

with vision by exerting pressure on the nerves. The individual may complain of blurred vision and headaches.

Although both these investigations are straightforward, women and their partners need careful explanations because the words 'tumour' or 'growth', especially in connection with the brain, are alarming. In addition, they may seem only remotely connected with the immediate problem of sub-fertility.

Elevated prolactin levels can also be detected by a blood test. Repeated tests may be necessary as prolactin levels are sometimes elevated by stress. This may help account for the amenorrhoea sometimes reported as one of the effects of chronic stress.

Hyperprolactinaemia is readily treated by the drug bromocriptine which is thought to act by stimulating an inhibitor in the hypothalamus, and preventing prolactin release. Bromocriptine slows growth of the tumour and surgery may not be necessary. However, bromocriptine can induce nausea and vertigo. It may be necessary to gradually increase dosage until 2.5 mg are taken three times a day.

Hypothyroidism

Subfertility may be caused by hypothyroidism but, in this case, the woman is likely to seek medical help for other symptoms (weight gain, feeling cold, tired, depressed) and diagnosis is readily suggested on clinical presentation. Other endocrine causes of subfertility are rare.

Failure to ovulate

Anovulatory cycles occur from time to time in many women, although they are naturally more frequent at the extremes of reproductive life. In some girls periods do not start at the expected time, a condition known as *primary amenorrhoea* (see Table 8.1.). Although primary amenorrhoea is an obvious cause of fertility problems, it is usually investigated when the girl is much younger (see Chapter 14). *Secondary amenorrhoea* is the disappearance of menstrual periods for more than six months after they have become established. The most common reasons are shown in Table 8.2. It may take a few months for ovulatory cycles to become re-eatablished once a woman has discontinued oral contraception, but the idea that the pill is a serious and common cause of subfertility by inducing secondary amenorrhoea is no more than a 'modern old wives tale'. Many women are surprised at the short time it takes to conceive once they have stopped taking the pill.

Even if periods are occurring they may be anovulatory if they are irregular or scanty, especially if accompanied by little pelvic pain or breast soreness.

Table 8.1 Causes of primary amenorrhoea

1. Constitutionally delayed puberty
2. Puberty delayed due to endocrine disorders, e.g. adrenogenital syndrome
3. Genetic abnormalities, e.g. Turner's syndrome
4. Cryptomenorrhoea
5. Anorexia nervosa

Ovulation

Clinical signs and symptoms

There are numerous clinical signs that ovulation is probably occurring:

- Pain in the middle of the cycle when the egg escapes;
- Cyclical changes in vaginal mucus (see Chapter 7);
- Cyclical changes in vaginal cytology;
- Cyclical endometrial changes;
- Cyclical temperature changes.

Table 8.2 Causes of secondary amenorrhoea

Defects of the pituitary and hypothalamus
1. Pituitary tumour and hyperprolactinaemia
2. Defective hypothalamus feedback mechanism
3. Premature menopause due to raised FSH levels
4. Anorexia nervosa
5. Anxiety
6. Pseudopregnancy
7. Oral contraceptives

Defects of the ovary
1. Premature menopause due to ovarian failure
2. Polycystic ovary disease
3. Tumours secreting androgens

Other endocrine disorders
1. Hypothyroidism
2. Hyperadrenalism

Systemic disease
1. Prolonged general ill health

Vaginal cytology
The cyclical effects of oestrogen and progesterone on the squamous epithelium of the vagina provide good presumptive evidence of ovulation, although they are insufficiently precise to time it. Before ovulation, cells sampled from the vagina lie flat on the microscope slide and there are few, if any, leucocytes (in the absence of infection or inflammation). Once ovulation has occurred, the rising levels of progesterone induce the edges of the cells to roll up in a distinctive fashion, and a shower of leucocytes (mainly neutrophils) is visible among them (see Fig. 8.2). Although vaginal cytology is rarely performed today, it was one of the standard methods of detecting ovulation prior to the wide availability of plasma hormone assay techniques. It is time-consuming for the woman who has to prepare daily smears, then take the batch of microscope slides preserved in fixative to the laboratory.

Vaginal cytology is also sometimes used to assess the effectiveness of hormone replacement therapy in the treatment of menopausal problems, since oestrogen withdrawal induces change in the vaginal epithelium.

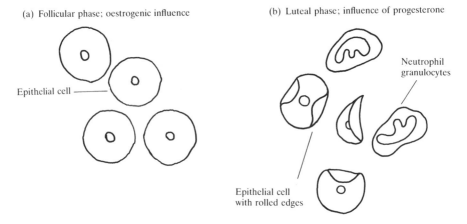

Figure 8.2 Cyclical changes in the vaginal epithelium.

Endometrial changes
Since the endometrium responds to cyclical variations in oestrogen and progesterone, a small quantity of tissue, aspirated at a known point in the cycle, can be used to detect characteristic changes (see Fig. 8.3). Endometrial biopsy can be performed by *Vabra curettage* (see Chapter 1), but this can be painful for a woman who has not had children. It is more usual for tissue to the obtained when the woman is anaesthetised to undergo laparoscopy to visualise the pelvic organs. This is an invasive procedure, carrying the same risks as other minor surgical operations and requiring admission to hospital. Laparoscopy is not usually planned until some of the more easily detected

reasons for sub-fertility have been ruled out. However, laparoscopy is valuable because the ripening follicles can be directly visualised. It has been suggested that failure to ovulate may sometimes occur because the egg is not released from the follicle. This condition, *ovum entrapment syndrome*, can only be diagnosed with the laparoscope. No stigma appears on the follicle, and the egg can retrieved in fluid aspirated from it.

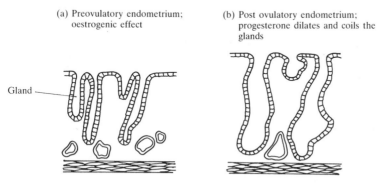

(a) Preovulatory endometrium; oestrogenic effect

(b) Post ovulatory endometrium; progesterone dilates and coils the glands

Gland

Figure 8.3 Cyclical endometrial changes.

Cyclical temperature changes

■   Christine showed her temperature charts to the nurse. Figure 8.4 suggests that, compared to a classic temperature chart for a woman ovulating normally, Christine's cycles may have been anovulatory. Temperature change was not readily detectable and did not bear much relationship to the time when the LH surge was supposed to occur.

The nurse explained these ambiguities but pointed out that temperature is difficult to record accurately and the results hard to interpret even when ovulation is occurring.

Traditionally, temperature charts have been used extensively during fertility investigations in the belief that they give clients opportunity to participate in meaningful investigations benefiting treatment. Some experts now suggest that temperature charting may not be helpful. Despite a high degree of commitment, the couple may feel disheartened when their carefully constructed graphs do not dip and peak in the classic way. Variations may occur despite ovulation or meticulous record keeping. Lenton *et al.* (1977) showed over ten years ago that time of ovulation, estimated from the temperature charts of 60 women, were accurate in only 34 per cent of cases according to the more accurate results of hormone assays. Today, experts recommend that temperature charting should not continue for longer than three months (Winston 1986).

■   Christine was told that she need not continue to record her temperature. She was pleased as she had found taking her temperature first thing every morning unbelievably tiresome. She and Kevin had also been discouraged by the need to have intercourse 'to order' at the predicted time of ovulation. The nurse explained that again this may be a myth which needs exploding. Sperms are known to survive for up to five days in cervical mucus and, if deposited during the follicular phase, the cervical mucus may act as a reservoir, releasing sperm when ovulation occurs. It may not be necessary therefore to time intercourse very closely to the time of predicted ovulation and, if couples feel distressed at having intercourse to suit the calendar, it is better for them to disrupt their sex lives as little as possible.

Hormone assays

The most accurate method of detecting the time of ovulation or its failure is by directly measuring plasma hormone levels. Since all the reproductive hormones are excreted via the kidneys, urinary hormone assays are also possible, although slightly less accurate. For many investigations and treatments, daily measurements throughout the menstrual cycle are necessary. Figure 7.4 (page 155) shows that oestrogen levels rise progressively as the follicle matures, stimulating the LH surge. Increase in FSH

(a) Normal temperature chart.

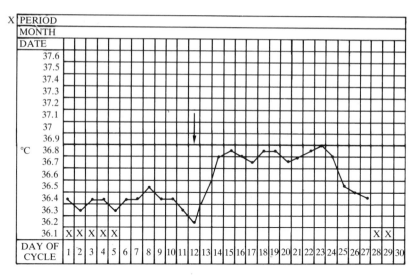

(b) 'Normal' chart, with slight fall in temperature at about the time of the LH surge. Ovulation occurs twenty-four hours later.

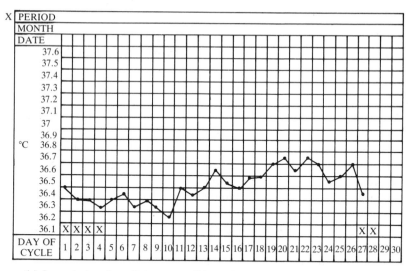

(c) Inconclusive chart. It is not possible to determine the time of ovulation.

Figure 8.4 Temperature charts.

occurring at the same time is used less often as a marker in fertility work, since it is less pronounced, but may help diagnose hypothalamic or pituitary failure (rare causes of infertility) or ovarian failure, since levels are elevated at the menopause (see Chapter 9).

Oestrogen and progesterone levels in urine collected continuously over a complete cycle, into twenty-four bottles, can give a reliable picture of the menstrual cycle, especially as the LH surge can very occasionally take place without ovulation. However, some doctors may wait until the results of semen analysis are available before proceeding with hormone assays. In the past women have been subjected to many uncomfortable and sometimes unnecessary procedures when an earlier examination of the semen might have suggested the reason for subfertility. Men often worry a great deal about these tests however, and must be reassured that, contrary to popular opinion, sperm count is not related to masculinity or potency. The endocrine cells which secrete testosterone, responsible for the male sexual characteristics and libido, are present in connective tissue between the seminiferous tubules and are not damaged by any of the agents which depress spermatogenesis.

Sperm count

Semen analysis

When semen analysis is performed the laboratory technician will make the following observations:

- *Total volume of ejaculate* – for optimum fertility this should be at least 2 ml. An unusually large ejaculate may also decrease fertility because sperm will be diluted in a larger volume of seminal fluid. If any ejaculate is lost during collection, another specimen must be obtained.
- *Sperm count* – this should be more than 20,000,000 per ml. Clients may find it difficult to accept this; after all, only one sperm is needed to fertilise one egg. However, a low sperm count means that fewer sperm are likely to succeed in the journey from the vagina to the uterine tubes where fertilisation takes place, and the statistical odds of a sperm meeting an egg at the optimum time for fertilisation are reduced if the count is low. (Nevertheless, doctors advise men who have had a vasectomy to avoid unprotected intercourse until *all* the sperms have disappeared from the ejaculate.)
- *Motility* – sperm become inactive below body temperature, but more than 40 per cent should remain active four hours after collection. Men who have low sperm counts are often encouraged to wear loosely fitting underwear and to spray the testes with cold water to encourage spermatogenesis.
- *Abnormal forms of sperm* – some abnormal sperm are expected in any ejaculate, but normal undamaged cells should constitute at least 70 per cent of the total. Some laboratories use the *swim-up test* which also helps to eliminate damaged sperm before *in vitro* fertilisation. The sperm are covered with a layer of medium in a test tube. Normal sperm swim into the medium, leaving damaged ones behind. It is acknowledged that, although some sperm do not look abnormal, they may be functionally damaged in a way not detectable at present except by this test.

- Coagulability – semen is of a jelly-like consistency when ejaculated, but it liquefies in the vagina. The technician will observe consistency, as this may affect sperm motility.

The specimen can be collected by coitus interruptus or masturbation, but not in a condom as most brands are impregnated with spermicide. For couples whose religious beliefs forbid these practices, information must be obtained from a post-coital test (page 205).

Instructions given for collection vary between one clinic and another, especially the maximum length of time allowed between collection and delivery, and whether or not the man should abstain for one or more days before the test is performed. Most fertility specialists agree that there can be considerable variation in the character of the semen and sperm counts for the same man on different occasions. Sperm are continually produced and rate can be influenced by a range of environmental factors. One or two unfavourable results are *not* cause for despair.

It is good practice for the couple to be asked to return to the clinic together for the results of semen analysis. Women report that telling their husbands about the unfavourable results of these tests is one of the most stressful experiences of fertility investigations (Pfeffer and Woolett 1983).

Treatment for low sperm counts

Low sperm counts (*oligospermia*) can sometimes be improved by giving testosterone or gonadotrophins (LH and FSH help to control testicular activity in men). Synthetic male sex steroids (Mesterolone) are sometimes given, or bromocriptine if there is a specific pituitary defect. The fact that so many different drugs have been tried indicates that success is variable. However, men who have low sperm counts *can* have children. No treatment is presently available for *azoospermia* (semen containing no sperm at all).

Other causes of male subfertility are shown in Table 8.3.

Immunological causes of subfertility

An antibody is a protein the body produces against harmful foreign materials called antigens (foreign cells, tissue grafts, transplants, micro-organisms, pollen). For every different antigen invading the body, the plasma cells (a special group of leucocytes) make specific antibodies. Antibodies combine with specific antigens in a lock and key mechanism see Fig. 8.5) rendering them inactive and therefore harmless. Eventually the antigen-antibody complexes are engulfed by phagocytic white blood cells (neutrophils or macrophages).

Scientists have known since the beginning of the century that men can sometimes develop antibodies which destroy their own sperm. Anti-sperm antibodies have been detected in up to 60 per cent of men following vasectomy. It is thought that antibodies escape from the vas deferentia into the blood during the operation when the vasa are divided. However, anti-sperm antibodies have been detected in men who have not

Table 8.3 Causes of infertility in the male

Testicular abnormalities
1. Varicocele
2. Damaged or infected testes

Endocrine abnormalities
1. Defective FSH/LH secretion
2. Hyperprolactinaemia

Other
1. Obstruction of the vasa deferentia
2. Prostatitis
3. Drugs e.g. Sulphasalizine

---

had a vasectomy although the mechanism remains obscure. Sperm develop from germ cells lining the seminiferous tubules (see Fig. 8.6). The tubule wall forms a barrier between the sperm and the blood. Male anti-sperm antibodies interfere with fertility by causing sperm to clump tail to tail (see Fig. 8.7) instead of swimming through the cervical mucus. However, this is not a common cause of subfertility.

Women can develop antibodies against their partner's sperm but again this is not a common problem. The antibodies are present throughout the plasma and tissue fluids, but are most strongly concentrated in cervical mucus where they immobilise sperm by agglutinating them head to head (see Fig. 8.8). The pattern of clumping can therefore

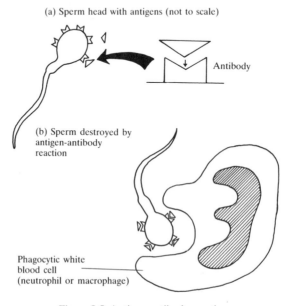

(a) Sperm head with antigens (not to scale)

Antibody

(b) Sperm destroyed by antigen-antibody reaction

Phagocytic white blood cell (neutrophil or macrophage)

Figure 8.5 Antigen-antibody reaction.

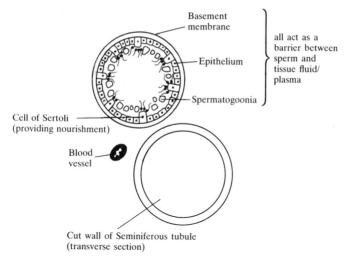

Figure 8.6 Sperm production (spermatogenesis).

help to determine the origin of the antibodies. Results can then be confirmed by blood test.

The first step towards diagnosing an immunological problem is to perform a post-coital test.

Post-coital testing (PCT)

A post-coital test demonstrates the ability of sperm to remain motile in ovulatory cervical mucus. Precise instructions must be given to clients because success of the test depends on careful timing as it must be performed at the predicted time of ovulation:

- The woman must wait until Day One of her next period, then calculate the date on which she expects to ovulate during the new cycle. She can then make the appointment for the test.
- The couple must have intercourse as near to the time of predicted ovulation as possible.

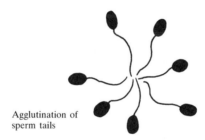

Figure 8.7 Anti-sperm antibodies (male).

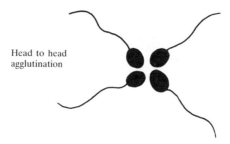

Head to head
agglutination

Figure 8.8 Anti-sperm antibodies (female).

- The woman should come to the clinic within a few hours (the time limit specified varies between one clinic and another). She should not have a bath.
- She should be told that a speculum is used to expose the cervix and a drop of cervical mucus is painlessly aspirated to be examined under the microscope.

At this time of the month the ovulatory mucus should lie in chains with sperm able to swim through it in straight lines (see Fig. 8.9). If the woman is not ovulating or releasing enough oestrogen, the cervical mucus remains thick and impenetrable to sperm.

■   Although post-coital tests can provide information about the quality of ovulatory cervical mucus, Christine's doctor decided to perform some hormone assays first as there was an indication that she might not be ovulating properly. Christine was glad. She knew from discussions with other women attending the clinic that post-coital tests are particularly disliked, because they are embarrassing, inconvenient, and represent the ultimate invasion of the couple's sex life. Some clients find themselves unable to have intercourse at the appropriate time.

Post-coital tests often have to be repeated; from time to time results may naturally be poor or inconclusive. Couples should be warned about this in advance.

Two other tests are sometimes performed on cervical mucus:

The sperm invasion test
This may be performed when the results of post-coital tests are repeatedly poor or negative. A drop of ejaculate and cervical mucus are placed adjacent to one another on a warm microscope slide. Under the microscope, sperm should be seen actively invading the mucus.

The cross-hostility test
This is performed to determine whether antibodies are present in the cervical mucus or semen. The ejaculate and ovulatory mucus are tested against each other, then

(a) Ovulatory mucus

(b) Hostile mucus

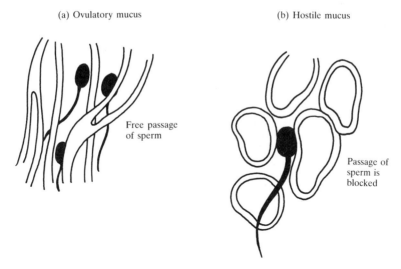

Free passage
of sperm

Passage of
sperm is
blocked

Figure 8.9 Cervical mucus.

against semen and mucus from donors of proven fertility, which are known not to contain antibodies.

Currently there is much debate about the importance of cervical mucus in promoting fertility. Some experts believe that it is the single most important factor, while others think that it is of no importance at all. Probably the truth is somewhere in between (Winston 1986).

Treatment for hostile mucus and anti-sperm antibodies

Steroids can be given to the partner producing the antibodies but this is not always effective and the dose required is sufficiently high to cause side effects. If the woman is producing antibodies, preventing sperm coming into contact with the mucus for several months may help to remove them from the bloodstream because the stimulus for antibody formation will no longer be present. This can be achieved by wearing a condom, but such advice may seem illogical to a couple trying to conceive and is not guaranteed to work. Artificial insemination directly into the uterus by-passes the cervix where antibodies are most concentrated, but may not work if systemic concentration is high. The best treatment for this uncommon problem is *in vitro* fertilisation.

If cervical mucus appears to be hostile without anti-sperm antibodies, little can be done at the present time. Often the problem is related to anovulation and the best treatment is directed towards promoting this.

Some couples worry because most of the semen drains from the vagina soon after intercourse. In the past women have been encouraged to adopt an array of postures to help maximise contact with the cervix. However, post-coital loss is normal. It has been calculated that, even if intercourse occurs at the optimal time, only one in 2,000 sperm penetrates the mucus. Most escape or are killed by the natural acidity of the healthy adult vagina. Steps to reduce acidity by douching (with mildly alkaline solutions like bicarbonate) are not only ineffective, they are dangerous because they destroy the natural vaginal defence against infection.

■   Christine and Kevin were relieved to hear that semen analysis was normal. The doctor explained that, according to her menstrual history, Christine might not be ovulating. She was asked to collect her urine every day to determine whether an egg was released. She found this most inconvenient, especially as she had been told that the assay might be necessary over several months, and every drop of urine must be included if the calculation was to be meaningful.

Anovulatory cycles: treatment

Hull *et al.* (1985) found that 21 per cent of the couples in their study were subfertile because of anovulation, but 96 per cent responded to treatment, conceiving within two years. This is the most responsive of all fertility problems to treatment.

Several drugs can be used to induce ovulation, but the first treatment of choice is clomiphene citrate (clomid).

Clomiphene therapy

Clomiphene is a non-steroid drug operating on the hypothalamus to stimulate ovulation. All cells which respond to oestrogen contain cytoplasmic oestrogen receptors to which oestrogen must bind before it can influence metabolic activity (see Chapter 1). The target cells of the hypothalamus contain receptor sites for oestrogen, as the hypothalamus is sensitive to the hormone, helping to monitor its level in the plasma. Although clomiphene is not identical to oestrogen, part of its molecule has a very similar shape so it can bind to cytoplasmic oestrogen receptors (see Fig. 8.10). Clomiphene-receptor complexes then move to the cell nucleus, leaving the cytoplasm empty of oestrogen receptors. The cell is able to replace its oestrogen receptors rapidly if normal binding with the hormone has occurred, but not if binding takes place with clomiphene because it is irreversible. The cell is no longer able to detect plasma oestrogen levels. Because this prevents the normal feedback control on oestrogen by the hypothalamus, there is release of gonadotrophin releasing factor, followed by FSH and LH surge from the pituitary. Ovulation follows the LH surge.

Clomiphene is given between Days Three and Seven of the cycle to promote ovulation between Days Twelve and Fourteen. Because the drug is anti-oestrogenic it

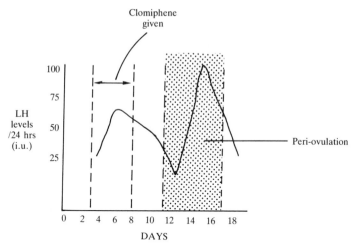

Figure 8.10 Ovulation induction by clomiphene.

has an unwanted effect on cervical mucus, making it hostile to sperm. Restricting drug therapy to the early days of the cycle helps to avoid this.

A woman should be given the following instructions:

- She should take one 50 mg tablet of clomiphene daily from Day Three to Day Seven of her next cycle (counting the first day of her period as Day One).
- Assuming a 28 day cycle, ovulation should occur between Day Twelve and Day Fourteen.
- On Day Nineteen she should come to the clinic for a blood test to estimate progesterone levels to check that ovulation has occurred.
- She may not conceive during the first treatment cycle but, if conception has not occurred within three or four cycles, clomiphene must be considered unsuccessful and another method of induction must be attempted.
- Clomiphene therapy causes numerous side-effects. These are unpleasant but do not persist once the course of tablets is complete and are not harmful. They include hot flushes (anti-oestrogenic effect, mild depression, nausea, and (rarely) transient visual flickering or blurring.

The results confirmed anovulatory cycles and clomiphene therapy was commenced – Christine and Kevin knew of the publicity surrounding fertility treatment and multiple births. They were reassured that, with carefully controlled clomiphene therapy, there is only a slightly increased risk of twins.

Christine was very disappointed when, after the first cycle of treatment, her period arrived at the expected time. At the end of the second cycle she waited forlornly for pre-menstrual symptoms to develop, but they did not. She bought a pregnancy testing kit, and the result was positive.

Gonadotrophin therapy

Gonadotrophins can be used to stimulate ovulation in women who have not responded to clomiphene, or who are thought to be unlikely to respond because their amenorrhoea is known to be due to low endogenous FSH, LH or oestrogen levels. Gonadotrophin therapy is seldom the first choice of treatment because:

- It requires close laboratory supervision and very accurate timing, and can therefore be inconvenient for clients;
- There is a greater risk of multiple pregnancy;
- It is expensive.

The object of treatment is to ripen a follicle by repeated injections of FSH, then stimulate ovulation by injecting LH. Two drugs are used: FSH and LH in a one-to-one ratio (marketed as Pergonal) and hCG, which is biologically the same as LH. The dosage suitable varies from one woman to another, and even between one cycle and the next. Urinary assays of oestrogen are necessary throughout treatment. A typical dosage scheme would incorporate 75 units of FSH, given on Days One, Three and Five of the cycle, followed by 5,000 units of hCG on Day Eight. However, gonadotrophins are very effective. Multiple ovulation can be detected by ultrasonography.

Other problems

Polycystic ovary disease (Stein Leventhal syndrome)

Polycystic ovary disease was first recognised as a possible cause of oligomenorrrhoea, secondary amenorrhoea and associated subfertility in the 1970s. It is thought to be caused by the ovaries producing excessive quantities of androgens.

Oestrogen and testosterone are synthesised from cholesterol via the same biosynthetic pathway (see Chapter 1). In the ovary, most of the testosterone is directly converted to oestrogen. The enzymes responsible appear to be deficient in women

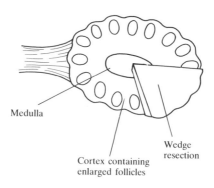

Medulla

Cortex containing
enlarged follicles

Wedge
resection

Figure 8.11 Wedge resection of the ovary.

with polycystic ovary disease. The high levels of testosterone inhibit maturation of the follicle and disrupt and FSH/LH ratio. The ovaries themselves undergo characteristic changes. They enlarge due to the development of many large follicles in the cortex. These changes can be detected on laparoscopy and confirmed by biopsy. Treatment is advisable even if the woman is not trying to conceive because elevated testosterone levels promote distressing virilisation, including hirsuitism. Often these symptoms are the main reason for seeking medical advice.

Treatment is by wedge resection of the ovaries (see Fig. 8.11). About half the tissue is removed from each. This reduces the amount of testosterone and oestrogen released, diminishing feedback stimulus to the hypothalamus. Care must be taken not to remove too much ovarian tissue to avoid oestrogen withdrawal and the formation of adhesions involving the uterine tubes.

Tubal patency

■   When Nigel and Cathy Day attended the fertility clinic there was nothing to indicate that Cathy might not be ovulating and, when the results of Nigel's semen analysis proved normal, the doctor decided that Cathy should be investigated for signs of tubal damage.

There are two methods of investigating tubal patency:

- *Hysterosalpingography* (HSG)
- *Laparoscopy* and *tubal insufflation*

Hysterosalpingography
This investigation permits X-ray examination of the female genital tract. Although some problems are better demonstrated by laparoscopy, HSG is still considered a valuable diagnostic aid because it is the best way of demonstrating internal uterine abnormalities and site of tubal occlusion, if any. Women require detailed explanations about HSG as it is usually performed in the Outpatient Department without general anaesthesia.

The following instructions may be helpful.

- The appointment for HSG should be made for the first day of the cycle (Day I of a period). HSG must be performed in the follicular phase as it could disturb a pregnancy if conception has occurred. Since dye will be injected up the uterine tubes, the test cannot be performed during menstruation or if there is evidence of active infection, as foreign material could enter the tubes by reflux.
- The woman will lie on the X-ray table in the lateral position. A speculum will be used to expose the cervix and radio-opaque dye will be injected into the cervical canal via a cannula. Progress of the dye through the uterus and uterine tubes can be followed on a television screen (see Fig. 8.12). Abnormalities such

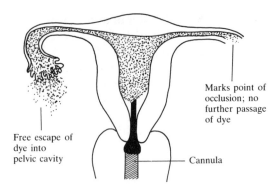

Marks point of
occlusion; no
further passage
of dye

Free escape of
dye into
pelvic cavity

Cannula

Figure 8.12 Passage of radio-opaque dye on hysterosalpinogram.

as fibroids or a bicornuate uterus will show up and, if the tubes are patent, dye will spill into the pelvic cavity. Over the next few days it will be harmlessly absorbed into the bloodstream and excreted via the urine. An HSG may need expert interpretation, but the woman herself will often be able to see defects shown on the screen.

- HSG can be painful because the uterine tubes may go into spasm as the dye travels upwards. The pain feels like severe menstrual cramping, and may sometimes be followed by vomiting. The reason is unknown.
- Because of the discomfort of HSG and the need in some cases for analgesia or sedatives, women should arrange for a friend to accompany them, or at least collect them at the end of the procedure, if at all possible. They may need to spend the remainder of the day resting in bed. Recovery should take place within twelve hours.

■   Cathy's HSG suggested some degree of fimbrial obstruction, but the X-rays were not definitive so she was asked to come into hospital for laparoscopy and tubal insufflation as HSG occasionally gives misleading results. Other disadvantages are failure to show up the ovaries or the presence of endometriosis.

Laparoscopy and tubal insufflation
Hospital admission is necessary for this procedure, which is superior to HSG because it permits visualisation of the ovaries. It is performed during the follicular phase, and the developing follicles can be viewed directly. Endometriosis and areas of pelvic sepsis show up, and the exit of dye passed through the uterine tubes can be viewed through the laparoscope. Endometrial biopsy performed at the same time can provide information about hormone levels. Physical preparation and after-care are the same as for laparoscopic sterilisation (see Chapter 2) but the woman must be warned that some of the dye may escape from her vagina after insufflation has been performed.

■   The morning after the operation Cathy felt tired and rather sore, but anxious to hear the results. Nigel came to the ward so he could be with Cathy when she was told the outcome.

Results confirmed that the fimbriae of both uterine tubes were scarred and narrowed, preventing the egg from entering the main part of the tube.

Types of tubal occlusion

There are four possible sites of tubal occlusion:

1. Blockage of the fimbriae. Surgeons can perform an operation called *fimbrioplasty* to reconstruct the outer end of the tube.
2. Adhesions around the tubes. This is thought to be the commonest problem, and can sometimes be corrected by an operation called *salpingolysis* (adhesiolysis).
3. Blockage of the outer end of the uterine tube, near the ovary, often due to infection. The operation performed to open such a tube is called *salpingostomy*.
4. Blockage of the cornua, where the uterus and uterine tube join, often following septic abortion or infection with an IUCD. If part of the tube is undamaged, the occluded section can be removed surgically and the tube can be re-implanted or re-anastomosed.

The uterine tubes may be occluded at any point along their length by lesions of endometriosis or because the woman has previously been sterilised.

Tubal surgery

Tubal damage is one of the major causes of subfertility. Treatment is often considered difficult, although this depends on the extent of damage which may be uni or bilateral. In the study by Hull *et al.* (1985) tubal damage was the cause of 14 per cent of all cases of subfertility and only 19 per cent of women conceived after surgery. Winston (1986) is more optimistic (see Table 8.4).

■   Cathy and Nigel were told that the most successful treatment would be tubal surgery, but they should think carefully before deciding to proceed since likelihood of success would probably be no greater than 50 per cent. Cathy asked about their chances of conceiving without surgery and it was gently explained that this was negligible. The doctor also pointed out that couples who decide against surgery may come to terms with their childless condition, while those who undergo it may still not conceive and find it difficult each month to accept that pregnancy has not occurred.

Cathy and Nigel needed some time to think things over. They were reassured that tubal damage could not jeopardise Cathy's general health and was not likely to become progressively worse over time. It was important for

Table 8.4 Success rates following tubal surgery (after Winston 1986)

Operation	Percentage success rate	Reasons for failure
Fimbrioplasty	40–45%	Often the tube itself has escaped damage so overall success rate is fair
Salpingolysis	35–60%	Success is much more likely if the adhesions surround the tubes, leaving them undamaged
Salpingostomy	18–40%	It is possible to unblock the tubes in 90 per cent of cases, but there is usually severe damage to the tubal epithelium and muscular wall
Tubal re-implantation and re-anastomosis	25–60%	
Reversal of sterilisation (if clips or rings were used)	90%	Results depend on the woman's age and the amount of damage sustained during surgery
Tubal ligation	75%	

them to realise that, following any kind of tubal surgery, there is some risk of ectopic pregnancy. They had heard the publicity about *in vitro* fertilisation (IVF) and were anxious to know whether this technique would be suitable for them. The success rate of IVF is generally lower than tubal surgery, especially in a case like Cathy's where the main part of the tube is not profoundly damaged and, although an operation is necessary, there is need for only one episode of surgery. If IVF fails, the entire procedure, which is highly stressful, must be repeated.

Cathy and Nigel eventually decided that even a slender chance of having their own baby was not to be missed and Cathy was admitted for fimbioplasty.

Nursing care of women undergoing tubal surgery
These operations involve complex micro-surgical techniques and the women may be in theatre for quite a long time, but members of this client group are young and fit. Pre- and post-operative nursing care are routine and complications few. There is usually a small Pfannenstiel incision, and the woman can expect to be in hospital no more than five or six days. However, nurses must think carefully about the possible reaction of patients to others undergoing abortions or sterilisation on the same ward. Both client groups may feel resentment towards one another and the atmosphere created can be damaging not only to the women concerned but to everyone else on the ward. In a modern ward, subdivided into bays and with single rooms, it is possible to keep women physically apart but they are very likely to meet in communal areas such as the day room and it is possible that conversation may develop before they become aware of the treatment which the other is receiving.

Rehabilitation

■   Cathy felt much better after the operation than she had expected, although rather tired. Before leaving hospital she was provided with the following information:

- She would need a period of convalescence at home, gradually returning to normal activities within three to four weeks. Most women feel able to return to work after this time although some, whose work is particularly strenuous, may need up to six weeks at home.
- Heavy lifting and vigorous exercise should be avoided for four weeks until the abdominal muscles have fully healed. Moderate exercise (walking, swimming) are helpful because they strengthen the muscles without straining.
- Cathy and Nigel should have intercourse as soon as Cathy felt comfortable. It is possible to conceive within a month of surgery.
- They would be seen at the clinic at regular intervals during the first year after surgery. Couples are often grateful for the continued support of the clinic staff once the woman has had surgery (this may vary between centres).
- If surgery was not successful (if Cathy had not conceived within eighteen months), she would be given the option of undergoing repeated laparoscopy to detect the reformation of adhesions. This is the most common reason for failure. However, tubal occlusions are less likely to reform after modern micro-surgical techniques, and the idea that unless conception occurs very soon after surgery it is unlikely to occur at all is a myth; if adhesions do re-form, the process begins within forty-eight hours of surgery (Winston 1986).

    Cathy asked whether she would be able to deliver normally after tubal surgery and was reassured that this should be possible. However, Caesarean section is sometimes necessary after tubal re-implantation since this procedure can weaken the uterine walls.

In vitro fertilisation (IVF) and embryo transfer

Few people today can be unaware of the advances in this field, especially those undergoing investigations for subfertility. IVF is an ideal topic for journalists because it combines sensational, highly technical, subject matter with issues that are emotionally laden, raising questions of ethics and morality. However, IVF is of no help to large numbers of infertile people. It is indicated only for the following circumstances:

- Couples where the man has a sperm defect, since only about 15,000 sperm are needed.

- Couples where the woman's cervical mucus is hostile to sperm, or where the woman is producing anti-sperm antibodies.
- Couples where the woman has severely damaged tubes especially when tubal surgery has failed. The success rate of IVF is presently 10 per cent – significantly less than any type of tubal surgery. It is unfortunate that publicity about IVF has not emphasised its relatively high levels of failure, although it is hoped that, with increasing expertise, treatment will be more successful in the future.

A mature egg is aspirated from a follicle under laparoscopic vision, fertilised with the partner's sperm, and the embryo returned to the uterus. Donor sperm or eggs may be used if necessary. Chances of success are increased if several eggs are fertilised at once, but this then results in the dilemma of what to do with the spare embryos generated – whether they should be destroyed, used for research, or whether they should ever have been created at all. Much depends on the point at which 'life' is considered to begin. Those in favour of IVF research programmes point to the large number of fetuses aborted spontaneously and artificially every year. Those against argue that deliberate destruction of any potential human individual is wrong, regardless of nature's profligacy. A more persuasive argument is probably that research into the mechanism of conception and early human embryonic development may, in the long term, benefit childless people, help develop new safer methods of contraception and provide information about spontaneous abortion and genetic and congenital handicap. Research with animal embryos will not provide information about exclusively human disorders, and there is evidence that early embryonic development proceeds differently between species.

The *Report of the Warnock Committee on Human Fertilization and Embryology* (1984) recommended that human eggs should not be used in experimental programmes after the fourteenth day of development, and made numerous suggestions to safeguard the handling of embryos. The Government acted swiftly to curb commercial surrogacy, but has not restricted any of the other activities recommended by the Committee, although at the time of writing there have been two unsuccessful Private Members Bills to restrict embryo research and IVF.

IVF is extremely stressful for the couple concerned. Treatment is available at only a few specialist centres around the country (Lovell 1986), and they may have to travel a considerable distance to obtain it.

Treatment schedule for IVF

IVF may be performed during the normal menstrual cycle, but it is more usual for the woman to receive Clomiphene because this allows more accurate prediction of ovulation and permits several follicles to mature. The couple must be fully aware of what the procedure will entail:

- The woman must notify the clinic on Day One of her period, and her FSH and LH levels are monitored. Clomiphene therapy is started as on page 208.
- At the approach of the LH surge the woman comes to the clinic and is injected with hCG to mature the follicles.

- The woman undergoes laparoscopy three days later so the eggs can be aspirated from the follicles. They are placed in a special culture medium and incubated.
- Semen (from the partner or donor) is used to inseminate the eggs five to six hours later. The eggs are incubated for several hours, exact time depending on the centre.
- There is still some disagreement about optimal time for embryo transfer, but it is considered to be at about the stage when the fertilised egg has divided into eight cells. It is transferred to the uterus via a fine catheter inserted through the cervix, two days after insemination.
- Pregnancy testing is possible two days later.

The present failure rate of IVF is high for several reasons. It may be impossible to collect any eggs, fertilisation may not occur *in vitro*, or the eggs may not develop properly afterwards. Even if transfer is possible, only about 25 per cent pregnancies occur, and some end in miscarriage. Although anaesthesia and laparoscopy carry some risks to health, most people agree that the greatest problem associated with IVF is emotional stress. It is a very expensive procedure, and as many couples seek private treatment they will have to bear the cost themselves.

Gamete intra fallopian transfer (GIFT)

GIFT is a recently developed technique in which eggs and sperm from respective partners are mixed, then transferred to the uterine tube, avoiding the complex laboratory facilities necessary for *in vitro* culture. Laparoscopy must be timed just before ovulation, as for IVF, and clomiphene may be used. A woman must have at least part of a uterine tube undamaged if GIFT is to be possible. It is helpful for some couples where there are problems with cervical mucus, and is said to be successful in about 25 per cent of cases.

Artificial insemination

Sperm may be used to inseminate the woman during the fertile phase of the cycle from her partner (artificial insemination by husband, AIH) or from a donor (artificial insemination by donor, AID).

AIH

AIH is recommended when sperm count is low. Semen is obtained by masturbation and transferred to the cervix or uterus via a cannula. AIH may be unsuccessful during the first cycle of treatment, and several inseminations are usually attempted during successive cycles to maximise chances of conception. Most couples find AIH very stressful: it represents a severe invasion of their sex life, necessitates precise timing of ovulation, and the process itself takes place in a clinical atmosphere.

Sperm can be frozen in nitrogen and stored for long periods without damage, although it is less potent than sperm in a freshly collected ejaculate. This technique is valuable for young men undergoing radiotherapy or chemotherapy likely to leave them azoospermic, and after spinal injury.

AID

AID is of value when the man is either azoospermic or oligospermic. Donor sperm is obtained from young, healthy volunteers, and every attempt is made to match race, skin colour, height and build, eye and hair colour, and blood group of the couple. Donors should have no known history of hereditable disease, but its incidence will be the same as for the general population. There must be no HIV infection in donors.

Winston (1986) argues that AID should not be looked upon as treatment for infertility, but as an alternative, to be regarded in the same light as adoption. In the past, social and emotional barriers prevented widespread acceptance of AID, but its stigma is now disappearing. Precise figures are difficult to obtain, but it is believed that more than 10,000 AID babies have been born in the UK, and few problems have been reported. At present, under English law a child born as a result of AID is illegitimate and must be adopted by its social father. Since birth certificates require the name of the biological father, who is unknown, couples may get round this by providing false information. This is perjury, but there are no records of anyone being prosecuted, and it is likely that with wider acceptance of AID the law will change.

Childlessness

Individuals writing about the experience of infertility, whether describing their own (Pfeffer and Woolett 1983) or that of their clients (Winston 1986), describe the grief which accompanies childlessness feelingly, pointing out a need for the couple to mourn for their 'loss'. A recent report commissioned by the Greater London Association of Community Health Councils (GLACHC) has not only drawn attention to the inadequacies of fertility services and the stresses placed on couples, but has also pointed to a need for services to be reoriented so that those for whom treatment is unsuccessful are helped to come to terms with childlessness – which is primarily a social, rather than a medical, condition.

■   As the months passed and Cathy Day had still not conceived, she and Nigel became more despondent as they realised that surgery had been unsuccessful. Eventually, Cathy gave up recording the dates of her expected periods and tried not to think about how or when she had developed the adhesions damaging her tubes. Guilt about past behaviour and possible source of an old infection were becoming corrosive: she and Nigel felt they had done everything possible to have a child of their own, and did not wish to damage their relationship, which had weathered the initial disappointment of subfertility, and subsequent invasion of their privacy during fertility investigations. For a time Cathy allowed herself to become very busy at work, but tried not to neglect her life at home and leisure activities shared with Nigel.

When they returned to the clinic, a year after surgery, they said they did not wish the operation to be repeated or to proceed with IVF. The nurse specialist asked them if they would like to see a professional counsellor, and they welcomed this opportunity to discuss their feelings away from the clinical situation where so many tests and medical discussions had taken place.

The counsellor believed that Cathy and Nigel were adjusting gradually but well to childlessness, but was not surprised when they asked about adoption.

Adoption

Advice about the decision to try to adopt a child must be given with caution as the number of young babies (less than six months) adopted each year does not presently number more than a thousand, although several thousand more older children are adopted annually (Winston 1986). Adoption agencies vary widely in their criteria for acceptance, but these are likely to be stringent as they are concerned with placing children in homes where they will be well provided for, both in emotional and material terms. Couples must be able to give evidence of sound health, stable marital relationship and financial security. Agencies may use other criteria, such as an upper limit on the couple's age. Some do not object if the couple wish to pursue fertility investigations, while others regard this unfavourably, as evidence that the couple have not yet come to terms with infertility.

■   The counsellor provided Cathy and Nigel with some factual information, but suggested that they should think carefully before deciding what to do, especially as all the intrusive probing into their social background which had taken place before fertility investigations would certainly be repeated. She also answered their questions about surrogacy.

Surrogacy

Surrogacy is a topical issue much publicised in the media. It means that a fertile woman has a baby for another woman who is absolutely infertile, and hands it over at birth. There are two types:

- The surrogate (woman who is to give birth) is inseminated with sperm from the male partner of the infertile woman, or actually has intercourse with him.
- An egg is taken from the fertile woman and mixed with her partner's sperm as in IVF. The embryo develops in the uterus of the surrogate mother.

Surrogacy is a legal and emotional minefield because of the risks of exploitation to the surrogate mother and child, and possibly also to those hoping to have a baby by this means; the father may, for example, develop an attachment to the surrogate mother because she has carried his child, especially if he has had a sexual relationship with her.

■ Cathy and Nigel knew that surrogacy is illegal in Britain (though not in the USA at present), but in any case considered it unacceptable. They felt that it would be unethical to expect another woman to have a baby on their behalf in view of possible emotional damage when it came time to hand the baby over, apart from their own unresolved legal rights if she refused to part with it.

Eventually Cathy and Nigel decided to proceed with adoption, even though they understood that this might result in disappointment and would involve individual approaches to each adoption agency. They knew that, in their favour, were youth, their involvement with the church (many agencies are run by religious bodies), and their willingness to accept a child of ethnic minority.

Resources

Books that can be recommended to clients:

Kovacs, G. and Wood, C. (1984) *Infertility. Patient Handbook No. 22*, Edinburgh: Churchill Livingstone.
Decker, A. and Loebl, S. (1980) *We Want to Have a Baby*, London: Penguin.

Associations

National Association for the Childless
318 Sumner Lane
Birmingham B19 3RL
Tel. 021 359 4887

Women's Reproductive Rights Information Centre
52/54 Featherstone Street
London EC1

References

Bresnick, B. and Taymor, M.L. (1979) 'The role of counselling in infertility, *Fertility and Sterility* 34(2), pp. 154–6.

Christianson, C. (1986) 'Support groups for infertile patients', *Journal of Obstetric, Gynaecological and Neonatal Nursing* 15(4), pp. 293–6.

Edelmann, R.J. and Connolly, K. (1986) 'Psychological aspects of infertility', *British Journal of Medical Psychology* 59, pp. 209–19.

Elkington, J. (1986) *The Poisoned Womb*, London: Pelican.

Hull, M.G.R. *et al.* (1985) 'Population study of causes, treatment and outcome of infertility', *British Medical Journal* 293, pp. 1693–7.

Laycock, J. and Wise, P. (1982) *Essential Endocrinology*, Oxford: Oxford University Press.

Lenton, E. *et al.* (1977) 'Problems in using basal body temperature recordings in an infertility clinic', *British Medical Journal* 284, pp. 803–5.

Lovell, B. (1986). *In vitro* fertilization: a way of hope', *Nursing Times* 82(44), pp. 26–9.

McCormick, T. (1980) 'Out of control: one aspect of fertility', *Journal of Obstetric, Gynaecological and Neonatal Nursing* 9(4), pp. 205–7.

Newill, R. (1974) *Infertile Marriage*, London: Penguin.

Oakley, A. (1979) *From Here to Maternity*, London: Pelican.

Pfeffer, N. and Quick, A. (1988) *Infertility Services: A Desperate Case*, London: GL ACHC.

Pfeffer, N. and Woolett, A. (1983) *The Experience of Infertility*, London: Virago Press.

Rosenfield, D. and Mitchell, D. (1979) 'Treating the emotional aspects of infertility', *American Journal of Obstetrics and Gynoecology* 135, pp.177–80.

Stanway, A. (1980) *Why Us? (Infertility)* London: Granada.

Warnock, M. (1984) *Report of the Committee of Inquiry into Human Fertilisation and Embryology*, London: HMSO.

Wilcox, A. *et al.* (1988) 'Caffeinated beverages and decreased fertility', *Lancet* 2, pp. 1453–5.

Winston, R.M.L. (1986) *Infertility. A Sympathetic Approach*, London: Martin Dunitz.

9　The Climacteric

Descriptions of the menopause date from 1857 when Tilt catalogued 105 different health problems among 500 women undergoing the change of life. Judging most to be psychological in origin, Tilt compared the emotional upheavals of the menopause to the disruptions of puberty.

In Eastern societies the menopause is welcomed because age enhances female status (Mead 1950), but in the West the menopause is viewed as a negative event, perhaps because the media is so concerned with portraying the attractiveness of youth. Older women are less favourably depicted and the menopause remains a taboo subject, rarely mentioned except as a target for insensitive jokes.

Tilt's observations were made at a time when poor living conditions and the undeveloped state of medical science prevented large numbers of women from reaching middle life. Today, the population includes far more women in this age group and the physical changes accompanying the menopause have been well documented. Controversy exists over the correct approach to the treatment of menopausal symptoms however, and the psychological impact of the menopause is often treated without sensitivity. Although menopausal problems seldom bring women into hospital wards, nurses need to know about the difficulties faced by women in this age group because they may use the health service for other reasons and will appreciate sympathetic understanding.

Definition and age of onset

Confusion exists between the terms *menopause* and *climacteric*. The menopause is the last menstrual period, while the climacteric refers to the physical and emotional changes occurring around this time. These definitions are used throughout this chapter, although lay people frequently refer to the menopause when they actually mean the time around it.

Although the menopause is associated with middle age, the time of the last menstrual period can vary enormously. Most women will have their last period when they are about 50, but a few may menstruate as late as 57 or cease to do so in their early thirties.

Menstruation does not end because the supply of eggs has run out. Usually follicles remain in the ovaries after the last period, but soon degenerate; women who begin their periods early usually have a late menopause.

Physiology of the menopause

The menopause occurs as a result of ovarian failure. This may be sudden, although it occurs gradually in most women. Menstruation becomes increasingly irregular and the last few cycles are usually anovulatory. Despite waning fertility there is no guarantee that ovulation has not taken place, however, and contraceptive precautions should continue until two years after the menopause. Irregular cycles may bring problems for couples who previously relied on natural methods of birth control.

At the menopause, the ovaries cease to respond to stimulation by gonadotrophins and ovarian follicles no longer ripen every month. Levels of plasma oestrogen and progesterone therefore decline. When levels fall below a critical threshold, the negative feedback system regulating release of gonadotrophins from the anterior pituitary breaks down. Levels of plasma FSH and LH then rise between five- and tenfold.

Measuring plasma gonadotrophin levels is the diagnostic test used to confirm that a woman is genuinely menopausal. This may be necessary to help exclude the possibility of pregnancy or when medical treatment of menopausal symptoms is contemplated. A woman who has had a hysterectomy conserving the ovaries will still experience the menopause even though she no longer menstruates.

Some oestrogen is released by the adrenal cortex after the menopause, but not in sufficient quantities to compensate for ovarian failure. Oestrogen withdrawal affects numerous body systems and is responsible for most physical changes encountered during the climacteric.

Physical changes

Cardiovascular system

The notorious hot flushes seem to be directly related to falling oestrogen levels, ex-plaining why they are often among the earliest signs of the menopause. Vasomotor changes cause sudden dilation of the capillaries supplying the skin, so the woman suddenly looks and feels hot. Not all women find hot flushes a problem but many feel embarrassed, particularly in public, because they think other people will notice. There may be palpitations and severe perspiration as the body's homeostatic mechanisms attempt to reduce temperature. Hot flushes may be experienced without warning at any time of day or during the night, disturbing sleep. They seem to coincide with surges of LH into the bloodstream, but LH does not appear to be directly responsible. Instead, some common factor appears to promote both the LH surge and vasomotor reaction.

Hot flushes and sweating are among the most common reasons for prescribing hormone replacement therapy (HRT) but, as they are due to *waning* oestrogen levels not absolute lack of oestrogen, they disappear as the body adjusts to the new lower hormone levels.

Up to the menopause, women have a lower incidence of cardiovascular disease than men possibly because oestrogen decreases the amount of cholesterol in the circulation (WHO 1981). After the menopause, this protective effect is lost. Cholesterol and triglyceride levels rise and arteriosclerosis begins to develop as rapidly as in men. Post-menopausal women are as vulnerable to cardiovascular complaints as men of the same age.

Skeletal system

Oestrogen increases activity of the osteoblasts, the cells which absorb calcium salts from the bloodstream and help build up bone. After the menopause, this effect is withdrawn and there is increased calcium resorption from the skeleton. The effect, over several years, is gradual decalcification eventually leading to osteoporosis. Osteoporosis accounts for much of the backache and arthritic pain experienced by older women as well as their higher incidence of fractures compared to men of the same age. Fracture of the neck of femur is one of the most common reasons for hospital admission in elderly women. For many, it marks the point when their health deteriorates to the stage when they can no longer cope independently at home. Although other factors may be influential in the development of osteoporosis, its progress appears to be slowed by oestrogen replacement providing it is started early enough (Nordin and Gallagher 1972). It will also prevent osteoporosis in women experiencing surgically induced menopause after oöphorectomy (Aitken et al. 1973).

Osteoporosis is one of the later effects of oestrogen withdrawal, and damage will not be apparent until many years after the menopause. This condition will *not* be corrected spontaneously over time.

Tissue atrophy

Oestrogen is mildly anabolic and is responsible for development of the breasts, female reproductive organs and secondary sexual characteristics at puberty. Not surprisingly, these tissues undergo a certain degree of atrophy when oestrogen production wanes. The breasts become pendulous due to loss of adipose tissue, pubic hair becomes scanty and the uterus becomes smaller and fibrous. The framework of connective tissue supporting the bladder and genital tract weakens, and this may contribute to the development of a prolapse (see Chapter 10). Adipose tissue is lost from the vulva and the vagina becomes drier, less vascular, and its pH rises (from 4 to 7.2). This can cause discomfort.

■   Joyce Kendall was exhausted looking after her elderly mother, who had had a stroke. Despite giving up the part-time job she enjoyed and reducing her social commitments, Joyce remained tired. She attributed loss of interest in sex to fatigue. Although her primary concern was the old lady, the district nurse felt perturbed when Joyce began to look unwell. Joyce confessed that she was not sleeping properly and hinted that she had a 'personal problem'. At first she was reluctant to disclose its nature but, with encouragement from the nurse, she explained that intercourse was now often painful. She also noticed a thick white vaginal discharge staining her clothes. In view of Joyce's age (51), and because she had not had a period for over a year, the nurse thought that the discharge was probably due to *Candida albicans*.

Atrophic (senile) vaginitis

Throughout the reproductive years the vagina is protected from many invading micro-organisms (see Chapter 6) by secretions from the cervix and Bartholin's glands. The superficial cells lining the vagina are constantly shed and release glycogen. This is metabolised by Lactobacilli making up the normal vaginal flora. Lactic acid is released, helping to keep vaginal secretions mildly acid (pH 4–5). At the menopause, oestrogen withdrawal causes vaginal secretions to become scanty. Lubrication is lost and the vaginal epithelium becomes thinner and prone to infection, particularly as the population of Lactobacilli becomes depleted. Foreign micro-organisms are now able to invade and establish infection.

Candidiasis is particularly common in women who have experienced the menopause, but even if infection does not occur, atrophic changes may still cause pruritus, inflammation and dyspareunia. Vulval atrophy can be successfully treated by applying oestrogen cream topically.

Hormone replacement therapy (HRT)

Since oestrogen withdrawal is responsible for the physical discomforts associated with the climacteric, they can be offset by hormone replacement therapy, but its use is controversial. Some authors take an extreme view, suggesting that the menopause should be regarded in the same light as any other deficiency state and oestrogen replaced as a matter of course (Wilson 1963). This idea has spilled into the lay literature. Medical journalists advocate treatment for all women approaching the menopause or earlier (Cooper 1976). However, HRT can be accompanied by a number of undesirable effects.

Although oestrogen replacement may reduce the danger of myocardial infarction, it increases risk of thrombo-embolism by increasing platelet aggregation and clotting time (Elkeles *et al.* 1968). There may also be slight risk of hepatitis, since oestrogen is metabolised in the liver. However, the long term effects of HRT receiving most publicity are the possible increased risks of endometrial and breast cancers. Many doctors are unwilling to prescribe HRT long-term, although they acknowledge that women often benefit over a defined, shorter period of time, providing progress is carefully monitored.

■   Heather Betts, aged 49, was troubled by backaches, headaches, hot flushes and night sweats. She found vasomotor symptoms particularly troublesome because her work as a sales representative involved long hours and the need to appear well-groomed. Deciding what to wear had become a problem. Heather worried in case the hot flushes were noticeable. She was often tired during the day and sometimes noticed an unpleasant tingling on her skin. This sensation, called *formication*, is frequently experienced by women during the climacteric, but its cause is unknown.

Heather had little support from her husband who was spending a year on business overseas. She thought she must be experiencing the 'change of life' since her periods were becoming erratic. Heather had heard about HRT and decided to consult her GP, who referred her to a Menopause Clinic.

The Menopause Clinic

Some GPs prescribe HRT themselves, while others prefer to refer women to Menopause Clinics which have become established in a number of hospitals throughout the country.

Menopause Clinics are usually organised by one or more gynaecologists with a special interest in the subject and may employ a nurse specialist whose role combines responsibilities for administration, clinical practice and research.

■   Heather's nursing assessment indicated that, clinically, she appeared to be experiencing the climacteric, while pressures of work and the absence of her husband seemed to be acting as further stressors with which she was less able than usual to cope. After a discussion of these problems, the nature of HRT was explained to enable Heather to make an informed decision about her treatment.

A sample of blood was sent to the laboratory to provide information about Heather's hormone levels. This confirmed a rising titre of gonadotrophins, indicating that the menopause had occurred.

Heather's care plan is shown on page 228.

Before HRT is prescribed there are several points that a woman must understand:

- HRT is not an elixir of youth. It will *not* prevent ageing, although it will ameliorate the immediate effects of oestrogen withdrawal.
- All women receiving HRT must be carefully monitored throughout treatment to identify any side effects. This will involve regular follow-up.
- Women should be warned about symptoms that need reporting. Their existing

state of knowledge must be carefully assessed before further information is provided. At one time it was thought that mentioning possible problems might have a detrimental effect, as prior warning could act as a self-fulfilling prophecy, encouraging women to 'notice' symptoms that would not have been troublesome before. However, there is no evidence that this occurs in women of this age group (see Chapter 7).

Side effects are minimised in a number of ways:

- Natural oestrogens are used for HRT. They are less potent than synthetic oestrogens, so many of the side effects associated with the oestrogen component of the combined oral contraceptive pill are avoided. Weight gain, nausea and increased vaginal secretion may occur in the early days, however.
- Each course of tablets incorporates progesterone to help prevent oestrogen over-stimulating the endometrium.
- Tablets are taken in the same way as the pill, missing out one week in every four. This helps to minimise the amount of oestrogen taken.

During the week when hormone tablets are withheld, women experience withdrawal bleeding, but this should not be confused with true menstruation; oestrogen replacement cannot restore fertility and pregnancy will not occur in women who have experienced the menopause. However, bleeding is sufficient to require sanitary protection and will last for several days. Women *must* be told about this in advance, since they may feel embarrassed buying towels or tampons as they get older. Some regard bleeding as more inconvenient than menopausal problems and may eventually wish to discontinue HRT because of it.

Many gynaecologists take a biopsy of the endometrium every six months, often by Vabra suction (see Chapter 1). Admission is not necessary.

All women will be happier if they feel well, so some health information particularly relevant to women in their middle years is given below.

Diet
Women need to know about the benefits of a well-balanced diet containing adequate vitamins and minerals, especially calcium. The dangers of sugar and saturated fats need to be emphasised now there is significant risk of cardiovascular disease. Fibre is an important constituent of the diet, but a component of green leafy vegetables, phytic acid, appears to interfere with calcium absorption so alternative sources such as wholemeal bread should be contemplated.

Exercise
This helps to improve the general circulation and burn calories. It stimulates the release of local hormones called endorphins which act as natural pain-killers, helping to relieve stiffness associated with muscular aches and pains. It strengthens the back and abdominal muscles, therefore reducing any tendency of the abdomen to sag and increases gut motility by massaging the abdominal organs, helping to prevent constipation. Exercise has social as well as physical benefits.

Care plan 9.1 (Orem's Self Care model)

Name: Heather Betts

Treatment/condition: Hormone replacement therapy (HRT)

Universal Self Care Requisites	Therapeutic Self Care Requisites	Self Care Deficits	Nursing Systems	Nursing Agency	Future
Universal self care requisite: Promote normalcy	Realistic self concept	Feels old, unattractive. Troublesome vasomotor symptoms, excessive tiredness. Demands of job currently seem excessive	Supportive/ educative	Discuss benefits of HRT realistically. Point out side effects, need for follow-up and explore reasons for tiredness. Suggest strategies for coping with fatigue and hot flushes. Suggest ways of modifying working day to reduce stress for the present and longer term	Good. Vasomotor effects are short term. HRT will control symptoms until body adjusts to lower oestrogen levels. Heather should be able to find ways of coping with job. Plans to join husband for short holiday
Development self care requisite: Maintain living conditions that promote maturation	Successful transition to post-menopausal status. Accept that she is growing older and will need to make adjustments	Concerned about appearance. Worried about weight gain, hot flushes	Supportive/ educative	Discuss Heather's concept of 'middle age'. Allow her to express her anxieties. Provide dietary advice. Explain effects of HRT	Good. HRT should help resolve physical health problems short-term. Body will adapt longer term. Vasomotor disturbance should cease

			Supportive/ educative		
Health deviation: Modify self concept to accept need for health care and appropriate medical and nursing assistance	Accept and actively participate in treatment. Understand need for HRT and how to take tablets. Recognise side effects requiring investigation	Worried about HRT. Does not understand reason for monthly breast self-examination. Worried about endometrial biopsy (previously had D & C and does not want to undergo this again)		Explain dose may be reduced as the body adjusts to new menopausal status – short-term treatment only is envisaged. Teach how to examine breasts, explaining oestrogenic stimulation of breast tissue. Clarify difference between endometrial biopsy and D & C	Will need encouragement to perform breast self examination and accept endometrial biopsy. Regular follow-ups necessary as long as HRT continues

The use of care plans for outpatients does not take place in all hospitals or clinics, but the need for an underlying philosophy of nursing care can clearly be seen here. Many of Heather's problems could have been overlooked if the nurse had not used a framework to document them comprehensively. *Orem's Self Care model* (1985) seems a good choice as it emphasises the need for changing outlook and approaches to care throughout the life cycle and Heather, experiencing the 'change of life', has entered a period of transition.

Many patients receiving gynaecological care are admitted to hospital only for brief periods or not at all. Is the use of a model always justified? Is there a place for standard care plans?

Weight
Weight is more likely to be maintained at a constant level with a healthy diet and regular exercise. There is no endocrine reason for weight gain to occur at the menopause.

Sleep and relaxation
Sleep and relaxation are improved with exercise. Boredom can result in fatigue through lack of stimulation.

Smoking
Cigarette smoking is an important contributory factor in the development of cardiovascular disease. Women may be encouraged to give up, or at least reduce, the number of cigarettes smoked.

Throughout the country a number of support groups for women in this age group have been established. These provide an invaluable source of comfort to many women (Drennan and McGeeney 1985). Nurses may establish and publicise groups as a forum in which they may act as facilitators, providing health information as well as counselling and support.

Other methods of providing HRT

HRT can be given as subcutaneous implants, renewed every six months under local anaesthetic. Oestrogen creams can also be applied locally to help reduce vulval atrophy. Topical oestrogen can be absorbed into the systemic circulation but in small amounts, so there are few, if any, risks.

Emotional, social and physical problems

The menopause often coincides with changes in lifestyle and family structure which may be unwelcome (Rose 1977). Evidence suggests that work outside the home helps to protect women from depression by providing a source of social support as well as enhancing self-esteem (Weiseman and Paykel 1974). Children grow up and leave home. The 'empty nest syndrome' described by Bart (1971) seems to be experienced by women who have enjoyed a traditional mothering role, never working outside the home. Diekelman (1975) describes numerous other changes which may culminate in 'mid-life crisis'.

Coinciding with the time when the woman perceives her role to be reduced, her husband may achieve seniority at work, spending less time at home. The woman may fear that he will be attracted to someone more youthful. There may be financial worries associated with children's higher education or care of elderly relatives. Adolescent children may cause concern. Career women may suffer because of the need to perform highly at work despite domestic worries and menopausal discomfort.

The menopausal syndrome

Despite the range of potential problems documented for women in this age group, the menopause has not been associated with any specific psychiatric condition such as depression. Most of the symptoms reported during epidemiological investigations can be traced to the effects of oestrogen withdrawal, exacerbated by difficulties in coping with adverse social conditions. Several authors have noted that women referred to specialist menopause clinics may not be experiencing the menopause at all, although they may appear depressed (Donovan 1951, Stern and Prados 1946). These early researchers linked psychiatric problems experienced during middle age to previous patterns of emotional expression. Women whose earlier reactions to unfavourable life events had been depression appeared to respond in the same way as they anticipated the menopause. Researchers concluded that menopausal symptoms form a continuum: at one extreme they provide a focus for life long problems, in the middle range the menopause is simply one stress among several that may occur in middle life, at the other extreme the menopause may cause particular distress to a group to women who are especially vulnerable.

More recently, these ideas have been developed by Greene and Cooke (1978) who showed that, in a population of 408 women drawn randomly from the electoral roll, there were increased trends of psychiatric and physical symptoms during the climacteric which appeared to be related to high levels of stress. From their data, these authors suggested that some women appear to cope less well with negative life events during the climacteric than if faced with the same problems at an earlier or later stage in the life cycle. Particular events, such as undergoing hysterectomy, may add to the stress experienced at this time (see Chapter 7).

The relationship between stress, negative life events and their possible effects on recovery, should be taken into consideration by nurses providing care for women in the middle years. Menopausal problems are common, so the next section discusses prevalence in the general population.

The prevalence of menopausal symptoms; epidemiological studies

Numerous investigators have attempted to assess the prevalence of menopausal symptoms. Many of these studies have been conducted on a large scale using interviews or questionnaire techniques, but there are two weaknesses in their research designs: researchers do not define the menopause accurately and leave women in no doubt about the purpose of the study, so results may contain bias. Observing these drawbacks, and the poor sampling techniques of older studies, Bungay et al. (1980) conducted a questionnaire survey in which women aged between 30 and 64 were asked about a range of physical, emotional and sexual problems *without* any mention of the menopause (the information included with the instructions explained that the research was concerned with general health). From the results, it appears that vasomotor symptoms, loss of confidence and ability to make decisions, gradually resolved over time. Other more general problems (headaches, fatigue, irritability, depression) seemed to occur before and after the menopause with much the same frequency. Low backache and aching breasts were usually first reported at the menopause, and resolved slowly.

Since diminishing oestrogen levels are responsible for so much discomfort at the climacteric, it is hardly surprising that women so often feel miserable. Emotional reaction can be unpredictable, and cannot be altered in a positive direction by HRT, although better health may improve outlook by providing a sense of well-being. Women should *not* believe that HRT will remove all their problems, and sympathetic nursing intervention may achieve much more than drugs. Self-help is an important aspect of care, especially at a time when women report decreased confidence, reported by Bungay's team. Few women will be sufficiently unfortunate to experience all the problems documented in this chapter, and many others will not find menopausal problems sufficiently worrying to constitute a 'mid-life crisis', but they may, nevertheless, diminish enjoyment of a stage in the life cycle which otherwise has much to recommend it.

Rather than mourning the loss of children from the home, some women find compensation in the extra time now available for themselves, which can be invested in new interests at home, at work, or with their partner. Finances may improve as children become independent. The arrival of grandchildren may be anticipated with pleasure.

The purpose of this chapter has been to emphasise the range of emotional as well as physical problems confronting women during middle life, and to point out that stress may generate problems or alter women's perception of these. Nolan (1986) argues that in the past most researchers in this field have taken a biomedical perspective, but suggests that more emphasis should be placed on social factors. Nurses can help women who require specific treatment and those they meet during routine work in hospital or the community.

Resources

A book that can be recommended to clients:

Bromwich, P. (1989) *Menopause*, London: British Medical Association.

References

Aitken, J.M. *et al.* (1973) 'Oestrogen replacement therapy for prevention of osteoporosis after oöphorectomy', *British Medical Journal* 3, pp. 515–18.
Bart, P. (1971) 'Depression in middle-aged women', In: Gornick, V. (ed.) *Women and Sexist Society*, New York: Basic Books.
Bungay, G.T. *et al.* (1980) 'Study of symptoms in middle life', *British Medical Journal* 228, pp. 181–3.

Cooper, W. (1976) *No Change*, London: *Arrow Books*.

Diekelman, N. *et al.* (1975) 'The middle years', *American Journal of Nursing* 75, pp. 995–1012.

Donovan, J.C. (1951) 'Menopausal symptoms: a study of case histories', *American Journal of Gynaecology* 62, p. 281.

Drennan, V. and McGeeney, S. (1985) 'Menopausal support', *Nursing Mirror* 160 (23), pp. 27–30.

Elkeles, R.S. *et al.* (1968) 'Effect of oestrogens on human platelet behaviour', *Lancet* 2, pp. 315–18.

Greene, J.G. and Cooke, D.J. (1978) 'Life stress and events at the climacteric', *British Journal of Psychiatry* 136, pp. 486–91.

Mead, M. (1950) *Male and Female: a Study of the Sexes in a Changing World*, London: Gollanz.

Nolan, J. (1986) 'Developmental concerns and the health of midlife women', *Nursing Clinics of North America* 21 (1), p. 155.

Nordin, B.E.C. and Gallagher J.C. (1972) 'Treatment with oestrogens of primary hyperparathyroidism in post-menopausal women', *Lancet* 1, pp. 503–6.

Orem, D.E. (1985) *Nursing: Concepts of Practice* New York: McGraw-Hill.

Rose, L. (1977) '*The Menopause Book*, New York: Hawthorn Books.

Stern, K. and Prados, M. (1946) 'Personality studies in menopausal women', *American Journal of Psychiatry* 103, p. 358.

Tilt, E. (1982, reissue) *The Change of Life in Health and Disease*, London: J.A. Churchill.

Weisman, M. and Paykel, E. (1974) '*The Depressed Woman: a Study of Social Relationships*, Chicago: University of Chicago Press.

WHO Scientific Group (1980) 'Research on the menopause', *Technical Report Series* 670, Geneva: WHO.

Wilson, P. (1963) 'The fate of non-treated post-menopausal women: a plea for the maintenance of adequate oestrogen from puberty to the grave', *Journal of American Geriatric Society* 11, pp. 347–59.

10   Pelvic support

Displacements of the uterus are common, especially in older women. Ninety per cent of those affected have had children, although it appears that the development of a prolapse depends more upon the quality of obstetric care than number of deliveries (Fergusson 1984). With improvements in obstetric practice, hopefully fewer women will be affected in future. Midwives and health visitors have a vital role in ante-natal and post-natal care, explaining how to prevent laxity of the pelvic floor muscles. Occupational health nurses can provide instruction about correct lifting techniques to women engaged in manual work. Effective teaching depends on sound understanding of the structures making up the pelvic floor and their contribution to pelvic support. This knowledge is also needed by nurses working with women who are to undergo gynaecological procedures, so they can provide appropriate information about the effects of surgery and after care.

The normal position of the uterus: anteversion and retroversion

Figure 10.1 shows that the normal adult uterus lies at an angle of 90° to the vagina, and is inclined forwards over the posterior wall of the bladder. In this position it is described as *anteverted*. In 15–20 per cent of women the uterus lies in the same plane as the vagina and points backwards towards the sacrum. In this position it is described as *retroverted* (see Fig. 10.2).

At one time it was believed that women with retroversion were infertile. Strenuous attempts were made to suture the uterus into the anteverted position by shortening the round ligaments (an operation called *ventrosuspension*). The effect was generally short-lived since the round ligaments are elastic and soon stretch again. Surgery is seldom attempted today, because it has become apparent that pregnancy can occur despite retroversion, although in the anteverted position it is probable that semen remains in longer contact with the cervix because it pools in the fornices. Any link between infertility and retroversion probably stems from the fact that women with this condition often have some underlying pathological condition which may lead to the formation of adhesions (endometriosis, pelvic inflammatory disease). These conditions may be responsible for the pelvic discomfort, backache and heavy bleeding previously ascribed to retroversion. Once a woman has been told that the uterus is displaced she may blame this for vague pelvic discomfort when there may be no association between the two.

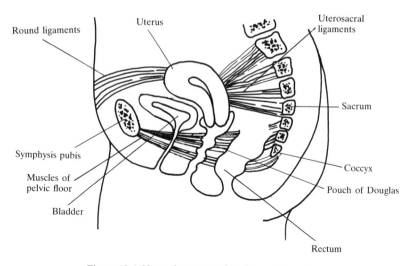

Figure 10.1 Normal anteverted position of the uterus.

It is now recognised that retroversion is often congenitally present or occurs temporarily after childbirth, when the pelvic ligaments become lax. Often there are no symptoms and no treatment is necessary. The uterus normally returns spontaneously to the anteverted position between one and two months after delivery. However, some women with retroversion complain of deep dyspareunia from pressure on the ovaries during intercourse. This occurs because the ovaries are pulled down into the pouch of Douglas when the uterus tilts backwards. The pain can be severe and persist for several hours. During pelvic examination the doctor can diagnose the condition by reproducing the pain. The uterus can be mainpulated into the anteverted position and held in place by inserting a Hodge pessary, allowed to remain in position for 8–10 weeks (see Fig. 10.3).

If a woman is fitted with a Hodge pessary to correct retroversion, the nurse must include the following explanations and information before she leaves the clinic:

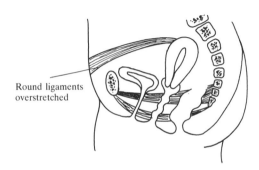

Figure 10.2 Retroverted uterus.

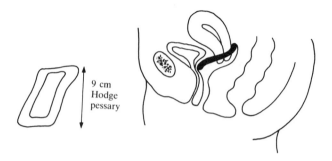

Figure 10.3 Uterus with Hodge pessary in position.

- The pessary will remain in place for a few weeks. During this time it should not be possible to feel it and it should not interfere with sexual intercourse.
- Personal hygiene is very important because the pessary acts as a foreign body, providing a possible focus for infection.
- The pessary must be removed at the time arranged by the doctor. If it is forgotten and remains in place too long it may irritate the vaginal walls, contributing to the development of infection and vaginal discharge. Over long periods of time ulceration may occur.
- If there is pain or vaginal discharge, the woman should contact the clinic or her GP.

Retroversion is possible because the fundus of the uterus is free to move in the pelvis since it must be able to enlarge during pregnancy. It is supported at the level of the cervix and vaginal vault, mainly by the underlying pelvic floor.

The pelvic floor

The muscles and ligaments of the pelvic floor provide support for the pelvic organs by acting as a sling, hitching them up from below. The account given below begins with a description of the deepest structures providing most support, and works to the exterior.

Levator ani muscles

The two levator ani muscles provide the strongest support to the pelvic floor, even though they are to some extent weakened by the passage of the urethra, rectum and vagina. They form a broad sheet running from the back of the symphysis pubis to the sacrum and coccyx, extending to the lateral pelvic walls (see Fig. 10.4).

(a) From above

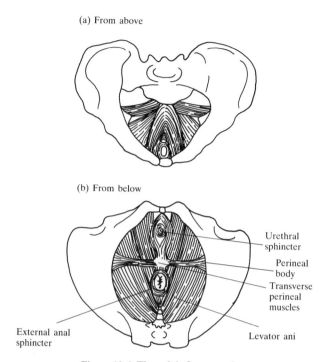

(b) From below

Urethral
sphincter

Perineal
body

Transverse
perineal
muscles

External anal
sphincter

Levator ani

Figure 10.4 The pelvic floor muscles.

Superficial perineal muscles

These two less powerful muscles run from the symphysis pubis, sacrum and lateral walls of the pelvis, uniting between the rectum and vagina (see Fig. 10.5). They form the superficial part of the perineal body.

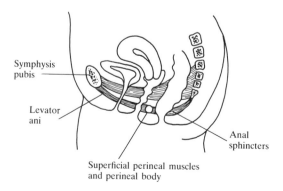

Symphysis
pubis

Levator
ani

Anal
sphincters

Superficial perineal muscles
and perineal body

Figure 10.5 Superficial muscles of the pelvic floor.

Perineal body

The perineal body is the wedge of muscular tissue between the vagina and rectum. It is made up of the junction between the levator ani muscles and the junction of the superficial cardinal muscles, providing less support than other muscles of the pelvic floor.

The uterus and its appendages are surrounded by a fold of peritoneum (the broad ligament) and held in place by the round ligament, uterosacral ligaments and the cardinal (transverse) ligaments.

Broad ligaments

The broad ligament is not really a ligament at all, but a double raised fold of peritoneum stretching over the uterus and running to the side walls of the pelvis (see Fig. 10.6). It does not provide much uterine support.

Round ligaments

The round ligaments were shown in Fig. 10.1. They run from each cornua of the uterus (point of junction with the uterine tube) to the subcutaneous fatty tissue of the labia majora. They hold the uterus in the anteverted position, but are elastic and therefore easily stretched.

Uterosacral ligament

The uterosacral ligament runs backwards from the cervix to the sacrum, dividing to pass the rectum, then re-uniting (see Fig. 10.7). Because it pulls the cervix backwards, it helps to maintain anteversion.

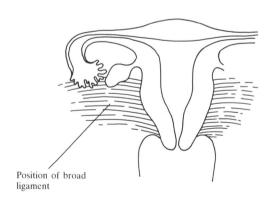

Position of broad
ligament

Figure 10.6 The broad ligaments.

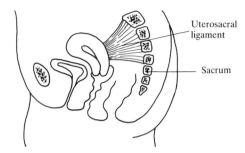

Figure 10.7 The uterosacral ligaments.

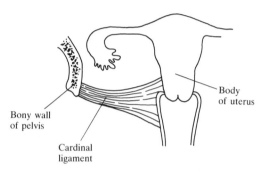

Figure 10.8 The cardinal ligaments.

Cardinal (transverse) ligaments

These two fibromuscular structures fan outwards from the cervix and run to the lateral pelvic walls (see Fig. 10.8).

Pubocervical ligament

This helps to support the bladder and urethra. It runs from the front of the cervix to the posterior part of the symphisis pubis, dividing to pass around the urethra.

The pelvic floor, and perhaps to a lesser extent the ligaments holding the uterus in position, must be strong:

- To provide continuous support for the pelvic structures despite the downward pull of gravity;
- To withstand the intermittent increases of intra-abdominal pressure exerted by coughing, laughing and defaecation.

Strength is combined with elasticity to permit the passage of a full-term baby. It is when the ligaments and muscles become over-stretched that the vagina, and sometimes the uterus, descend (*prolapse*) through the gap between the muscles. It is obviously much better to prevent prolapse, and to this end women should be taught about pelvic support when they are young, certainly before the first confinement.

Utero-vaginal prolapse

Prevention

One of the most important measures in the prevention of utero-vaginal prolapse is good management of labour. Midwives are taught accordingly:

- Not to let the woman push until the cervix is fully dilated.
- To avoid a prolonged second stage of labour whenever possible.
- To repair perineal tears or episiotomy incisions so that the healing wound regains maximum strength (scar tissue is never quite as strong as intact tissue). Infection further reduces strength because pathogenic bacteria release an enzyme, collagenase, which disrupts collagen fibres, the toughest fibres present in connective tissue from which scar tissue is formed.

The pelvic floor muscles atrophy from lack of use within a very short period of time (Montgomery 1986) so women should be encouraged to return to normal activities as soon as possible after delivery and to perform pelvic floor exercises. Ideally, these exercises will have been learned already, during the ante-natal period. There is evidence, however, that some women feel poorly motivated to attend ante-natal classes, may encounter practical problems which prevent regular attendance, or find classes of limited value (Gould 1986b).

Even when women have been taught how to do exercises they may lack motivation because the benefits are not immediately obvious, and because practise and feedback are necessary to ensure that the technique has been perfected. Many women are unaware that the muscles of the perineal area can be moved independently, and will probably be unable to continue exercises for more than a few minutes at first.

Montgomery (1986) suggests that the midwife performing an ante-natal examination has the ideal opportunity to teach pelvic floor exercises. The gloved index finger is introduced into the vagina, and the woman instructed to grip, then relax, noticing how the tissues around the birth canal draw up, then become soft and elastic again. During relaxation the space inside the vagina increases. The woman should be told that relaxation during labour makes passage of the baby easier. Montgomery emphasises that the aim of ante-natal exercises is to develop the woman's perception and control of her pelvic floor, not to stretch the muscles or make them more powerful at delivery. Contraction of the gluteal and abdominal muscles and breath holding should not occur. Once the technique has been mastered, the woman can practise several times a day during normal activities when she is sitting or standing.

After delivery, gently performing the exercises helps to stimulate blood flow to the sore, congested perineum, improving healing and reducing the chances of infection. Pressure on the local nerve endings decreases, so perineal discomfort is relieved.

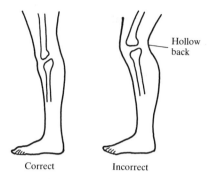

Hollow
back

Correct   Incorrect

Figure 10.9 Correct and incorrect standing postures.

Pelvic floor exercises should be continued into the post-natal period, when their aim is to redevelop strength, promote effective use of the pelvic floor and prevent genito-urinary problems. The same exercises are beneficial for women who have developed stress incontinence (see Chapter 11). Damage to the pelvic floor muscles can be reduced by avoiding obesity, prolonged unnecessary periods of standing, adopting the correct standing posture (see Fig. 10.9) and using the correct technique when lifting heavy objects. Although women are usually given this advice routinely after gynaecological surgery, there is evidence that it is of limited value unless the nature of a heavy weight is specified (Gould 1986b).

Unfortunately, many women now reaching the menopause develop a prolapse because they have not received this essential health teaching.

■   Mary Craddock, aged 75, had lived alone since she was widowed. She occupied a flat on the fifteenth floor of a council building, and sometimes had to climb several flights of stairs with laundry or shopping bags as the lift was often broken. She was an active person who made a major contribution to the housework of her disabled brother living alone nearby.

Mary's concern for her brother caused her to disregard her own increasing health problems for quite some time. Over a period lasting several months, she gradually became aware of a dragging sensation in the vaginal area. It was most noticeable when standing, and tended to disappear when she lay down. Walking became uncomfortable and soreness developed in the vaginal area, sometimes accompanied by a slight, but offensive, discharge. Mary had always suffered from constipation. Now she became aware of the need to pass urine very frequently, and she occasionally passed small amounts involuntarily, especially when she coughed or laughed. Eventually, micurition was accompanied by pain and the urine looked cloudy. Mary visited her GP. She told him that she felt as though 'something was coming down' her vagina.

Risk factors for utero-vaginal prolapse

■   Mary had all the risk factors predisposing to utero-vaginal prolapse. Mary had five children who had all arrived over a very few years, in the days before ante-natal exercises were widely taught. Family circumstances had not been good, so Mary had always worked, usually cleaning jobs involving lifting and carrying. This had weakened her pelvic floor when she was quite a young woman. At 75 Mary smoked twenty cigarettes a day and had a smoker's cough. She was overweight and suffered from chronic constipation. All these factors placed extra strain on her pelvic floor.

The symptoms of prolapse normally develop gradually, as a consequence of damage accumulating over the years. At the menopause, when plasma oestrogen levels fall, the muscles and ligaments undergo a degree of atrophy, contributing to prolapse. Uterine descent seldom occurs in nulliparous women. Once damage has begun following a prolonged or difficult labour, further descent occurs due to the human upright stance; prolapse is virtually unknown among quadrupedal animals.

Degrees of uterine prolapse

There are three degrees of uterine prolapse.

First degree
The uterus becomes retroverted and descends into the axis of the vagina, pulling the vaginal wall with it (see Fig. 10.10). The body of the uterus and the cervix remain in the pelvic cavity.

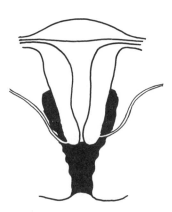

Figure 10.10 First degree prolapse.

Second degree
The uterus descends further into the vagina and the cervix appears at the introitus (see Fig. 10.11).

Third degree (procidentia)
This is complete prolapse. The vaginal walls invert completely and the uterus now lies outside the vulva (see Fig. 10.12). The prolapsed area becomes sore, ulcerated and often infected. Walking is very uncomfortable and life becomes restricted.

When the uterus prolapses, the vagina always descends with it. Sometimes, however, vaginal prolapse may occur without uterine descent.

Vaginal prolapse

Reference to Fig. 10.1 shows that the vaginal walls lie in close association with the bladder (in front) and the rectum and pouch of Douglas (behind). Prolapse of the vagina will therefore cause herniation of the adjacent organs, depending on whether the anterior or posterior walls are affected.

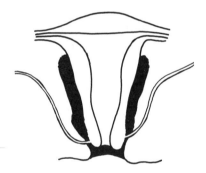

Figure 10.11 Second degree prolapse.

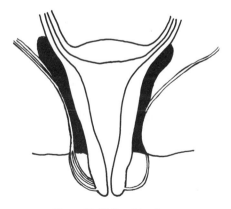

Figure 10.12 Procidentia.

Anterior vaginal wall prolapse

If the upper part of the anterior vaginal wall prolapses, it carries the wall of the bladder down with it. The bladder wall herniates into the vagina. This is called a *cystocele* (see Fig. 10.13). If prolapse involves the lower part of the vaginal wall, the urethra descends with it (*urethrocele*). Cystocele and urethrocele are often accompanied by urinary problems (frequency, stress incontinence).

Posterior vaginal wall prolapse

If the upper third of the posterior vaginal wall descends, it causes a length of small bowel or *omentum* to herniate into the Pouch of Douglas. This is called an *enterocele* (see Fig. 10.14). Prolapse of the middle third of the posterior vaginal wall causes herniation of the rectum (*rectocele*). Descent of the lower third of the vaginal vault is

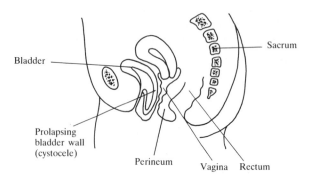

Figure 10.13 Anterior vaginal wall prolapse.

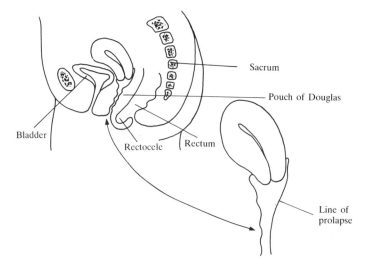

Figure 10.14 Posterior vaginal wall prolapse.

only possible if the perineum has been weakened by trauma or childbirth, because the last part of the vagina is normally held in position by the perineal body.

Prolapses of the posterior vaginal wall generally cause fewer symptoms than cystocele unless they become large enough to interfere with bowel functioning. However, many women develop anterior and posterior prolapses simultaneously.

Two avenues of treatment are possible: correction by ring pessary or surgery.

Treatment of vaginal prolapse

The outpatient appointment

■ Mary was referred to the gynaecologist. She was very anxious because she had not been examined by a doctor since the birth of her children. She was embarrassed and afraid that the examination would be painful. When she arrived at the clinic, she was reassured by the nurse who told her what to expect during the examination and gave her the opportunity to ask questions before helping her to undress. The nurse knew that many women in this age group feel reluctant to seek medical help for genito-urinary and gynaecological problems. She spent some time with Mary beforehand, to give her the opportunity to disclose her fears. People attending outpatient clinics commonly express non-verbal cues of distress which nurses do not always recognise (Maguire 1980).

The nurse was present while Mary saw the gynaecologist to provide support, and to enable her to go over the information afterwards if Mary had not been able to absorb all that was said. On examination, Mary was found to have an anterior and posterior prolapse, with a cystocele, rectocele and a degree of stress incontinence. Stress incontinence is demonstrated by inserting Sim's speculum (page 7), designed to hold back the posterior vaginal wall, then asking the woman to cough so that any escaping urine can be seen.

Treatment depends on the degree of prolapse, the woman's general health and her preference, so careful medical and nursing assessments must be made before the appropriate choices can be offered.

Non–surgical intervention

A ring pessary can be inserted to distend the vaginal walls so they no longer prolapse, providing the perineal muscles are strong enough to hold the pessary in place. Initially, the gynaecologist fits the pessary, but it may be changed later and re-fitted by the nurse who will also have to teach the woman about personal hygiene and self-care.

All the points about the Hodge Pessary discussed in this chapter (page 235–6) are relevant, but the ring pessary will be in place long term, and must be checked and changed regularly, probably about every six months.

Although modern types of pessaries, made of vinyl, reduce the chances of trauma and infection, the most effective treatment today is surgery. With modern anaesthesia many very elderly women prefer to have a repair operation (*colporrhaphy*) rather than wear a pessary permanently.

Surgical treatment

Anterior colporrhaphy
The anterior vaginal wall is incised, followed by excision of redundant tissue. The surgeon exposes the *vesico vaginal fascia* (connective tissue between bladder and vagina) and sutures the edges more tightly together to provide increased support for the bladder and urethra. The incision is then repaired.

Posterior colporrhaphy
The rectocele is obliterated by tightening the fascia between rectum and vagina, followed by excision of excess vaginal tissue, then the perineal muscles are sutured over the incised area. The wound is closed in a 'Y' shape to avoid narrowing the introitus. The *levator ani* and perineal muscles are brought together with sutures. This procedure is often more painful than anterior repair.

Buttressing of the bladder neck
Non-absorbable sutures (three or four) are inserted into the fascia surrounding the bladder neck to elevate, tighten and support the urethral sphincters, helping to relieve stress incontinence.

The nurse's role

■   Before Mary left the clinic, the nature of the operation was explained to her and she was given some information about the expected events during recovery in the ward and later when she left hospital. It is important to provide women coming into hospital with this kind of practical information so they can make plans for discharge. Mary had no immediate worries because she had discussed the possibility of admission with her daughter. They had decided that it would be best if she went to stay at her daughter's house. Mary's main concern was returning to her own flat, carrying shopping up all those flights of stairs, and that her brother, who relied on her visits for company, would miss her while she was away. Mary's social circumstances had contributed to the development of her prolapse and it was evident that they could impede long term recovery. The nurse arranged for her to be visited by a social worker from the Social Services Department *before* admission, to see if there was any possibility of re-housing.

The nurse discussed with Mary how she could help herself make a good recovery. Research has shown the difficulty of categorising recovery as 'good' or 'poor', because every woman is an individual and, particularly with older women, there is the difficulty of concomitant deterioration in health (Gould 1986a). However, much can be done to maximise the potential for return to normal levels of functioning if the woman can be assessed before she reaches the ward, and if some health teaching is undertaken. Guided by the nurse, Mary was helped to recognise that healing would take place more swiftly if she could reduce weight (adipose tissue is poorly vasculated) and reduce the number of cigarettes smoked. Smokers often have low levels of ascorbic acid (vitamin C) needed to enhance connective tissue repair and their tissues have poor oxygen perfusion due to the increased ratio of carbon monoxide to oxygen in the blood. Smoking increases the risks of anaesthesia, predisposes to chest infection and, like obesity, puts a strain on sutured tissues. Women undergoing repair procedures need to be told about the internal sutures since no external wound is visible after the operation and they may wonder why precautions are necessary, and feel surprised they are so tired. Figure 10.15 shows the suture line after repair.

Mary was asked about her diet to identify any faulty eating habits. It was evident that she needed fewer sugary foods and more fibre to help her lose weight and to re-educate her bowels. Hospital, with its strange environment and unfamiliar routines, is *not* the place to learn new bowel habits (Wright 1974). Health education must be accompanied by practical and realistic advice. Many older people eat inappropriately because they lack motivation or have poorly fitting dentures (DHSS 1972). Mary was asked about her teeth. Finance can be a problem: some vegetables, fruits, and wholefoods

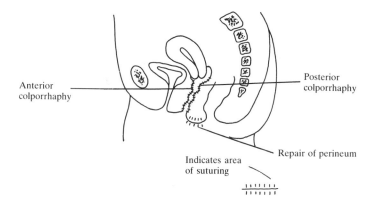

Anterior colporrhaphy

Posterior colporrhaphy

Repair of perineum

Indicates area of suturing

Figure 10.15 Anterior and posterior repair, showing suture lines.

may be considered expensive compared to starchy, refined products and need more preparation to make them palatable (Hunt 1985). They may also be bulky to carry home from the shops. Fortunately, Mary could enlist the help of her children. They were always offering her vegetables from the allotment which she refused as she generally preferred pre-prepared convenience foods.

Finally, as Mary obviously had a urinary tract infection, she was asked to provide a mid-stream specimen of urine so that the bacteria responsible could be identified and their antibiotic sensitivities checked. Meanwhile Mary was instructed how to take the broad-spectrum antibiotic tablets prescribed by the doctor, and reassured that the burning, and probably some of her frequency and incontinence, might clear up spontaneously when the infection had been cured. She was told to return to her GP when the antibiotics had been taken. He would test her urine again just in case the antibiotics had not been fully effective.

Pre-operative care

The pre-operative care of a woman who is to undergo a repair procedure is very similar to that before any major gynaecological operation (see Chapter 7), except that she will probably return to the ward with a catheter *in situ* and must be warned about this in advance.

A urine specimen must be sent for microbiological examination before surgery.

Post-operative care

Mary's post-operative care was based on the model by Roper *et al.* (1985). Webb (1986) justifies the use of this model with the older woman, since its straightforward terminology makes it a good choice for someone whose previous experience of nursing care, many years previously, may be different from the approach today. Mary's care plan for the first few days is shown in Care plan 10.1 (page 249).

Longer term recovery and planning discharge

■   Before leaving the hospital Mary was warned that she would feel tired at first, and might like to rest in the afternoons while she was staying with her daughter. She was reminded not to lift or stand for long periods and to avoid constipation or straining at stool. Vaginal discharge should be slight (brown or pink, not bright red) and should disappear gradually after the first week or two. The nurse checked to ensure that Mary could recognise the symptoms of urinary tract infection since this can often happen after vaginal surgery and needs prompt treatment. Mary had seen the gynaecologist before discharge and he had performed a vaginal examination to ensure that no adhesions had formed in the vagina and there was no haematoma. If vaginal adhesions form they must be gently separated because intercourse is otherwise difficult. If women have been having intercourse prior to the operation, they are advised

Care plan 10.1 (Roper, Logan and Tierney: Activities of Living model)

Name: Mary Craddock

Treatment/condition: Anterior and posterior repair

Assessment and care plan:

Activity of Living	Date & Time of Assessment	Assessment	Problems	Goal	Nursing Intervention	Evaluation
Providing a safe environment	20.02.89 Three days post-operatively	*Vital signs:* Temperature 36.8°C Pulse 70 beats per minute BP 130/90 Intravenous fluids discontinued	These are all dealt with under appropriate headings			
Eating and drinking	20.02.89	Overweight for height (75 kg; 5′ 3″). Information about healthy eating was provided before admission. Says she knows she 'eats the wrong things'. Drinking 2.5 litres of fluid daily in hospital. Wears dentures – reports no problems	(1) Obesity (actual) (2) Trying to lose weight during post-operative recovery when normal activity will be reduced (potential) (3) Poor dietary habits despite some health education and apparent knowledge (actual)	(1) Receive further information about diet (2) Discuss the practical difficulties of losing weight during recovery	Discuss suitable foods, draw attention to fibre content and calorific value. Discuss financial implications. Provide handbook of suggested recipes and menus compiled by hospital dietician. Point out suitable dishes on hospital menu – ask Mary whether these are to her taste and check that her dentures are in sufficiently good repair for her to eat the food	25.02.89 Mary has read the diet handbook and feels encouraged about weight loss. She finds some wholefoods palatable (brown rice, wholemeal bread, beans), while others are definitely not (wholemeal pastry)

Activity of Living	Date & Time of Assessment	Assessment	Problems	Goal	Nursing Intervention	Evaluation
Communication	20.02.89	Mary is a sociable and talkative lady who enjoys the company of the nurses and of all other patients, regardless of their ages. She is persistently cheerful, and it is not always easy to determine whether, underneath, something may be worrying her	Outward demeanour may hide some underlying worry either to do with health, her housing situation or her disabled brother	Mary will feel able to express her feelings	Give Mary the opportunity for private conversation so that, if necessary, she may voice her fears	25.02.89 Mary feels that her recovery so far has been favourable, considering her age and chest problems. She feels sad about not visiting her brother, but has made up for this by phoning every day. She tries to be realistic about the chances of having a new flat. Her main anxiety was expressed to the night Sister – 'I'm 75, and really I should make a will'
Breathing	20.02.89	Smoked 20 cigarettes daily before admission. Now smokes five daily. Smoker's cough. Expectorating 15 ml grey sputum daily – always 'coughs up phlegm' in the morning.	(1) Smoker's cough (actual) (2) Expectorating tenacious mucoid sputum (actual) (3) Chest infection (potential) (4) Lack of motivation to	(1) Will not develop chest infection (2, 3, 4) Will be given further information about giving up smoking if she wishes	(1) Monitor respiratory rate four hourly (2) Give steam inhalations twice daily to liquefy pulmonary secretions and aid expectoration – Send specimen of sputum for bacteriological monitoring (4) Provide further	25.02.89 Mary is still coughing, but her general condition seems better. She has not developed a chest infection. She does not want to reduce cigarette consumption further at present, because she is also restricting her diet

	Assessment	Problem	Goal	Nursing intervention	Evaluation
	Respiratory rate – 20 breaths/minute. Not cyanosed. Normally becomes breathless easily on exertion (two flights of stairs)	reduce smoking further (actual) (5) Mobility restricted by breathlessness (actual)		health education as requested (5) Encourage early ambulation (see mobilising) – Encourage deep breathing exercises taught by physiotherapist	
Elimination 20.02.89	Tends to be constipated. Bowels last opened 19.02.89 (before surgery). Indwelling Foley catheter *in situ*, to be removed 22.02.89. Previous urinary tract infection resolved prior to admission. Drinking 2.5 litres fluid daily	(1) Constipation (actual – has not opened bowels since surgery) (2) Urinary tract infection due to catheter (potential)	(1) Alleviate constipation and prevent in future (2) Avoid urinary tract infection	(1) Advise high fibre diet (see eating and drinking) – Give two glycerine suppositories to avoid straining at stool (2) Monitor urinary output. Send urine specimen for bacteriological monitoring – Teach and encourage Mary to look after her own catheter and empty the drainage bag to avoid risks of cross-infection (1, 2) See also 'Eating and drinking'	25.02.89 Bowels last opened 24.02.89 (suppositories). Catheter removed 23.02.89. No evidence of urinary tract infection. Not in negative fluid balance

Activity of Living	Date & Time of Assessment	Assessment	Problems	Goal	Nursing Intervention	Evaluation
Personal cleansing and dressing	20.02.89	Wearing night-dress and dressing gown. Finds this most comfortable and convenient in view of catheter and vaginal loss. Daughter does laundry. Helped to bath daily by nurse	None identified			No problems reported throughout admission
Controlling body temperature	20.02.89	Oral temperature – 36.8°C	(1) Infection of urinary tract (potential) (2) Infection of vaginal wound (potential) (3) Pyrexia resulting from infection (potential) NB older people may not respond to infection with pyrexia as readily as younger adults	Will not develop infection	(1) Prevent urinary tract infection – maintain high fluid intake and teach Mary how to look after her own catheter (2) Prevent infection of vaginal wounds. Observe condition of external suture line daily. Provide Mary with sterile sanitary towels. Observe vaginal loss four hourly. Report changes to medical staff.	25.02.89 Temperature 38.6°C. Vaginal loss slight, pink. No evidence of infection

Activity of living	Date	Assessment	Problem	Goal	Nursing action	Evaluation
					Maintain good hygiene. Encourage use of bidet twice daily and after opening bowels (3) Monitor temperature four hourly	
Mobilising	20.02.89	Does not walk far without becoming breathless (length of ward only). Problem climbing stairs to flat before admission. Social worker contacted re housing 23.01.89 (before admission). Movement since operation restricted by catheter	(1) Breathlessness restricts mobility (actual) (2) Difficulty climbing stairs (actual)	(1) Breathlessness – see breathing (2) Rehousing if possible in long term. Appropriate plans for convalescence short term	(1) Explain reason for breathlessness (smoking, obesity). Offer appropriate health teaching (2) Liaise with social services department concerning rehousing. Discuss convalescence with Mary and her family.	25.02.89 Mary will stay with her daughter to convalesce. She is able to relate her breathlessness to smoking and has expressed a desire to lose weight. The social services hope to rehouse her in a smaller flat, but no date is yet available. At her daughter's she will be able to sleep on the ground floor, but will have to climb one short flight of stairs to bath (WC is downstairs)
Working and playing	20.02.89	Mary is retired and has been widowed for many years. She visits her brother 3 or 4 times a week to do his	None identified			Mary seems happy in the ward throughout her stay in hospital

Activity of Living	Date & Time of Assessment	Assessment	Problems	Goal	Nursing Intervention	Evaluation
		washing, general housework and to provide company (he has had a mild stroke). For recreation she likes to knit, watch television and do crossword puzzles. She has adjusted well to the ward and says she enjoys the company of other women				
Expressing sexuality	20.02.89	Five children. Widowed many years. No longer sexually active. Likes to 'look nice'. Very distressed about urinary incontinence and vaginal discharge – prevented her from feeling clean	Altered body image, especially until vaginal discharge has resolved and catheter is removed (actual)	Mary's self-esteem will not be damaged. She will understand the temporary nature of vaginal loss and catheterisation	Provide information about expected course of recovery. Give Mary the opportunity to voice her feelings	25.02.89 Mary accepts that bleeding may continue for a while after leaving hospital, but that her catheter will soon be removed. She knows what to expect during longer term recovery at home
Sleeping and resting	20.02.89	Normally sleeps well (10.30 pm –	None			25.02.89 Says she has slept much

| Dying | 20.02.89 | Aged 75. Appears fit despite breathlessness. Has made good recovery so far. Told night sister that coming into hospital has made her think about the future, when she will no longer be so well | Beginning to think of her own mortality | Mary will feel able to express her thoughts and discuss them with family and members of the caring team with whom she feels comfortable | Give Mary the opportunity to initiate discussion as she chooses, and to plan to put her affairs in order | 25.02.89 'When I go out of here I must make a will. I've been putting it off. I haven't much to leave, but I know it leaves a whole load of trouble for people's families when they don't put their house in order' |

5.30 am), but has had to get up at night to pass urine in recent months (3–4 times). Since coming into hospital she has adapted to sleeping in a strange bed better than anticipated

better since surgery than in recent months, because she is no longer afraid of wetting the bed

---

The model developed by Roper et al. (1985) proved a successful approach for planning Mary's care, as it was possible to identify physical, psychological and social problems with achievable nursing aims. Longer term recovery and discharge planning are discussed on page 248. You could use the same model, or Orem's model (1985) (see page 86) to develop a care plan for Mary after the immediate post-operative phase. Does the lack of nursing and medical research concerning the success or otherwise of repair procedures influence the advice you would give to Mary?

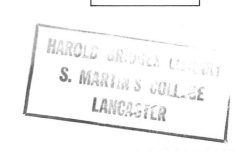

to refrain for four or six weeks (depending on the consultant) to avoid trauma to the sutured area. When a woman is in the older age group, advice may still be necessary, and the nurse should remain alert to this possibility, since many older women may feel too shy to ask. Women who drive are asked not to do so for six to eight weeks to avoid muscular effort.

Mary and her daughter both knew that Mary would need to attend the clinic in six weeks to have the wounds examined and ensure that all was well.

The success of vaginal repair procedures does not appear to be well documented. Fergusson (1984) claims recurrence in up to 20 per cent of cases, but provides no figures to support this. In the study by Gould (1986a) eleven women, in a sample of eighty-five, had had a repair procedure in conjunction with vaginal hysterectomy. This number was too small for meaningful comparisons to be made with other women undergoing abdominal surgery, but the data suggested overall less satisfaction with the effects of surgery. In one case repair was definitely unsuccessful, while for another woman there was some return of stress incontinence. Two women developed dyspareunia. In one case this was due to the development of vaginal adhesions which were later broken down under anaesthetic and, in the other, sutures had been inserted too tightly reducing the size of the introitus.

Vaginal hysterectomy

When the uterus is well descended or prolapse is complete, it may be removed via the vagina, followed by a repair procedure. Some gynaecologists favour vaginal hysterectomy rather than abdominal surgery because of the cosmetic effect and because some authors have reported lower levels of morbidity (Porges 1980, Gudex 1965, Hawksworth 1965, Ellenborgen 1981). This is, however, debatable since bleeding is more difficult to control during the operation, increasing the chances of a haematoma developing in the vaginal vault. Once the uterus has been removed, there is a risk of distorting the ureters if the bladder fascia are tightened too much when the cystocele is repaired. Some surgeons (Wilson 1963) believe the uterus should always be removed once childbearing is complete to avoid risk of cervical carcinoma. This fails to take into consideration the desires of women who do not wish to part with their reproductive structures in the absence of pathology.

Pre- and post-operative care of women undergoing vaginal hysterectomy does not differ much from repair, and they require the same counselling and support as women who undergo abdominal hysterectomy (see Chapter 7).

Manchester (Fothergill) repair

This operation is sometimes used to treat first degree prolapse. The cervix is partially amputated and the stretched cervical ligaments are divided, then joined again in front

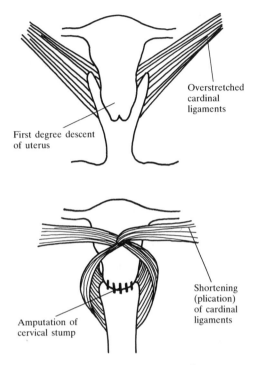

First degree descent
of uterus

Overstretched
cardinal
ligaments

Amputation of
cervical stump

Shortening
(plication)
of cardinal
ligaments

Figure 10.16 Manchester repair.

of the remaining cervical stump (see Fig. 10.16). A cystocele or rectocele can be repaired at the same time. After-care is similar to that for vaginal hysterectomy and repair.

Inversion of the uterus

This condition occurs very rarely as a complication of the third stage of labour (acute) or when the uterus is contracting to extrude a fibroid or polyps (chronic). The uterus turns inside out so the fundus passes through the cervix into the vagina. Hysterectomy is usually necessary.

References

DHSS (1972) *Nutrition and Health in Old Age*, Report No. 16, London: HMSO.
Ellenborgen, A. *et al.* (1981) 'The Role of Vaginal Hysterectomy in Aged Women', *Journal of American Geriatrics Society* 29 (9), pp. 426–8.
Fergusson, I.L.C. 'Genital Prolapse' (1984) In: Chamberlain, G. (ed.) *Contemporary Gynaecology*, London: Butterworths, pp. 211–19.

Gould, D.J. (1986a) 'Hidden problems after a hysterectomy', *Nursing Times* 82 (23), pp. 43–6.
Gould, D.J. (1986b) 'Locally organised ante-natal classes and their effectiveness', *Nursing Times* 82 (12), p.59–62.
Gudex, R.G. (1965) 'Pelvic floor repair with or without hysterectomy', *Journal of Obstetrics and Gynaecology of the British Commonwealth* 72, pp. 864–5.
Hawksworth, W. (1965) 'Indications for vaginal hysterectomy', *Journal of Obstetrics and Gynaecology of the British Commonwealth* 72, pp. 847–50.
Hunt, S. (1985) 'Below the breadline', *Nursing Times Community Outlook* (October), pp. 19–21.
Maguire, P. *et al.* (1980) 'Effect of counselling on the morbidity rate associated with mastectomy', *British Medical Journal* 1 (281) 1454–6.
Montgomery, E. (1986) 'Pelvic Power', *Nursing Times Community Outlook* (September), 33–4.
Porges, R.F. (1980) 'Changing indications for vaginal hysterectomy', *American Journal of Obstetrics and Gynaecology* 2, 153–8.
Roper, N., Logan, W.W. and Tierney, A.J. (1985) *Using a model for nursing*, Edinburgh: Churchill Livingstone.
Webb, A. (1986) 'Care plan for a woman having a vaginal hysterectomy based on Roper's Activities of Living' In: Webb, C. (ed.) *Using Nursing Models: Women's Health Care*, Sevenoaks: Hodder and Stoughton, pp. 171–6.
Wilson, R. (1963) 'The fate of the non-treated pre-menopausal woman – a plea for adequate oestrogen from puberty to the grave', *Journal of the American Geriatric Society* 11, 347–62.
Wright, L. (1974) *Bowel Function in Hospital*. London: Royal College of Nursing.

11   Urinary Problems

Although urinary problems are not inevitably related to pelvic pathology, the two frequently co-exist. The organs of the lower urinary tract are anatomically in close association to the reproductive structures, and many women come to gynaecology wards and departments for treatment. Urinary symptoms are a common source of distress to women, contributing to loss of dignity and often to significant reduction in quality of life (Tattersall 1985). Of the large number of people in the community thought to experience urinary incontinence, only a small proportion are known to health care professionals, often because they are under the misapprehension that little can be done for them (Smith 1982). This is no longer true. Urinary incontinence may still rank among those topics considered unmentionable by the layperson, but the promotion of continence is now recognised by nurses as one of their major professional responsibilities, and is an area that has attracted considerable attention and research in recent years (*King's Fund Project Paper* 1983). However, before abnormal physiology can be appreciated, an understanding of normal function is essential.

Nursing responsibilities

■   Hazel Novak and Pat Cohen were health visitors attached to a busy health centre in an inner city area. During their day to day visits to women at home they were often asked about urinary problems, sometimes by young and otherwise fit women. When they established a Well Woman Clinic, they were not surprised to find that many clients were specifically worried about urinary problems or mentioned them when they completed a general health question-naire. Invaluable help was provided in the clinic by a number of women working as lay volunteers, especially with clients otherwise unwilling to seek advice about health. To help increase their knowledge, Hazel and Pat invited the Continence Adviser Nurse to visit their clinic to discuss normal bladder function and its disorders.

Physiology of micturition

The bladder

The bladder is a hollow organ with a normal capacity of about 400 ml (see Fig. 11.1). It is highly distensible. Stretching is possible because the detrusor muscle making up its walls consists of closely interwoven involuntary (*unstriated*) muscle fibres instead of clearly defined muscular layers. The detrusor is lined by a water-resistant transitional epithelium. When the bladder is empty the epithelial cells overlap, but as it fills they stretch increasing capacity. The *fundus* (main body of the bladder) is mounted on the *trigone*, a triangular area defined by the two ureteric orifices and the internal urethral meatus.

The urethra

The female urethra is aproximately 4 cm long, much shorter than in the male. The relatively short distance which bacteria have to migrate before gaining access to the bladder is considered to be one of the main reasons for the much higher incidence of urinary tract infections in women compared to men.

The urethral wall consists of an outer layer of smooth (*involuntary*) muscle with fibres arranged longitudinally around an inner, circular layer (see Fig. 11.2). The upper two thirds of the urethra are lined with transitional epithelium, but immediately before the urethral orifice this changes to stratified squamous epithelium similar to the cells lining the vagina. This tissue is under the cyclic control of oestrogen, so women may experience urethral soreness and dryness at the menopause when oestrogen is no

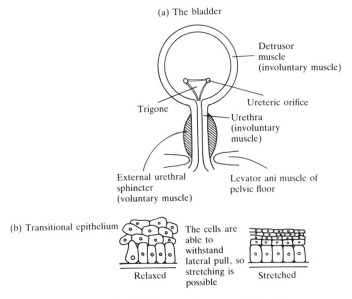

Figure **11.1** The lower urinary tract (female).

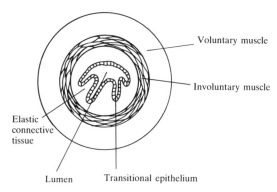

Figure 11.2 The urethra: transverse section.

longer secreted, an effect open to correction by hormone replacement therapy. The outermost tip of the urethra is colonised by the same bacteria as those normally living on the vulva, but in health the rest of the urinary tract is free of micro-organisms and, before it leaves the urethra, urine is sterile.

The urethral sphincters

Exit of urine from the urinary tract is controlled by two muscles, the external and internal urethral sphincters. The external sphincter consists of voluntary muscle and is therefore under conscious control. It encircles the urethra midway along its length, exerting pressure so the urethral orifice is kept closed. The internal sphincter consists of longitudinal and circular involuntary muscle fibres with elastic connective tissue.

The action of the following structures also help to keep the urethra closed during coughing, sneezing and laughing, when intra-abdominal pressure is raised:

- The levators ani muscles;
- Voluntary muscle in the pelvic floor;
- Perineal muscles.

The ureters

The two ureters (see Fig. 11.3) descend from the pelvis of each kidney and enter the bladder obliquely, near its base, helping to define the trigone. Their position helps prevent reflux of urine to the kidneys.

The micturition cycle

Feneley (1986) believes that normal micturition and maintaining continence should be viewed as a cycle of events, rather than a series of discrete acts, as follows:

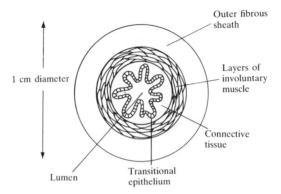

Figure 11.3 Structure of the ureter (transverse section).

- Ability to store urine;
- Ability to void urine voluntarily in a suitable place at a convenient time.

Much of our knowledge comes from urodynamic studies conducted in the 1960s. These techniques are now important as clinical diagnostic tests. However, micturition is highly complex, and there is much that physiologists have yet to explain. Fundamentally it appears to be a reflex arc on which the higher centres of the brain are able to impose control in individuals after about two years of age. Events in the micturition cycle are outlined below:

- The bladder gradually distends as urine enters (phenomenon of *compliance*).
- Intravesicular pressure remains below 10 cm Hg until 400–500 ml of urine are present (see Fig. 11.4).
- Meanwhile, stretch receptors in the bladder wall trigger nervous impulses which travel along sensory (*afferent*) nerve fibres to the sacral region of the spinal cord.
- Once critical capacity (400–500 ml) has been reached, impulses return to the bladder along motor (*efferent*) nerve fibres, causing the detrusor to contract (see Fig. 11.5).
- The urethral sphincters now relax and the bladder empties.

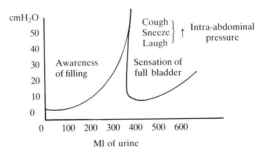

Figure 11.4 Mechanism of compliance.

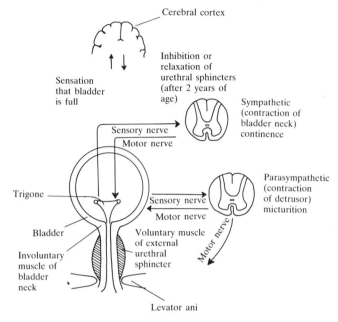

Cerebral cortex

Inhibition or
relaxation of
urethral sphincters
(after 2 years of
age)

Sensation
that bladder
is full

Sympathetic
(contraction of
bladder neck)
continence

Sensory nerve

Motor nerve

Parasympathetic
(contraction
of detrusor)
micturition

Trigone

Sensory nerve

Motor nerve

Bladder

Voluntary muscle
of external
urethral
sphincter

Involuntary
muscle of
bladder
neck

Motor nerve

Levator ani

Figure 11.5 The micturition cycle.

- When voiding is complete, the urethral sphincters return to their formerly contracted state which, in health, they are able to maintain over prolonged intervals of time.
- The stretch receptors in the detrusor wall now cease to relay impulses and the detrusor relaxes.

After the age of approximately two years, this reflex arc can be voluntarily inhibited by the influence of higher centres in the brain. It is then possible to delay micturition until a convenient time and place present themselves.

Nervous control of the bladder is mediated by the sympathetic, parasympathetic and voluntary systems. This is summarised in Table 11.1.

Mechanism of voiding

The technique of *cystometry* (see page 272) has helped to demonstrate the timing of events when voiding occurs:

- First there is an increase in intra-abdominal pressure;
- The detrusor muscle then contracts so that intravesicular pressure rises;
- The urethral sphincters relax;
- Urine begins to flow.

When micturition is not occurring, the urethra and bladder neck are kept closed by contraction of the muscle at the base of the bladder (*trigonal base plate*) and the

Table 11.1 Nervous control of micturition

Autonomic nervous system (involuntary control)	{ Parasympathetic: stimulates detrusor contraction { Sympathetic: contracts bladder neck and urethra
Voluntary nervous system (external urethral meatus)	Contracts under conscious control to resist micturition until convenient time and place are found
Involuntary control	Present at birth. Reflex mechanism operating in infants, after damage to brain or spinal cord (stroke, spinal injury, etc)
Voluntary control	Develops at approximately two years of age. Varies from one individual to another and in the same individual at different stages in the life cycle. Usually over-rides involuntary control

urethral sphincters. When micturition occurs the detrusor contracts and the bladder neck relaxes (*funnelling*).

The urethral sphincters simultaneously relax and voiding is initiated. As flow continues the neck of the bladder moves downwards and backwards and the angle between the urethra and bladder (*urethral-vesicular angle*) is lost (see Fig. 11.6).

The micturition cycle is possible because a synergistic relationship exists between the bladder and urethra. Leakage is prevented because intravesicular pressure is normally lower than the pressure offered by urethral resistance. When voiding occurs this situation is reversed; the detrusor muscle contracts and the urethral sphincters relax, allowing urine to escape.

Urodynamic studies indicate that voiding proceeds more rapidly for women than for men. Average voiding rate for women under 50 is 25 ml/second, falling to about 18 ml/second as they grow older.

Once voiding is complete, the urethral sphincters contract and the pelvic floor

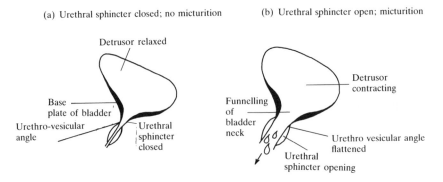

(a) Urethral sphincter closed; no micturition   (b) Urethral sphincter open; micturition

Figure 11.6 Micturition.

muscles help the basal plate to rise again, restoring the original urethral-vesicular angle. The dynamic equilibrium is reversed, and the micturition cycle recommences.

Normal micturition

'Normal micturition' should be viewed in the same light as 'normal menstruation' (see Chapter 7): there is such enormous variation between women of the same age that a nursing assessment should focus on what the individual woman considers usual for herself. Comparisons are not possible between one woman and another. At Well Woman Clinics questionnaires may help women identify actual and potential urinary problems (see Fig. 11.7), or a nurse or counsellor may feel more happy using a less structured approach to obtain the assessment.

Common urinary problems

■   Rajinder Patel came to the Well Woman Clinic for a health check shortly before her wedding, as she hoped to start a family as soon as possible. Rajinder seemed happy until Hazel began to ask questions relating to urinary function. It emerged that Rajinder had had several episodes of frequency and dysuria, but had not seen her GP because there was no female partner attached to the practice. Such problems were not readily discussed in Rajinder's family but, from friends in the factory where she worked, Rajinder had heard several alarming stories about 'honeymoon cystitis'.

Hazel asked about fluid intake, remembering to include questions about type as well as quantity. Tea and coffee are diuretics: women, especially those in sedentary occupations, may consume large quantities during the day. Diuresis is particularly likely if they are taken last thing at night because glomerular filtration is speeded in the supine position. This is because glomerular filtrate increases (see, for example, Hinchliff and Montague 1986, p. 328). Rajinder said that she drank a great deal of coffee during the day at work, but not at home. She had heard that maintaining high fluid intake helped prevent urinary tract infections by flushing out the bladder. Hazel explained that, although the mechanical action of voiding helps to keep the bladder free of bacteria, Rajinder's problem might be more effectively treated if she drank clear fluids without diuretic action (water, unsweetened fruit juices). She was not surprised when Rajinder said that, generally, her frequency became more troublesome before menstruation. The action of progesterone during the second half of the menstrual cycle has a relaxant effect on involuntary muscle (including the pelvic ligaments), so many women notice increased frequency at this time.

CONFIDENTIAL
Name   Age
Clinic No.   GP
Date   Health worker

HEALTH PROFILE

1. Have you come to us for a general health check, or is there a special reason?
   General health check
   Special reason
   Details

2. If for a special reason: Have you seen anyone else about this?
   Yes
   No
   Details

3. Are you taking any pills or medicines at present?
   Yes
   No
   Details

4. Are you receiving any treatment at present?
   Yes
   No
   Details

5. Do you get cystitis?
   Yes
   No
   If yes:
   About how often does this happen?

   Do you get pain passing water?
   Want to pass water often?
   Have you seen anyone else about this?
   Any treatment given?
   How much do you have to drink each day?
   Preferred beverage (tea, coffee, water etc.)

Figure 11.7 Well Woman Clinic questionnaire (extract).

Frequency

Frequency is defined as the need to pass urine more than seven times a day, and/or the need to wake up and pass urine more than twice during the night. It is an extremely common problem which may reflect some underlying urinary or gynaecological problem, or may be associated with nothing more complicated than excessive fluid intake.

Frequency is common in the following conditions:

- As an accompaniment to urinary tract infections;
- During the first trimester of pregnancy, when the enlarging uterus is still contained in the pelvis and exerts pressure on the bladder;
- As a pressure effect of tumours, particularly ovarian cysts;
- As a result of local irritation from other inflammatory conditions in adjacent organs (endometriosis, ectopic pregnancy, pelvic inflammatory disease, appendicitis, radiotherapy to the pelvic area).

All these conditions may also be accompanied by dysuria.

Dysuria

Dysuria is defined as painful micturition. It can be caused by any condition resulting in irritation or inflammation of the bladder and urethra, including infection, and is usually accompanied by frequency. Typically women describe 'burning' or 'scalding' pain on micturition which may last several days, which tends to recur, and is sometimes accompanied by surprapubic pain. They may notice that the urine is cloudy and offensive during attacks. Cloudiness is due to the presence of leucocytes (*pyuria*). Offensive odour indicates that inflammation is due to bacterial infection. Most urinary pathogens are Gram-negative, and many are associated with a typical odour. *Pseudomonas*, for example, has a characteristic fishy smell. Severe inflammation may be accompanied by frank bloodstaining (*haematuria*).

Urinary tract infection

■   Hazel agreed that Rajinder appeared to have experienced several episodes of urinary tract infection which should be investigated as soon as possible. Although she was unable to persuade Rajinder to visit her own (male) GP, she was able to arrange for her to be transferred to another practice where she could see a female doctor. Since Rajinder was hoping to become pregnant soon, it was appropriate that she should receive professional advice from someone with whom she felt comfortable, whether discussing her health needs or receiving physical care. Hazel arranged for her to return to the Well Woman Clinic to discuss the care she would receive during pregnancy and how best to prepare for it (preconceptual counselling). A specimen of Rajinder's urine was sent for bacteriological screening.

Bacteriological investigations

Although bacteriological investigations are so commonly performed, collecting an uncontaminated specimen of urine from a female subject is often poorly executed. It may require a considerable degree of ingenuity if the woman is bedbound or otherwise unco-operative and, even if she is able to assist, much will depend on clear instructions. The nursing actions and rationale are shown in Table 11.2.

Interpretation of the findings of bacteriological investigation frequently seem to cause problems, especially as any contaminating bacteria may rapidly multiply in warm urine and result in a false positive result.

A result is more likely to reflect a genuine urinary tract infection rather than contamination if the patient complains of the classic symptoms of urinary tract infection, and if the specimen contains leucocytes indicating that inflammatory response has occurred. If the infection is genuine, it is more likely that the specimen will contain large numbers (at least 10^5 per millilitre of urine) of bacteria of *one* kind rather than fewer bacteria of several different kinds (see Fig. 11.8). The presence of

Table 11.2 Collecting a clean catch specimen of urine

Nursing action	Rationale
1. Use a sterile receptacle and specimen container	To avoid growth of extraneous bacteria that may confuse diagnosis
2. Cleanse (or ask the woman to cleanse) the external genitalia with sterile water or normal saline	To reduce the likelihood of contamination of the specimen. Disinfectants must *not* be used as they may irritate the delicate urethral and vulval mucosa
3. Ask the patient to micturate with the labia separated, catching the middle part of the specimen in the sterile receptacle	Avoids contamination of the specimen
4. Send to the laboratory immediately or store at 4°C for a few hours if necessary before dispatch	Many bacteria can divide once every thirty minutes; delay results in false positive diagnosis

large numbers of epithelial cells from the urethra suggests that cleansing was probably inadequate before the specimen was obtained. This is further evidence of possible false positive diagnosis.

Nurses may give women experiencing dysuria the following information:

- Drink at least three litres of clear fluids every day – different flavours are important to help give variety.
- Take paracetamol for pain.

CLINICAL MICROBIOLOGY			
SURNAME PATEL	FIRST NAME RAJINDER	DATE COLLECTED 20.02.1988	TIME COLLECTED 14.30
D.O.B. 1.5.68	Mr. Mrs. <u>Miss</u>	DESTINATION OF REPORT Well Women Clinic	LAB. REF: XY002 FE
~~CONSULTANT~~/G.P. WWC	WARD/G.P. PRACTICE Well Women Clinic	SIGNED. APK.	
INVESTIGATION Microscopy, culture and sensitivity please			
CLINICAL DETAILS Complaining of episodic dysuria and frequency urine sometimes offensive. Appearance today – cloudy.		Is patient taking antibacterial drugs? YES (NO) During previous week? YES (NO) If Yes, supply details below: —	

		RESULT White blood cells + + +
		        Epithelial cells –
		        E. coli 10^5/ml.
		        sensitive to gentamycin,
		        nitrofurantoin, co-trimoxazole.	

Figure 11.8 Bacteriology form and result.

- Avoid acidic foods and fluids (citrus fruits, vinegar, cola and most carbonated drinks) as these make dysuria worse (NB aspirin is acidic).
- Mild alkalis can help relieve the burning discomfort. Mixture of potassium citrate (*Mis. Pot. Cit.*) is a mildly alkaline suspension which can be purchased without prescription, but many women object to its bitter taste. This can be overcome by taking a proprietary medicine such as cymalon, specially designed to help relieve dysuria. In an emergency a solution of sodium bicarbonate (one teaspoon in a glass of water) will help.
- Go to the GP as soon as possible.

Urinary tract infections are extremely common in women because of the female anatomy (short urethra opening close to the perineal area) but, in both sexes, the bladder has remarkably few defences against invading pathogens. Its immune defence mechanism is weak because glomerular filtration in the nephrons prevents large, complex molecules entering the urine. This means that antibodies, which help the body destroy foreign proteins, are prevented from entering the urinary tract. A bladder damaged by surgical instrumentation (including catheterisation) or radiotherapy is even more likely to become infected.

Although urinary tract infections are common, they should not be dismissed lightly, especially if recurrent. There is a danger that bacteria may migrate up the ureters to the kidneys resulting in *pyelonephritis* and permanent renal damage. Women who experience recurrent episodes of urinary tract infection require full urological investigation, including intravenous urogram and cystoscopy. In severe cases renal function tests may be necessary. Many people admitted to hospital each year develop urinary tract infections as a result of catheterisation (Meers *et al.* 1981). A small but significant proportion die from septicaemia as a direct consequence and many others suffer prolonged ill health (Clifford 1982). The urine of all pregnant women is screened for urinary pathogens to help detect potential problems early.

Urethral syndrome (honeymoon cystitis)

Women often develop dysuria after their first experience of sexual intercourse, partly due to local trauma and partly because the friction of the penis on the female urethra forces bacteria upwards into the bladder. Sometimes discomfort persists for 24–36 hours and pain accompanies micturition after repeated attempts at coitus, even though the results of bacteriological investigations are negative.

Women may find the following advice helpful:

- Drink three or four glasses of clear fluids just before intercourse is expected;
- Empty the bladder immediately after intercourse;
- Always maintain a good fluid intake (two to three litres daily) and empty the bladder every four hours so that bacteria cannot multiply in the collecting urine;
- Follow guidelines for self-care during urinary tract infection if an acute attack results (see page 268).

If the problem is recurrent, an anti-bacterial drug, nitrofurantoin, may be taken on a permanent basis. However, women with urinary tract infections should do as much as possible to help themselves in order to avoid any need for antibiotics as these destroy the body's natural microbiological flora. A woman given antibiotics to treat the burning pain of a urinary tract infection may well develop candidiasis instead. Nitrofurantoin avoids this problem because it is a urinary disinfectant, not an antibiotic. Women with dysuria deserve sympathy and prompt treatment, even if bacteria cannot be isolated from their urine, but indiscrimate antibiotic therapy may cause additional problems without doing much that is positively helpful.

Loss of continence

Loss of continence is thought to be a common problem in the general population as a whole, but especially among women. The practical difficulty of organising research studies and collecting data from large numbers of people about a socially unmentionable and unacceptable subject make precise figures difficult to document. However, a postal survey by Thomas et al. (1982) indicated a prevalence of 8.7 per cent in women between 15 and 64 years compared to only 1.6 per cent in men in the same age range. Among older women, incontinence seemed more likely to be regular than occasional. Only 0.2 per cent of the people who reported themselves incontinent in this study were known to the health or social services, although the provision of pads and other aids represent a major part of their expenditure. Older studies have reported a much higher prevalence of incontinence. Wolin (1969) found that in a sample of over 4,000 student nurses at least 50 per cent reported occasional stress incontinence on physical exertion, and for 16 per cent urinary leakage was a daily occurrence. It is therefore likely that during their professional lives nurses will meet many women who experience this problem. Many feel too ashamed or embarrassed to admit that they have urinary incontinence, and do all they can to hide it. This may result in the woman becoming afraid to venture into society. She may be afraid to sit in public for fear of wetting the seat, and wear dark colours to hide stains (Norton 1986).

■ When Lucy Moss visited the Well Woman Clinic it was apparent that she was worried about a specific problem. She told Freda, one of the lay volunteers, that she had experienced episodes of urinary incontinence since the birth of her last child, sixteen years previously. Coming to the clinic had required all her courage; she had never mentioned her problem to anyone before.

Initially there had been little to discuss, as Lucy leaked urine only occasionally when she coughed, laughed or took vigorous exercise. However matters had become worse over the years and now Lucy seldom went out socially. She no longer participated in active sports and avoided running for the bus. She was concerned about coping with incontinence at work, but could not afford to stop as she was divorced and bringing up two children now in their teens.

Freda recognised that Lucy would definitely require specialist medical help and, as well as detailing the frequency of Lucy's incontinence, she asked her permission for the GP to make a more detailed assessment. She explained to Lucy that information would be asked about the following:

- Past and present medical conditions;
- Surgery, especially gynaecological and urological operations;
- Obstetric history;
- Contraception;
- Her symptoms and their duration in as much detail as she could provide.

Women often find it beneficial to prepare for interviews with health care professionals in this way. Freda suggested that Lucy should write down some of the main points to act as an *aide-mémoire* during the consultation.

Lucy was referred to a urodynamic clinic. Although Freda impressed the importance of this visit upon Lucy and reassured her as far as possible, she was concerned that Lucy might not attend, and she was worried that as a lay helper she had limited information to provide as she had never been to the clinic herself. However, Freda knew from the information given by the Continence Adviser that many qualified and experienced health care professionals know little about this specialist field, a fact that is not surprising as urodynamic investigations are expensive and the service tends to be organised on a regional basis. Remembering that the work of the Continence Adviser involves considerable responsibility for the education of both clients and staff, Freda approached her with a request that Lucy should be visited at home.

The Continence Adviser was able to explain to Lucy that the urologist would perform a full physical examination, including abdominal and pelvic examinations, before urodynamic studies were performed. This is to establish any underlying pathology. Urinary incontinence is sometimes an early indication of a neurological disorder such as multiple sclerosis, which will require further but different investigation. She spent some time explaining the nature of urodynamic investigations as Lucy's co-operation would be required throughout.

Investigations

Videocystogram and micturating cystograms

These are X-ray investigations where use of a radio-opaque medium permits visualisation of bladder functioning (Booth 1983). It is possible to measure pressures outside and inside the bladder as it fills and empties. These pressures are monitored on a graph and the filling bladder is visualised on a television screen (see Fig. 11.9). It is also possible to determine the effectiveness of the internal and external urethral sphincters. From the results it is possible to find the precise cause of urinary incontinence so these tests are regarded as an invaluable diagnostic aid, but they are much

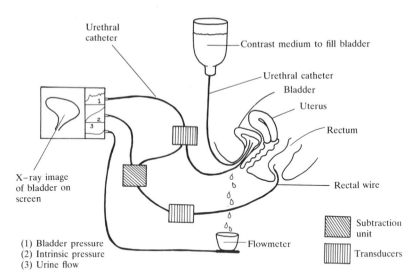

Figure 11.9 Videocystourethrography.

too expensive and invasive for normal screening. They are often distressing for the woman who will have to micturate in front of other people (urologist, nurse, technician) when standing as well as sitting. Success is unlikely unless she can be put at ease.

It is important to provide as much privacy as possible, and to explain clearly what will happen.

Three basic procedures are usually performed:

- Uroflometry (urine flow studies);
- Cystometry (studies of bladder filling and emptying);
- Urethral pressure studies.

Videocystourethrography (synchronous cystometry and urethral pressure studies with video recordings) now combines the two latter procedures.

Uroflometry
When she arrives in the X-ray room, the woman will be asked to pass urine so that the urologist can obtain information about rate of flow. This will involve micturating into a special receptacle with a weight transducer attached to allow electronic recording of rate, volume and pattern of micturition.

Cystometry
The woman will then be helped onto a table and a urethral catheter will be inserted to introduce radio-opaque medium. A fine rectal wire will be introduced to measure pressures inside the rectum. This is necessary because intra-abdominal pressure is transmitted to the bladder, and must be estimated and deducted from the total bladder

recording to give a valid result. The bladder will be filled with medium via the catheter, and the woman asked to say when her bladder feels full or uncomfortable. The amount of medium will be measured and the urologist will observe the filling process on the television screen (*videocystogram*).

Urethral pressure studies

Next the table will be tilted until the woman is standing in a vertical position. She will then be asked to relax, allowing the medium in her bladder to flow out again. Pressures will be recorded during micturition. Bladder neck competence will be assessed by asking her to cough, strain and reproduce any other activity which she has found to accompany incontinence. The catheter and rectal wire will then be removed and the investigations will be complete.

As urodynamic studies involve catheterisation there is some risk of infection, and trauma may cause the urine to appear bloodstained. The woman should be intructed to drink copiously (at least a litre during the twelve hours immediately following the investigation), taught to recognise the symptoms of infection and informed about what action to take if they occur.

Urodynamic studies permit the urologist to distinguish between genuine stress incontinence, which is open to surgical correction, and detrusor instability which is not. In some women the two conditions may co-exist, and the results of urodynamic studies will influence choice of treatment, so their invasiveness and the discomfort caused are justified.

Urinary diaries

The classic definition of urinary incontinence as 'any involuntary loss of urine which constitutes a social or hygienic problem' is difficult to demonstrate objectively because one woman may be able to tolerate a situation that another would regard as unbearable. Although any complaint of urinary incontinence must be regarded seriously, treatment will depend on the extent of the problem since there is no value in exposing the woman to the risks of anaesthesia and surgery if her symptoms could be treated effectively by less drastic measures. Much valuable information can be provided if she keeps a 'urinary diary' (see Table 11.3) which combines an input and output chart with spaces to record frequency, urgency and their association with particular activities.

Table 11.3 Urinary diary

TIME	FLUID DRUNK	URINARY OUTPUT	ACTIVITY
01			
02			
03			

Table 11.3 (cont.)

TIME	FLUID DRUNK	URINARY OUTPUT	ACTIVITY
04			
05			
06			
07			
08			
09			
10			
11			
12			
13			
14			
15			
16			
17			
18			
19			
20			
21			
22			
23			
24			
	TOTAL	TOTAL	

NAME
UNIT/WARD   COMMENTS
HOSP No.
AGE
DATE
DAY OF INVESTIGATION

Types of incontinence

In women these include the following:

- Stress incontinence;
- Detrusor instability;
- Retention of urine with overflow;
- Urinary fistulae.

Stress incontinence

Genuine stress incontinence is defined as the involuntary loss of urine when intra-abdominal pressure is raised as a result of coughing, laughing or any other physical exertion. It is caused by a leakage in the absence of detrusor contraction, and usually occurs due to displacement of the bladder neck which becomes unable to respond normally to sudden increases in intra abdominal pressure (see Fig. 11.10). This may

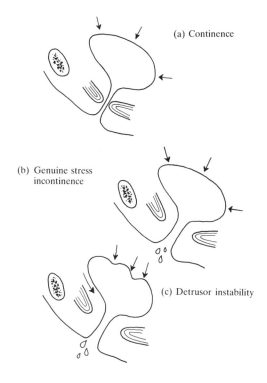

(a) Continence

(b) Genuine stress incontinence

(c) Detrusor instability

⟶ Arrows indicate direction of intra abdominal pressure exerted on the bladder

Figure 11.10 Mechanisms of normal continence and incontinence.

be due to weakening of the pelvic floor during childbirth, urogenital prolapse, ageing or a combination of all three. The following complaints are typical:

- Gradual onset of incontinence after childbirth;
- Leakage after effort;
- Leakage of only a few drops of urine irrespective of the fullness of the bladder.

Available treatments include physiotherapy, drugs and surgical correction.

Physiotherapy
This approach combines exercises (see Chapter 10) to strengthen the muscles of the pelvic floor with electrical stimulation (*faradism*), and is no longer used much today. Kegel (1951) reported that in a series of 500 women with genuine stress incontinence, 75 per cent experienced complete relief of symptoms after 7–8 weeks of physiotherapy. These results are supported by a more recent study of eighteen women in whom physiotherapy was combined with faradism (Moore and Schofield 1967). The beneficial effects can be monitored with a *perineometer*, an instrument consisting of an air-filled balloon placed in the vagina which measures the woman's ability to contract her vaginal muscles. However, longer term studies to evaluate results are lacking. Numerous drugs may help to relieve frequency and mild cases of incontinence. Information is provided in Table 11.4.

Surgical correction
Surgical correction is the treatment of choice for women with severe stress incontinence that has been an increasing problem for some time. Its aim is to elevate the bladder neck above the level of the pelvic floor and increase urethral resistance by giving support to the urethrovesicular junction. Any co-existing uterovaginal prolapse can be corrected at the same time.

Table 11.4 Drugs used in the treatment of urinary frequency and incontinence

Drugs

Propantheline bromide	(Pro-banthine)
Emepronium bromide	(Ceteprin)
Flavoxate hydrochloride	(Urispas)
Terodiline hydrochloride	(Terotin)

Action
All these drugs are anticholinergic. They increase bladder capacity and therefore reduce frequency and incontinence by diminishing unstable detrusor contractions

Side effects
Dry mouth
Thirst
Constipation
Dilated pupils with loss of accommodation

Note: The above list is not exhaustive. For further information and details consult the British National Formulary (new editions published twice-yearly).

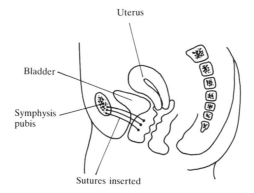

Figure 11.11 Marshall-Marchetti Krantz repair procedure.

Marshall-Marchetti Krantz repair

This operation is performed through a suprapubic incision. The surgeon inserts a
Foley Catheter into the urethra to help identify the bladder neck, then cuts into the
retropubic space. The urethra is dissected free of the surrounding connective tissue
and sutures are inserted on either side through the paraurethral tissues, but not
through the vaginal wall (see Fig. 11.11). The sutures are anchored to the periosteum
behind the symphysis pubis, so the net effect is re-elevation of the bladder neck above
the urethrovesicular junction.

Nursing care

■   Lucy was admitted to the ward the day before surgery to be prepared physically
      and emotionally for a Marshall-Marchetti Krantz repair. During her initial
      nursing assessment, it became apparent that she was concerned about her two
      daughters, aged 16 and 18, who had never been left alone before, and her
      care plan was designed so that she was able to discuss those anxieties.
          Pre-operative care for a woman undergoing a Marshall-Marchetti Krantz
      procedure is similar to that for any major gynaecological operation. However,
      particular care must be taken to warn the woman that she will return to the
      ward with a catheter *in situ* and a wound drain (redivac type). This will drain
      the retropubic space for 24–48 hours, as there is risk of haematoma formation
      and infection. Orem's Model (1985) was used to provide the framework under-
      pinning Lucy's care. Her care plan (Care Plan 11.1, page 278) reveals the
      importance of catheter care, especially the prevention of urinary tract infec-
      tion, one of the major hazards following urological surgery.

Catheter management after urological surgery

Women who have had urological surgery may have a urethral Foley or a suprapubic
catheter *in situ*, although suprapubic catheters are now more widely used as they avoid
the infection risks associated with urethral catheterisation.

Care plan 11.1 (Orem's Self Care model)

Name: Lucy Moss

Treatment/condition: Focus on two problems identified after Marshall-Marchetti Krantz Repair

Developmental Self Care Requisites	Therapeutic Self Care Requisites	Self Care Agency	Self Care Deficits	Nursing Systems	Nursing Agency	Future
(*Universal*) Provision of care associated with elimination	(1) At risk of urinary tract infection (2) Dislikes feeling dependent on nurse for catheter care – says she finds this embarrassing	Understands reason for catheterisation. Would like to be less dependent on nurse. Willing to maintain own fluid balance chart, and has had previous experience with 'urinary diary'	Needs to be shown how to empty drainage bag. Must understand the need for strict hygiene during these procedures. Needs equipment for catheter care	Compensatory/ educative	(a) Supply with equipment for catheter care (b) Demonstrate all aspects of catheter management (c) Monitor Lucy's record keeping daily (d) Obtain catheter specimen of urine for routine bacterial culture and sensitivity	Self caring

(Developmental) Maintain living conditions that promote maturation. Prevent or mitigate conditions that affect human development	Concerned about daughters who have never been left alone at night before. Anxious that she will be regarded as an 'over-protective' mother	Knows that daughters are responsible young adults. Needs to come to terms with their increasing independence	Attitude deficit	Supportive	(a) Allow Lucy to explore her feelings. Identify the main focus of her anxiety (b) Encourage socialisation with other women on the ward with children of the same age (c) Find out from Lucy's daughters how they are coping (visiting time) (d) Offer intervention from social worker as appropriate	Difficulties should resolve

---

Orem's model (1985) seems the most appropriate for planning Lucy's care, given her readiness and ability to participate in her own care. Only two problems have been examined in depth here, to illustrate the special nursing care required following a Marshall-Marchetti Krantz repair, and the particular social problems of this patient. For practice you could complete a full care plan for Lucy, identifying other potential problems. What information would you provide for longer term recovery at home?

Table 11.5 Preventing urinary tract infection in a patient with an indwelling urethral catheter

1. Avoid introducing infection at the time of catheterisation by:
   - Choosing small size catheters with small capacity balloons (avoids irritation of bladder, detrusor contractions and possible expulsion)
   - Aseptic technique during insertion
   - Avoiding recatheterisation (by choice of suitable long-term catheter if necessary, e.g. silastic variety)

2. Avoid introducing infection once the catheter is *in situ* by:
   - Avoiding disconnection of catheter and drainage bag (no spigots, no clamping, no bladder irrigation except to remove debris, specimens taken only from the special sleeve)
   - Ensuring good drainage (no kinking or twisting of tubing, drainage bag always allowed to hang clear of the floor).
   - Minimising risk of ascending infection (empty drainage bag frequently into a clean or sterile receptacle, choose a system with a valve to prevent backflow, never allow the drainage bag to become inverted)
   - Teaching the patient/family to look after the catheter, avoiding pulling, need to perform perineal toilet. Ensuring patient/family can recognise the signs and symptoms of urinary tract infection and know what action to take

3. Encourage adequate fluid intake. Monitor amount and character of urinary output (patient/family can be taught this)

Whichever regime is employed, the risk of cross-infection can be reduced if the woman is taught to clamp her own catheter and empty her drainage bag. Most need little encouragement to become responsible for their own fluid balance measurements because of their previous experience with the urinary diary.

During surgery the bladder neck is bruised, resulting in loss of tone and loss of desire to micturate. Several days may pass before voiding can occur normally and the catheter can be removed. Women need a great deal of encouragement and support, especially as they may see others admitted for different operations on the same day progressing more rapidly.

The site of insertion of the suprapubic catheter into the abdominal wall is a surgical wound and should be treated as such. The catheter is either taped or stutured into position and the area is covered with a sterile keyhole dressing.

Besides the Marshall-Marchetti Krantz repair, several other operations may be attempted to relieve stress incontinence. Two of these – repair of uterovaginal prolapse and buttressing of the bladder neck – have already been discussed (see Chapter 10).

Burch's colposuspension
This is similar to the Marshall-Marchetti Krantz repair procedure, except that the utures inserted on either side of the bladder neck and urethra are passed through the ravaginal fascia, then anchored into the ileopectinal (Cooper's) ligaments (Fig. 2). As well as raising the urethra and bladder neck to restore the urethrovesicular ion, this procedure elevates the vaginal vault, so any co-existant anterior vaginal prolapse is simultaneously repaired.

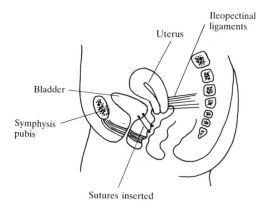

Figure 11.12 Burch colposuspension repair procedure.

Aldridge's sling operation

This classic sling operation (Fig. 11.13) is employed mainly when earlier attempts at surgery have been unsuccessful because it combines suprapubic and vaginal approaches. The surgeon incises the anterior vaginal wall, and dissects the urethra and bladder neck free of their surrounding connective tissues. A suprapubic abdominal incision then gives access to the two rectus abdominis muscles, and a strip of fascia is raised from each. These are threaded through the incision in the anterior vaginal wall and sutured together, forming a sling to support the bladder neck. Anterior and posterior repair may be performed at the same time if necessary.

The success rate of these operations is variable. Stanton (1986) claims an 86 per cent success rate for women followed up for two years after colposuspension procedure.

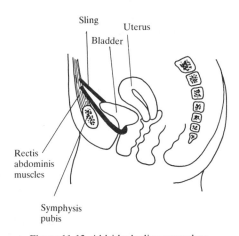

Figure 11.13 Aldridge's sling procedure.

Detrusor instability

Detrusor instability incontinence is caused by muscular irritability of the bladder wall. The woman is unable to control the resulting powerful contractions and, typically, she will complain as follows:

- *Urgency* – the sudden, irresistible desire to empty her bladder;
- *Urge incontinence* – voiding of the complete bladder contents, day or night, with little warning;
- *Frequency* – which she often imposes on herself in an attempt to keep her bladder as empty as possible to avoid 'accidents';
- *History of a weak bladder* – possibly with enuresis since childhood.

Full urological assessment is indicated because mild cases may initially be difficult to distinguish from genuine stress incontinence as the leakage may at first occur only in response to increased intra-abdominal pressure. Detrusor instability often develops in association with disorders of the nervous system, which must be ruled out, and as the problem becomes worse the woman may become housebound through the need to keep her bladder perpetually empty.

Bladder drill

The treatment of incontinence due to detrusor instability aims to break the cycle of urgency, frequency and urinary leakage, by increasing the woman's ability to postpone voiding and give her more confidence in her bladder control.

■ Mabel Attley was admitted to the cottage hospital for bladder training on the recommendation of the urologist and Continence Adviser nurse. Mabel was 78, and had been prone to urge incontinence since childhood, although it was now more a problem than formerly. She was mentally and physically alert, but episodes of incontinence restricted her activities inside as well as outside her home. She was widowed and for several years had lived in sheltered accommodation for the retired, where she was very happy. However, Mabel knew that to continue living in her flat she must remain fit and continent. Loss of continence is often the symptom which precipitates hospital admission to long stay wards.

The Continence Adviser visited Mabel at home, helping to prepare her for urodynamic assessment and admission. Her nursing assessment was made with the help of a urinary diary and included details of Mabel's short term memory (which was good), absence of sensory deficits, and the fact that Mabel had no problems with mobility or undressing herself, although she was understandably flustered when she felt the sudden need to void.

The aim of Mabel's treatment was to gradually increase the time between each episode of voiding. The chart used to document her progress was the same as the urinary diary with which Mabel was already familiar, except that her nurse marked the times at which she was permitted to void in big red letters every day. Each day the times were slightly further apart. Mabel's nurse pointed out the changes each morning, making sure that she knew how far she had progressed the day before. This evaluation had not proved successful at the end of the day, for Mabel found the hospital routine tiring and had difficulty concentrating in the evening.

Orem's Model (1985) was used to plan Mabel's care, and part of her assessment and nursing actions are shown on Care Plan 11.2 (page 284).

Mabel stayed in hospital for ten days. Although her condition showed marked improvement, she was grateful for the continued support of the Continence Adviser, as she needed to persevere with a modified regime at home.

The Continence Adviser plays an invaluable role, liaising between hospital and community staff so that clients receive continuity of care. The Continence Adviser was able to inform the district nursing service that Mabel was entitled to supplies of pads and garments and to the services of the Incontinence Laundry should she need them. Although Mabel continued to benefit from her treatment, she felt more confident if her clothes were protected when she was out for any length of time. A wide range of protective garments and appliances are now commercially available, and much of the market research has been conducted by Continence Advisers in association with manufacturers, so that products can be developed to meet consumers' needs.

Retention with overflow

This occurs without detrusor contractions when intravesicular pressure exceeds maximum urethral closing pressure. Urine is lost without warning, especially when the woman is standing or bending. Voiding tends to be followed by a sensation of incomplete emptying and, if performed at this time, catheterisation would reveal the presence of residual urine.

Retention with overflow most commonly results from neurological damage or as a complication of radical pelvic surgery such as Wertheim's hysterectomy (O'Laughlin 1986). Despite episodes of incontinence, the woman may find great difficulty voiding and only small amounts are passed at any one time.

The aim of treatment is to improve bladder function and to eliminate residual urine stagnating in the bladder, where it may lead to recurrent urinary tract infections. Management depends on the cause underlying retention. If incontinence has followed surgery, the problem may be short-lived, improving spontaneously. However, drugs which stimulate detrusor contractions may help (myotonine, distigmine). In cases where detrusor underactivity persists or the urethra proves to be obstructed urethral dilatation or internal urethrotomy may be attempted to increase the diameter of its lumen.

If these measures fail, or if the woman has a neurological disorder, she may learn to manage retention with overflow by a regime of intermittent self-catheterisation. This procedure carries a much lower risk of infection when performed by the woman

Care plan 11.2 (Orem's Self Care model)

Name: Mabel Attley

Treatment/position: Bladder training for detrusor instability

Universal Self Care Requisites	Therapeutic Self Care Requisites	Self Care Agency	Self Care Deficits	Nursing Systems	Nursing Agency	Future
Provision of care associated with elimination	Bladder retraining programme commenced. Occasionally fails to contain urine until appropriate time – sometimes needs to void earlier than planned	Embarrassed about possible incontinence. Understands bladder drill and does believe that bladder retraining is beneficial	Needs emotional support and reassurance	Supportive/ educative	Ensure that Mabel is shown and understands the goal for each day of bladder training programme and can see the times she is allowed to void. Provide encouragement by ensuring that she knows about progress made daily	Modified bladder training programme will be necessary under supervision of Continence Adviser at home

Maintain sufficient intake of fluids	Has asked whether she should decrease fluid intake to avoid episodes of incontinence	Does not appreciate need to maintain adequate hydration. Requires teaching	As above	Supportive/ educative	Check that Mabel has drunk at least two litres of clear fluids daily and understands rationale	Must continue to drink two litres of fluid daily at home

Bladder training is unlikely to be successful unless the patient is able to co-operate and understand the rationale for nursing interventions. Orem's model (1985), with its emphasis on self care, seems a good choice for Mabel – providing she is able to understand and participate. As bladder training will continue at home, longer term evaluation by the Continence Adviser will be important.

Turn to page 287 where the case study of Rose Boxall is presented. You could develop a care plan for her continued care at home having read this material carefully. Would Orem's model be appropriate? Give reasons.

herself outside the hospital environment, and it is then regarded as a clean rather than an aseptic procedure. The woman learns to identify the urethral orifice with the aid of a mirror and to introduce a fine gauge catheter which is afterwards rinsed with tap water and stored dry between use. Once the technique has been mastered, the incidence of complications are few, and the woman may well find that her personal life is minimally disrupted compared to the effects of sudden incontinence.

Urinary fistulae

A fistula is an artificial opening between one hollow *viscus* (internal organ) and another. Fistulae may develop between the vagina and urethra or bladder and ureter, leading to continual urinary leakage. Vesicovaginal fistulae are often the consequence of poor obstetric care, especially in developing countries. In the West they may also arise through the unchecked spread of malignant pelvic tumours or following radio-therapy or surgery to remove a malignant growth.

Very small fistulae may heal spontaneously but large defects must be surgically repaired. Success depends on the woman's general condition since healing is impaired by malignancy and inadequate nutrition. Much will depend on general improvement of overall health, including a good diet, bedrest and the provision of continuous bladder drainage until tissue repair is complete.

Congenital deformity is a rare but more easily treated cause of urinary incontinence via vesicovaginal fistulae.

The Urilos test of bladder function

This sytem is used to make objective measurements of the amount of urine lost when quantity is small and otherwise difficult to demonstrate. The equipment consists of a pad applied to the vulva inside a tight-fitting undergarment. It contains electrodes connected to a circuit energised by a low voltage current. A dry electrolyte impregnated in the pad dissolves any urine passed. The woman is asked to simulate normal activities while she is wearing the pad, particularly those resulting in leakage, so that the amount of leakage, if any, can be quantified.

Care of permanent indwelling urethral catheters

A high percentage of patients receive an indwelling urethral catheter at some stage during hospital stay, although the dangers of long-term catheterisation are now widely publicised. They include leakage, blockage, encrustation, bladder spasm and genital oedema (Ferrie *et al.* 1979), all problems related to infection or exacerbated by it. The best way of preventing them is to avoid catheterisation whenever possible, but there are still a few people for whom this may raise more problems than it can solve, and the supervision of patients with indwelling catheters still occupies a great deal of the district nurse's time (Roe 1989).

■   Rose Boxall had a cerebrovascular accident which left her permanently incontinent of urine. Despite the efforts of the staff on the geriatric assessment ward to which she was transferred, Rose was permanently wet and clearly distressed about it. Her husband, Maurice, felt that both he and Rose would prefer to cope with a catheter on a permanent basis than perpetually wet clothing and furnishings when Rose was discharged, so a catheter was reinserted and Maurice learnt to look after it while Rose was on the ward. When she went home, the district nurse supervised Rose's care. She liaised with the ward and, as soon as Rose was at home, explained to Maurice how the care he had given to Rose in the ward could be modified.

In hospital, where several patients on one ward may have a catheter, the risks of cross-infection are much greater, especially as the catheter and drainage system will inevitably be handled by more than one person. In the community, risks of cross-infection are greatly reduced and, if infection does occur, the chance of it being caused by a multi-resistant bacterial strain – difficult to treat with the usual range of antibiotics – is much less.

Resources

Books that can be recommended to clients:

Evans, P. (1979) *Cystitis and How to Cope With It*, London: Granada.

Feneley, R.C.L. and Blannin, J.P. (1984) *Incontinence: Help for an Unmentionable Problem*, Patient Handbook No. 18, Edinburgh: Churchill Livingstone.

References

Booth, J. (1983) *Handbook of Investigations*, London: Harper and Row.

British National Formulary No 14 (1987) London: British Medical Association and Pharmaceutical Society of Great Britain.

Clifford, C.M. (1982) 'Urinary tract infection. a brief selective review', *International Journal of Nursing* 19, pp. 213–22.

Feneley, R.C.L. (1986) 'Normal micturition and its control' In: Mandelstam, D. (ed.) *Incontinence and its Management*, London: Croom Helm, pp. 16–34.

Ferrie, B.C.T. *et al.* (1979) 'Long term catheter drainage', *British Medical Journal* 286, pp. 1946–7.

Hinchliff, S. and Montague, S. (1988) *Physiology for Nursing Practice*, London: Ballière Tindall.

Kegel, A.H. (1951) 'Physiological therapy for urinary stress incontinence', *Journal of American Medical Association* 146, pp. 915–17.

King's Fund Project Paper (1983) *Action on Incontinence*, London: King's Fund Centre.

Meers, P.D. *et al.* (1981) 'Report of the national survey of infection in hospitals', *Journal of Hospital Infection* 2, pp. 23–8.

Moore, T. and Schofield, P.F. (1967) 'Treatment of stress incontinence by maximum perineal electrical stimulation', *British Medical Journal* 3, pp. 150–1.

Norton, C. (1986) 'Care plan for an incontinent woman, using Orem's self care model' In: Webb, C. (ed.) *Using Nursing Models: Women's Health*, Sevenoaks: Hodder and Stoughton, pp. 112–26.

O'Laughlin, K. (1986) 'Changes in bladder function in the woman undergoing radical hysterectomy for cervical cancer', *Journal of Obstetric, Gynaecological and Neonatal Nursing* 15(5), pp. 380–5.

Orem, D.E. (1985) *Nursing Concepts of Practice*, 3rd ed. New York: McGraw-Hill.

Roe, B. (1989) 'Catheters in the community', *Nursing Times* 85 (36), pp. 43–4.

Smith, J. (1982) 'Editorial: the problem of incontinence', *Journal of Advanced Nursing* 7, pp. 409–10.

Stanton, S.L. (1986) 'Gynaecological aspects' In: Mandelstam, D. (ed.) *Incontinence and its Management*, London: Croom Helm, pp. 55–75.

Tattersall, A. (1985) 'Getting the whole picture', *Nursing Times* 81 (14), pp. 55–8.

Thomas, T.M. *et al.* (1982) 'Prevalence of urinary incontinence', *British Medical Journal* 281, pp. 1243–5.

Wolin, L.H. (1969) 'Stress incontinence in young, healthy, nulliparous female subjects', *Journal of Urology* 101, pp. 545–9.

12   Neoplasms of the Female Genital Tract

This chapter is divided into two parts: a general introduction explaining the behaviour and nature of neoplastic diseases, then a section demonstrating the treatment and nursing needs of women with specific malignant disorders.

Neoplastic disease

The word *neoplasm* ('new growth') is used by pathologists when referring to *any* swelling or tumour, whether malignant or not. Traditionally, however, tumours have been classified according to whether they are malignant or benign, although these groups may overlap. In time a benign tumour may undergo malignant change. Even if it does not, it may destroy its victim by exerting pressure on vital structures, disrupting normal functions. Nevertheless, a number of distinctions can be made between malignant and benign lesions, summarised in Table 12.1. It is important to remember that most of these differences are relative. The critical distinction is that malignant growths have the ability to develop secondary deposits (*metastases*) in distant parts of the body, whereas benign tumours do not (Petot 1986, page 28).

Although this chapter is concerned with benign as well as malignant neoplasms, much of the discussion will focus upon the care of women who have developed malignant disease, because numerous benign conditions have been described in earlier chapters (for example: *polyps*, Chapter 1; *fibroids*, Chapter 7).

The incidence of malignancy

In the Western world the most common cause of death is cardiovascular disease (heart attack and stroke). Mortality from malignant disease is second only to these. The latest statistics of incidence in the UK are for 1983 (HMSO 1986). They reveal that in 1983, 242,540 cases of malignancy were diagnosed. On this basis it can be forecast that one in three people will develop cancer at some time in their lives. However, cancer is mainly a disease of old age, and more than 70 per cent those diagnosed in 1983 were already at least 60 years old. Only a few cancers account for more than 50 per cent of all new cases but those affecting the breast and female reproductive tract feature prominently among them. Table 12.2 shows the incidence of cancers in the female population for 1983, mortality and five-year survival rate.

Table 12.1 Comparison of the characteristics of benign and malignant tumours

Benign	Malignant
Usually surrounded by a discrete capsule. May therefore be 'shelled out' of surrounding tissues	Not usually encapsulated. Not easily 'shelled out' of surrounding tissues
Usually non-invasive	Invasive
Highly differentiated	Poorly differentiated
Little evidence of recent cell divisions	Considerable evidence of cell divisions
Slow growing	Often rapidly growing
No metastases	Metastases

In general, the earlier malignancy is detected, the greater the chance of surviving five years or more. It is sometimes argued that the high incidence of cancers of the breast and female reproductive tract reflect changing patterns of childbearing and lactation in developed countries, since these tumours are often hormone dependent.

Many women who have developed malignant disease are nursed each year on gynaecology and general surgical wards, so nurses who work in these areas require sound knowledge of neoplastic disease and the principles underpinning treatment. Even larger numbers of women are bound to encounter others who have malignancy

Table 12.2 Cancer statistics in the UK

	Incidence (%) 1983		Rank incidence in female population	Mortality (%) 1984		Rank mortality in female population	Rate per million in UK	Five year survival rate
BREAST	24410	20	1	15070	20	1	844	64%
OVARY	5130	4	6	4290	6	5	177	27%
CERVIX	4400	4	8	2200	3	8	152	57%
UTERUS	3720	3	9	1143	no figs provided	15	128	72%

Notes: Total incidence of malignancy in the female population in the UK (1983) = 124,170. Total mortality from malignant disease in the female population in the UK (1985) = 75,970.

Information in this table is obtained from Cancer Registries set up by the DHSS in 1962, which report annually. However, there is no statutory requirement to report details of cancer registrations so the incidence of malignancy seen here may be under-estimated. Mortality statistics may also be unreliable because it is often difficult to determine the exact cause of death, especially in older people who are likely to suffer from several degenerative conditions simultaneously, of which cancer may only be one.

Sources:
1. HMSO (1986) *Cancer Statistics: Registrations. England and Wales 1983.*
2. HMSO (1985) *Mortality Statistics: Cause. England and Wales 1984.*
3. Cancer Research Campaign (1987) *Facts on Cancer.* Collates figures from England and Wales with those from Scotland and Northern Ireland, citing sources of all figures.

or hear of somebody who has died of it, and may be reminded of their own susceptibility when they attend cervical or breast screening clinics. Nurses working in a variety of different settings must remain alert to their fears and be able to provide information and reassurance realistically in terms women can understand.

Aetiology

Lay people, and sometimes health professionals, talk about 'cancer' as though referring to a single disease, but many different types are known, and it is now accepted that malignancy constitutes a group of different conditions rather than one single disease entity. A 'cure' for cancer cannot and should not be expected since the causative agent(s) in each case is likely to be different. It is now thought that the particular predisposing factors which may combine to increase the chances of developing a given type of cancer in one particular organ system may have little if any influence on the development of another kind of malignancy elsewhere. Just as the causes, treatment and prevention of infectious diseases must be considered separately, so must cancers (Doll and Peto 1981).

Numerous theories of carcinogenesis have been proposed. Malignant change is a complex process, probably dependent on the interplay of several triggering agents rather than one single factor.

Theories of carcinogenesis

Malignancy arises as a genetic change in a single cell, transmitted to its daughter cells when it divides. Scientists have therefore focused considerable attention on factors known to influence genetic material.

Viruses
Viruses are minute obligate parasites consisting of a core of genetic material (DNA or RNA) surrounded by a protein coat. Ability to survive outside host tissues is variable, but none are active or able to reproduce unless within a living cell. The old theory of viruses as a cause of cancer is as follows. When a virus attacks a host cell, it injects its genetic material into the cell, leaving its protein coat redundant on the surface. The viral genetic material then attaches to the host DNA and assumes control of the cell. Sometimes the host is directed to synthesise new viruses. When they mature, the host cell dies and they are liberated to infect new ones. In other cases, viral genetic material remains locked into that of the host, controlling the cell but not destroying it. Newer theories suggest that virus DNA may activate *oncogenes*, sequences of DNA already in the host (Clarke 1987).

In many laboratory animals injections of filtrate containing virus particles have resulted in the development of cancer over a period of weeks or months. Although this direct cause and effect relationship has never been verified in human subjects (for obvious ethical reasons), and it is apparent that no cancer can be transmitted in the same way as the classic infectious diseases, virus particles have been isolated from malignant cells. There is some evidence to suggest that women who have previously been infected with the herpes virus and human papilloma virus are at greater risk of later developing carcinoma of the cervix, for example.

Chemical agents

Exposure to carcinogenic agents has long been recognised as a potential cause of cancer. In many instances these have proved to be industrial chemicals (dyes, solvents) excreted via urine, increasing risk of carcinoma of the bladder. Once these noxious agents have been identified, steps can be taken to control or eradicate them or screen the population at risk. In other cases, the carcinogen is a recreational substance such as tobacco, and attempts to reduce public exposure have met with significantly less success, even though there is now evidence that at least one other malignancy, carcinoma of the cervix, may develop in addition to lung cancer (Trevathan *et al.* 1983).

Occasionally clinical treatment has resulted in malignancy. Adolescent daughters of women given the synthetic hormone diethystilboestrol in early pregnancy to avert miscarriage later developed vaginal cancer.

Radiation

The incidence of leukaemia in radiologists in the first half of the century demonstrated the carcinogenicity of ionising radiation. There are recognised sources of this hazard today:

- Natural sources (cosmic rays, etc.);
- Radioactive contamination due to nuclear explosions and nuclear plants;
- Medical irradiation (radiotherapy, radiological investigations).

Cells are damaged because radioactive particles disrupt DNA. Today every care is taken to ensure that the public is not exposed to dangerous levels, especially people undergoing medical treatments and those responsible for their care. Nevertheless, there is some evidence that breast and uterine cancers may be at least partly dependent on exposure to ionising radiation (Petot 1986).

Heredity

Few cancers are inherited in the same predictable way as eye colour (Mendelian inheritance) or blood clotting disorders (sex-linked inheritance), but there is some evidence that members of particular families stand greater than average risk of developing malignancy. A woman is more prone to breast cancer if another female blood relative (especially her mother) is affected, but the relationship is by no means clearcut and impossible to disentangle from other risk factors in the environment to which members of the same family may all have been exposed.

Harsanyi and Hutton (1983) suggest that one possible risk factor may result from over-active secretory glands, presumably because this results in over-production of some carcinogenic substance. Women who develop breast cancer often have profuse bodily secretions, especially cerumen. Runny ear wax, a harmless trait, is therefore said to be a 'genetic marker' for breast cancer but this does *not* indicate that every woman with the genetic marker will develop the disease.

Race and geographical factors

Race and country of origin have some influence on predisposition to certain cancers, but these effects are difficult to disentangle from heredity. Japanese women have a much lower incidence of breast cancer than those born in Britain or the USA, but the reason is obscure. Diet or some other factor related to lifestyle may be implicated as incidence is seen to increase among Japanese immigrants in the USA. There is an extremely low incidence of cervical carcinoma among orthodox Jews, perhaps because men are circumcised and number of sexual partners restricted (Priden and Lilienfield 1971). As viral transmission is believed to be a major factor in the development of this disease these factors may operate by reducing women's chances of encountering possible transmissible agents. Other influential behaviour possibly includes strict hygienic practice. Intercourse is forbidden within seven days of menstruation and for a specified length of time after parturition.

Injury and inflammation

Years ago, before the availability of effective treatment, it was not uncommon for cancers to ulcerate through the skin, giving rise to offensive discharge. Not surprisingly, malignancy became associated with inflammation, but genuine relationship is hard to establish, especially as chronic tissue damage is much less likely to be allowed to proceed unchecked today. There is a myth that knocking or otherwise damaging the breast could result in cancer, but this has never been verified and seems unlikely.

Immunity

It is widely believed that the immune system protecting the body against infection and other extraneous harmful substances may also provide some measure of protection against cancers. According to this hypothesis, potentially malignant cells are continually produced but destroyed by 'killer' cells circulating in the blood. Presumably malignancy develops when exposure to a carcinogen is so great that the immune response is overwhelmed, in the same way that individuals are able to withstand infection on some occasions but not others. Victims of HIV develop characteristic malignancies as well as infections and it is known that the virus directly attacks T helper cells of the immune system.

Hormones

It has been known for many years that the spread of some cancers could be checked by hormone manipulation, especially if the primary growth involved the breast or genital tract. More recently, it has become apparent that these neoplasms grow only in the presence of hormones, yet the idea that hormones, given therapeutically to menopausal women and as contraceptives, may increase the risk of developing malignancy has been acknowledged only slowly.

Exogenous and endogenous carcinogens
By now it should be apparent that many malignant diseases are at least triggered, if not entirely dependent, upon environmental factors referred to as *exogenous carcinogens*. Cigarettes, industrial chemicals and hormone therapy fall into this category. Internal factors predisposing to malignant change (heredity, defective immune system, hormones secreted by the body itself) are said to be *endogenous*.

Heath education: avoiding cancer

Doll and Peto (1981) point out that as so many cancers depend at least to some extent on exogenous factors, they should in theory be avoidable. Epidemiological studies can help identify individuals at risk and precautions are often possible before the long battle to identify the causative agent has been won; for example, those whose work brings them into contact with large numbers of different chemicals can wear protective clothing. The whole topic of cancer prevention is highly emotive and politically charged. Many people would argue that no member of the public should be expected to work in *any* environment even remotely likely to promote carcinogenesis (Mitchell 1984). Unfortunately, new potential carcinogens are continually identified. Even so, governments to date have had more success in promoting safer conditions in industry than in persuading the public to abandon equally harmful recreational practices, especially smoking. In view of this, Doll and Peto (1981) wisely point out that although many cancers are theoretically avoidable, this is not the same as claiming that at present they are preventable.

Since cancer represents a group of diseases, with manifestation in any given subject likely to be caused by a number of interacting factors, it is not logical to talk about 'preventing cancer' or searching for a universal cure. Methods of detection also vary, but if the tumour is to be eradicated and the individual is to recover, the growth must be discovered early, while it is still pre-invasive. Potentially screening programmes could do much to reduce the incidence of some cancers. The principles behind screening have already been outlined (see Chapter 1) taking cervical cancer as an example. Screening for breast cancer is discussed in Chapter 13.

Having considered the incidence and aetiology of cancers in general, it is now possible to consider the natural history of neoplastic disease. It is important for nurses to have this knowledge, as it is not otherwise possible to understand principles of treatment and therefore provide information to patients and their families. The behaviour of malignant cells is more readily appreciated given an understanding of the growth and development of normal tissues.

The structure of normal cells

The cells of all living organisms (excluding bacteria) contain a nucleus enclosing the genetic material (DNA) which exists in the form of long strands tightly coiled to form chromosomes (see Fig. 12.1). DNA controls all cellular activities by directing protein

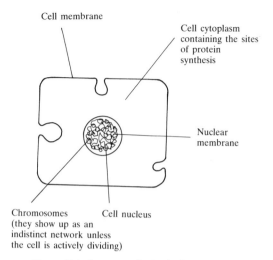

Cell membrane

Cell cytoplasm
containing the sites
of protein
synthesis

Nuclear
membrane

Chromosomes   Cell nucleus
(they show up as an
indistinct network unless
the cell is actively dividing)

Figure 12.1 Structure of a 'typical' normal cell.

synthesis. As proteins make up the structural elements of the cell (the membranes and organelles in its cyptoplasm, as well as all the enzymes it is able to secrete), DNA is responsible for both appearance and cellular behaviour. The vast amount of information required to exert control is coded by the arrangements of chemical units making up the long DNA strands.

Protein synthesis takes place in the cytoplasm, but DNA never leaves the nucleus. Its information is transferred to the cytoplasm by a second type of molecule, also large and complex, called ribonucleic acid (RNA, see Fig. 12.2).

Cell growth

The cell is the basic unit of all living organisms. Growth begins at fertilisation when the nuclei of the egg and sperm unite. The fertilised egg grows by a process of cell division called mitosis, in which the total number of chromosomes and DNA remain the same for every new cell. At each division the parent produces two identical daughter cells because DNA duplicates beforehand. Half the new chromosomes go to each daughter. The growing embryo therefore increases both in size and total cell number.

Differentiation

The cells of the developing embryo begin to take on specialist functions, giving rise to tissues and organ systems. Cellular specialisation, called *differentiation*, is controlled by mechanisms exerted on DNA; some parts are depressed so they become non-functional, while others are activated to initiate RNA synthesis and generation of new proteins. Thus erythrocytes are activated to produce haemoglobin, but are unable to secrete digestive enzymes because this part of their DNA has been repressed. The mechanisms responsible for repression and activation in human cells are not understood at present.

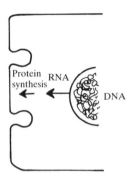

Figure 12.2 Pathway of cellular control mechanisms.

Up to this point, discussion has proceeded for a 'typical' cell, but there is no typical cell in the entire human body. All the cells of an individual are genetically identical, but activity varies according to the state of the DNA. However, some cells are more highly differentiated than others: a nerve cell, for example, has become much more specialised than a skin cell.

Cells divide very swiftly in the embryo, as this is the most rapid period of growth in the life of the individual. Frequent divisions continue as the child grows, but gradually cease as maturity is reached, except in those tissues perennially subject to wear and tear where replacement is continually necessary (skin, gut lining). Differentiation also continues in some tissues throughout adult life: cells in the bone marrow continually divide to give rise to different classes of blood cells. Cells, eternally capable of giving rise to new progeny, are regarded as relatively undifferentiated. Highly differentiated cells such as neurones lose ability to divide in the embryo. The tragic consequences of brain and spinal cord lesions occur because of the inability of neurones to replace themselves.

Malignancy: differentiated and undifferentiated cancers

Malignant cells seem to escape from the normal repression control mechanisms exerted on their DNA. Instead of orderly divisions and differentiation, they reproduce haphazardly and may eventually cease to resemble the original parent tissues. Degree of differentiation has important bearing on the patient's outlook. Cancers that are similar to their parent tissues (*highly differentiated*) are usually of lower grade malignancy than those which have become dissimilar (*poorly differentiated*). A poorly differentiated (*anaplastic*) tumour generally carries a poor prognosis. DNA in such cells may behave inappropriately; hence cancer cells in the lung may release hormones normally released by the anterior pituitary.

The manner in which these abnormalities arise can only be speculated upon at the present time, but the behaviour of normal cells during periods of rest and activity

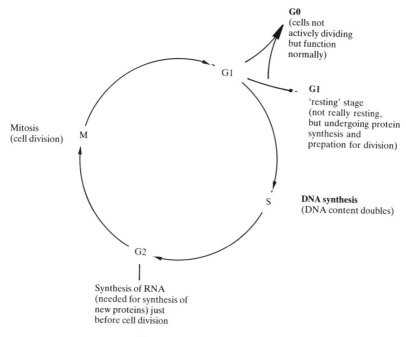

Figure 12.3 The cell cycle.

enhance understanding of the principles behind cancer treatment, especially radio-therapy and chemotherapy.

Cell kinetics

Cells do not begin and cease activity in a random fashion. Figure 12.3 shows that bursts of intense activity are followed by quiescent periods, a sequence of alternating events referred to as the cell cycle.

The time of cell division (*mitosis*) is called the *M phase*. It is followed by the *Gl phase*, described as the 'resting phase', although far from being inactive the cell is synthesising new proteins. DNA content doubles during the subsequent *S phase*, and in the *G2 phase* RNA is generated, ready to promote renewed protein synthesis in the daughter cells once mitosis has again taken place.

Different phases of the cell cycle require variable lengths of time for completion. Some, particularly the Gl phase, vary considerably according to the type of cell concerned. Those dividing slowly (whether malignant or normal) tend to have an extended Gl phase, whereas those dividing rapidly have brief Gl phases, sometimes none at all.

Returning to Fig. 12.3, it is seen that some cells are in a *GO phase*, temporarily outside the cell cycle. They are not actively dividing although they continue to function normally. Length of time spent in the GO phase is variable. Some cells (neurones, striated muscle) remain in the GO phase throughout their entire adult life, while others (bone marrow, skin) scarcely enter it.

Methods of treating malignant disease

For many years it was believed that cancer cells grew at the expense of normal tissues because they were able to divide more rapidly than non-malignant ones. This is now known to be erroneous. In adulthood, normal cells divide only to replace those that have died or become damaged, so the population of normal cells will always remain constant. Cancer cells divide *irrespective* of need for tissue replacement or repair because they have lost the cellular control mechanism that would ordinarily keep them in check. The cell population of a malignant growth therefore increases.

Chemotherapy and radiotherapy have the capacity to destroy all living cells, whether normal or malignant, by disrupting DNA. However, malignant cells take longer to recover than normal ones, so with repeated carefully monitored exposures the number of malignant cells should decline while normal ones return to pre-treatment levels. Some types of malignancy are most responsive to radiotherapy, others to chemotherapy. In many cases it is, of course, possible to remove cancers surgically and, depending on location and extent of the disease, this may be the primary choice of treatment. The particular treatment regime decided by the surgeon or oncologist will therefore be affected by a number of factors, not least by the patient's general health, age and outlook. Although several women with the same type of cancer may be admitted to the same ward, it is likely that they will receive different treatment protocols, reflecting individual need. Unless nurses understand factors influencing choice of treatment, they will be unable to provide women with information and education.

Natural history of pre-malignant and malignant disease

Observation of cellular behaviour has shown that cells undergo a series of alterations in appearance and behaviour before they can be regarded as overtly neoplastic. These have been classified as *hyperplasia*, *metaplasia* and *dysplasia*.

Hyperplasia
The term hyperplasia is used to describe excessive cellular proliferation. It is, however, clearly distinguishable from normal cellular increase (such as wound repair, or breast development during pregnancy). The main causes appear to be chronic irritation and hormonal imbalances.

Metaplasia
Metaplasia is change from one type of differentiated tissue to another, usually from high to low differentiation. In smokers, for example, mucus-secreting cells lining the respiratory passages are replaced by flattened squamous epithelium similar to the oral mucosa.

Hyperplasia and metaplasia frequently accompany one another, especially in cases of chronic irritation and occasionally when there is nutritional deficiency.

Dysplasia

Dysplasia is regarded as disordered cellular development, often accompanying metaplasia and hyperplasia, involving certain changes:

- Increased cell divisions;
- Disordered, irregular cellular arrangements.

Although the significance of dysplasia is not fully understood, it does appear to predispose the individual to malignant change, for dysplasic and malignant cells have been observed to share many similarities. However, malignant change is not inevitable as spontaneous return to the normal condition has been observed.

Pre-invasive and invasive cancers

At first malignant cells remain in the tissue of origin and growth remains localised. This represents the pre-invasive stage of malignancy. If change is detected early and surgical excision is possible, recovery may be absolute, at least in theory. In practice, metastases may already have occurred, even though secondary deposits may not become apparent for months or years.

Ability to metastasise appears to result from loss of a property of normal cells called *contact inhibition*. Cancer cells do not adhere closely together as do normal cells and, because of the ease with which they become detached, they escape from their site of origin. Patients may therefore receive radiotherapy or chemotherapy as an 'insurance policy' against recurrence.

Eventually the cancer begins to behave like an aggressive parasite, demanding more and more of the body's resources for its own development. A scaffolding of connective tissue develops to support it, and local blood supply increases to provide oxygen and nourishment. If the cancer grows very rapidly, it may outstrip its blood supply and the centre of the tumour will then undergo necrosis.

Dividing malignant cells gradually infiltrate normal tissues, including capillaries, and are carried by the bloodstream to new sites as metastases. The lungs, liver and brain, which receive rich blood supplies, are among the most common sites for the development of secondary deposits. Some malignant cells may leak into lymphatic ducts draining tissue fluid from the site of the primary growth, leading to metastatic involvement of the adjacent lymph nodes. The lag phase before development of metastases is very variable.

Patients known to have metastases may receive radiotherapy or chemotherapy as adjuvant therapy (adjuncts to excision of the primary growth). If the disease is progressive, it may not be possible to remove all the primary or hope for 'cure', but quality of life may be improved and sometimes considerably extended by palliative surgery, or by administering radiotherapy as the primary treatment to reduce size of the tumour and relieve symptoms. All methods of treatment have acknowledged side effects, but today they are considerably reduced compared to the situation only a few years ago, and can be even further diminished by resourceful nursing interventions. Moreover, the development of clinical 'staging systems' to relate extent of the disease to likely prognosis has helped oncologists decide the course of treatment likely to be most effective in each individual case.

Nursing care

In the second part of this chapter the care of women with particular types of neoplastic disease will be discussed.

Carcinoma of the vulva

■   Florence Lamb had a hard lump on her vulva which the district nurse noticed when she was helping her into the bath. Florence's husband persuaded her to see the GP but Florence was embarrassed and several weeks passed before she went. The GP arranged for a biopsy to be performed. Its result indicated that the lump was a squamous cell carcinoma.

Incidence and aetiology

Carcinoma of the vulva is a disease of older women – average age of presentation is over 60 years. Some women delay seeking medical help through embarrassment or failure to realise that the problem is serious. A pre-cancerous condition called *leucoplakia* is often associated with the disease, and it is believed that over 50 per cent of women who develop leucoplakia will develop malignancy (see Chapter 6). The most common site for the lesion to develop is on the labia majora, followed by the clitoris, then the vestibule. Lymphatic spread occurs via the inguinal lymph nodes to those in the pelvic cavity, but rate of progression is so variable that there may be little correlation between size of the primary and lymphatic involvement.

Treatment

Pre-invasive lesions may be effectively treated by laser (Brannigan and McCullough 1987). For a slightly larger but localised growth simple vulvectomy may be adequate, but if there is lymph node involvement radical vulvectomy is necessary. This operation involves removal of skin covering the vulva, subcutaneous fat and deep incisions into the groins to dissect out lymphatic tissue. Figure 12.4, which shows the extent of tissue loss, gives some indication of the mutilating nature of this operation. The surgeon may be unable to close the wound completely unless plastic surgery is possible and, as the raw area left (see Fig. 12.5) may take several weeks to heal, risk of infection is considerable. If the woman is too frail to undergo anaesthesia and major surgery, radiotherapy may be performed, but is less effective.

■   Sadly, in Florence's case the extent of lymphatic spread was such that the gynaecologist recommended radical vulvectomy as the most effective treatment option.

    Carcinoma of the vulva is uncommon, so the ward sister organised a

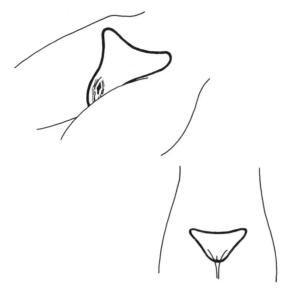

Figure 12.4 Radical vulvectomy: extent of the tissue removed.

teaching session to ensure that staff were familiar with the principles of treatment and nursing care. The effects of radical vulvectomy are such that it is vital for the woman to understand its nature and implications fully before it is performed. The nurse who had looked after Florence in the Outpatient Deparment had already broached this topic, explaining that intercourse is usually still possible, but removal of the clitoris will result in loss of sensation.

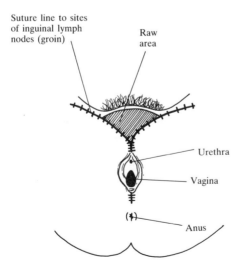

Figure 12.5 Position of the suture line following radical vulvectomy.

When Florence was admitted, the nurses were aware of her need for further information, and alert to recognise her possible reluctance to ask for it spontaneously. One of the student nurses asked if there was a special association to provide help for women undergoing vulvectomy, on the same lines as the Mastectomy Association, but was told by the sister that there is not. The rarity of the disease, perhaps coupled with the age of most sufferers, has failed to attract public attention. Women and their partners rely entirely on the support of health care professionals when vulvectomy is performed, and both require sensitive nursing care.

Florence would remain in hospital for about four weeks after the operation, in the company of women who would in most cases be much younger than herself. She would see them recover and go home long before she was ready to be discharged. A second factor requiring consideration was her reduced mobility due to osteoarthritis. She would therefore require more physical nursing care than the majority of women admitted to gynaecology wards. During their the teaching session, the nurses indentified the following possible post-operative problems for Florence:

- *Shock* – because radical vulvectomy is a long and complicated operation;
- *Pulmonary embolism* related to lack of mobility;
- *Increased risk of wound infection* owing to the site of the wound, the raw area left open and the body's decreasing ability to defend itself against infection with age. The wounds would require drainage for several days, and this also tends to increase the risk of infection. Dressings are difficult to apply in this area and, even if they are highly absorbant, they may rapidly become soaked and have to be re-applied.
- *Urinary tract infection*. The periurethral tissues would be traumatised during surgery and Florence would have difficulty with micturition. She would return from theatre with an indwelling urethral catheter *in situ*.
- *Constipation* as a result of local trauma and reduced mobility.
- *Discomfort from the wound site* which, added to the existing pain of her stiff joints, would further increase reluctance to move.
- *Pressure sores* – with a wound at this site it is extremely difficult to permit adequate pressure relief for the buttocks and sacrum.
- *Local swelling*; following the removal of inguinal lymph nodes tissue fluid cannot drain from the area, especially during periods of inactivity, leading to localised oedema.

Florence did not smoke and would be taught to perform deep breathing exercises, so the students did not feel she would be at particular risk of developing a post-operative chest infection. The sister was not so optimistic, given Florence's probable reluctance to move. She pointed out that Florence would probably be in considerable discomfort, and would need to be convinced of the need to comply with nursing interventions through careful explanation if she was to participate in her own care.

Evaluating their care, the nurses felt that, despite all the problems anticipated, Florence made a good recovery. She accepted the need for early ambulation despite the inconvenience of dressings, drains, catheter and intravenous infusion, and was willing to experiment to find the most effective way of holding the dressings in place so she could walk around the ward. She enjoyed the company of other patients but was grateful for the privacy of her own room as she disliked talking about her illness or the nature of her treatment.

As Florence's recovery progressed, plans were made for her continued rehabilitation at home, using Orem's Model (1985); see Care Plan 12.1 on page 304)

Tumours of the vagina

Primary tumours of the vagina are rare, although invasion may occur directly from a tumour of the cervix or as metastases from distant sites. Until recently, most primary vaginal neoplasms were squamous cell carcinomas mainly in older women, but in recent years malignancy has been reported in young girls whose mothers received hormone therapy during pregnancy. Most reported cases of incidence in very young women have occurred in the USA (Elkington 1986).

Outlook depends on the site of malignancy as this influences metastatic spread. Prognosis is least favourable for those lower in the vagina because malignant cells are more likely to be carried to other sites via the lymphatics. The *Clinical Staging System* (see Table 12.3) shows that very early non-invasive tumours can be completely cured providing they are detected by colposcopy (see page 311). The effects of synthetic hormones given during pregnancy have been well publicised in the medical press, so family doctors are in a good position to identify girls at risk and arrange screening. Older women may be less likely to seek help, especially as vaginal cancer is usually painless until advanced. The most effective treatment combination is then surgery followed by radiotherapy.

Tumours of the cervix

The cervix is affected by two types of cancer: *squamous cell carcinoma* (95 per cent) and *adenocarcinoma* arising from glands lining the cervical os (5 per cent). Figures from OPCS (1986) show that about 4,000 women develop the disease every year and, in 1984, 2,200 died (*Cancer Research Campaign* 1987). Both types of malignancy are detectable by cervical cytology (see Chapter 1) and deaths may therefore be regarded as avoidable. According to the British Medical Association (BMA 1986), rate of cure could reach 100 per cent providing pre-invasive and early malignant lesions are detected sufficiently early.

It is possible to predict those women at particular risk, and an effective screening programme theoretically exists in Britain, but there is evidence that it does not

Care plan 12.1 (Orem's Self Care model)

Name: Florence Lamb

Treatment/condition: Rehabilitation after vulvectomy

Universal Self Care Requisites	*Therapeutic Self Care Requisites*	*Self Care Agency*	*Self Care Deficits*	*Nursing Systems*	*Nursing Agency*	*Future*
Maintain sufficient fluid intake	Will remain at risk of urinary tract infection. When discharged must plan to drink two litres of fluid daily every day	Has been drinking two litres of fluid every day in hospital. Knows how to recognise symptoms of urinary tract infection. Will be able to supply self with fluids at home	Needs to understand the continuing need for high fluid intake at home	Educative	(1) Instruct Florence about the need to maintain high fluid intake at home (2) Review knowledge before discharge (3) Include husband in teaching	Self caring
Maintain sufficient intake of food	Dislikes many high fibre foods (cereals, wholemeal bread). Unlikely to eat these after discharge. Therefore danger of constipation	None at present. *On discharge:* Will need motivation to purchase and prepare appropriate food. Will need knowledge to choose high fibre products she can tolerate	None at present. *On discharge:* Will need to choose appropriate diet	Educative/ supportive	Dietary consultation to include both Florence and husband	Choosing appropriate diet will remain a continuous demand but Florence has capacity to be self caring

Goal	Assessment	Problem	Nursing diagnosis	Nursing system	Nursing action	Expected outcome
Maintain balance between rest and activity	(1) Mobility impaired by longstanding osteoarthritis (2) Further mobility impairment due to bulky dressings (3) Will not acknowledge lack of mobility as a problem. Refuses home help	Finds movement painful, but determined to mobilise. Gradually able to use lighter dressings as wound discharge decreases. Willing to contemplate paid help in the home for 'heavy housework' – shopping/lifting – cleaning floors – washing Husband agrees they can afford to pay	*In hospital*: limited mobility *On discharge*: limited mobility interfering with normal household activities	Supportive/ educative	Explore with Florence and her husband alterations in former lifestyle and changes they will need to make. Ensure Florence receives analgesia to reduce arthritic pain	Help in the home needed indefinitely
Maintain balance between solitude and social interaction	Will miss companionship of nurses and other patients when she goes home	Reduced social interaction on discharge	Potential loneliness	Supportive	Discuss social and recreational opportunities available at home. Plan for discharge appropriately	Has made new friends in hospital, but has never relied on people other than husband for companionship. Does not anticipate problems
Promote normalcy	Visible alteration in body structure. Impact on self concept. Grieving for self and husband. Loss of sexual functioning	Afraid to look at wound or touch it. Distressed for husband to see her disfigurement. They no longer have intercourse often but would like to express affection, and both	Permanent change in body image and sexual functioning	Supportive	Allow Florence to express her feelings to her nurse and her husband. Give both the opportunity to see	Acceptance of loss

grieve that this
operation was necessary

wound when they
feel ready and
come to terms
with effects of
surgery before
discharge

Orem's model (1985) proved a suitable choice for Florence's care after the immediate post-operative period was over. However, the use of a self care model during the earlier stages of recovery might be problematic, especially in an elderly woman, physically very dependent and possibly confused for some days as a result of anaesthesia. A better alternative in this situation might be the model by Roper et al. (1985). Florence's immediate post-operative problems have been highlighted on page 302, although no model has been used. Try developing a care plan for this period using Roper's model. Remember that some objective method should be used to assess Florence's pain and susceptibility to pressure sore development.

This situation tends to suggest that the same model may not be appropriate throughout all the stages of hospitalisation or recovery, especially if rehabilitation is likely to be protracted. The danger of using no model at all is that some aspects of care may be overlooked.

Table 12.3 Clinical staging for vaginal carcinoma

Stage	Clinical presentation	Five year survival rate
0	Confined to epithelium	Curable
1	Confined to vaginal wall	70–80%
2	Invading subvaginal tissue	30–40%
3	Extending to pelvic wall	20–40%
4	Extending to other organs	0–30%

reach women most in need (Yule 1984). However, evidence from other countries with more rigorous, highly organised services suggest that mortality could be reduced considerably.

Griffiths (1983), examining Scandinavian statistics, observed a 30 per cent decline in mortality once women aged 25–70 years had been advised to have smears every alternate year. Evidence collated by the BMA (1986) revealed that in Canada, where annual screening is recommended for those aged 18–35, then at five-yearly intervals until the age of 60, mortality fell by over 25 per cent. The key to success appeared to be development of an adequate recall system. British nurses concerned about cancer prevention and women's health argue that the UK is now lagging behind other Western countries in its endeavours to prevent deaths from cervical cancer (Borely 1985). Several reasons have been suggested:

- Women may be embarrassed or afraid to present themselves for routine smear tests. Knowledge that cervical cancer can be associated with promiscuity is now widely disseminated among the lay public; this may reduce acceptability of the service because stigma is becoming attached to the disease.
- Women may not know that the service is available, or have difficulty locating it.
- The recall system is ineffective.
- Other deficiencies exist within the service, related to finance and disagreement about the optimal frequency for repeating smears.

There is little agreement about the frequency with which smears should be performed. Spriggs and Hussain (1977) suggest that for those under 25 the first smear should be taken during initial consultation for contraception, pregnancy or visit to a special clinic. Sexually active women not in these groups should have their first smear aged 30. According to the National Cancer Control Campaign for Women, smears should be repeated every two or three years until the menopause, and at five-yearly intervals thereafter. However, if time intervals are this long, early manifestations of the disease may be missed as there is evidence that its epidemiological pattern is changing.

Peak age incidence, once 50 years, has now fallen to 35 (Parkin *et al.* 1985). Figures from OPCS (1986) show that incidence and mortality are now increasing among younger women, although overall incidence remains constant. Cervical carcinoma also appears to take a more virulent form in young women, with a shorter lag period

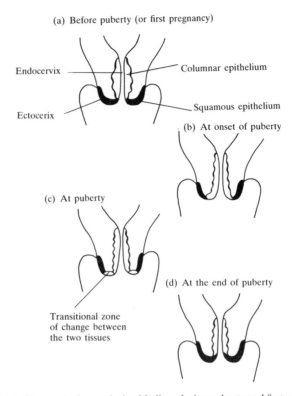

(a) Before puberty (or first pregnancy)

Endocervix

Columnar epithelium

Squamous epithelium

Ectocerix

(b) At onset of puberty

(c) At puberty

(d) At the end of puberty

Transitional zone
of change between
the two tissues

Figure 12.6 Changes in the cervical epithelium during puberty and first pregnancy.

between pre-cancerous lesions and those which are frankly malignant (Wolfendale *et al.* 1983). Screening may begin too late and be repeated infrequently among the young, while older women may be having smears unnecessarily.

Nurses need to be aware of these differences in opinion and provision, because they are very likely to be approached for advice by a public confused by all that has been written and said.

Natural history of cervical cancer
The natural history of cervical cancer has been well documented and helps nurses to understand why some women appear to be more at risk than others.

The cervical canal (*endocervix*) is lined with columnar epithelium, giving way to squamous stratified epithelium over the portion jutting down into the vagina (*ectocervix*). At puberty, under the influence of oestrogen, the zone of columnar epithelium moves outwards to cover the ectocervix, but as adulthood approaches it is again replaced with squamous epithelium (Fig. 12.6). This sequence of events recurs during the first pregnancy and it is at these times of transition that the cervix seems to be most susceptible to damage, explaining why exposure to a potentially carcinogenic agent is then more likely to result in malignant change although it may not manifest immediately.

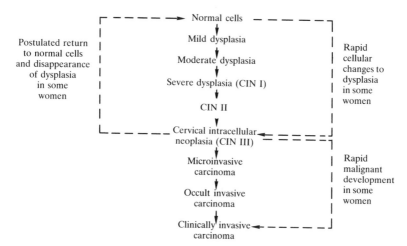

Figure 12.7 Possible natural history of cervical cancer.

Pre-cancerous changes of the cervical epithelium appear to form part of a sequence preceding the development of a frankly malignant lesion, although it appears that return to the normal condition is possible spontaneously (Fig. 12.7).

Cervical intracellular neoplasia (CIN)
In some women, epithelial cells covering the ectocervix begin to divide more often than usual. Microscopic examination reveals abnormally large, dark nuclei and disordered cellular arrangement but clinically no change is apparent and there are no symptoms. This condition cervical intracellular neoplasia, denotes a continuum as follows:

- Mild dysplasia CIN I – return to normal possible;
- Moderate dysplasia CIN II – condition more likely to persist;
- Severe dysplasia CIN III – pre-malignant (see Table 12.4).

Invasion
Once cells have undergone full malignant change (CIN III) they creep over the ectocervix in a thin carpet, but invasion does not occur immediately and the woman is still asymptomatic (Fig. 12.8).

At first invasion is limited, and the disease is described as *micro-invasive*, but the lymphatic and capillary networks gradually become infiltrated, leading to formation of distant metastases and a gradually deteriorating prognosis. Locally, the rectum, vagina and bladder may become infiltrated (Fig. 12.9).

As malignancy progresses clinical symptoms appear, although the disease is usually painless until considerably advanced. Micro-organisms which normally exist harmlessly in the vagina infect the damaged tissues, leading to offensive discharge. Bleeding is also common, especially after coitus. On clinical examination, the cervix now feels hard and stony.

Table 12.4 The cervical intraepithelial (CIN) staging system and the clinical staging system for cervical carcinoma CIN system (premalignant)

Stage	Histological change	Treatment	
CIN I	Mild dysplasia (reversible)	Laser	Completely curable
CIN II	Moderate dysplasia	Laser	
CIN III	Severe dysplasia grading into overt early malignancy, not yet invasive	Laser/cone biopsy	

Stage	Clinical staging malignant	Treatment	Five year survival rate
0	Malignancy not yet invasive	Cone biopsy	Curable
1	Limited to cervix		81%
2	Spread to upper third of vagina/ lower part of uterus	Wertheim's hysterectomy	60%
3	Involvement of parametrium	Radiotherapy	30%
4	Infiltration of bladder/rectum/ distant metastases	Sometimes with palliative surgery	8%

Note: CIN III and Stage 0 of malignant disease overlap.

Once a woman has a positive smear test, she should undergo colposcopy to determine extent of the disease and plan treatment.

■   Sally Carder had a smear taken routinely at the Family Planning Clinic. A few weeks later, she was contacted by her GP to make an appointment to discuss the result, which suggested CIN III. The smear was repeated as false positive results are occasionally given. Meanwhile, Sally was referred to the gynaecologist so that colposcopy could be performed.

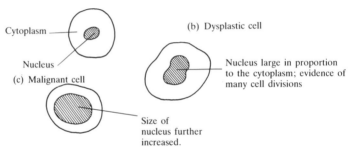

(a) Normal cell (squamous epithelium)

Cytoplasm

(b) Dysplastic cell

Nucleus

(c) Malignant cell

Nucleus large in proportion to the cytoplasm; evidence of many cell divisions

Size of nucleus further increased.

Figure 12.8 Cells from the cervix.

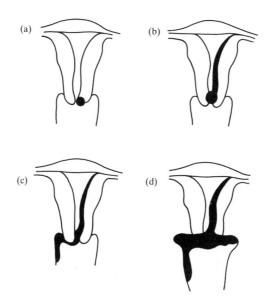

Figure 12.9 Spread of malignant cells in cervical carcinoma.

Colposcopy

The colposcope is a binocular magnifying instrument (increasing vision approximately twenty-fold) used to examine the cervix. The affected area is painted with iodine to help the doctor identify malignant cells, as they stain a different colour from normal tissues. The cervix has a poor nerve supply so it is possible to obtain biopsies without causing undue discomfort.

Although colposcopy is usually painless, women require a great deal of supportive nursing care. As well as worrying about the possible results of investigation, they may feel embarrassed and undignified.

■   Before Sally was examined, the nurse explained that the procedure might be uncomfortable but was not likely to hurt. Sally would be asked to lie on an adjustable table which could be tilted to give different views of the cervix. The doctor would insert a speculum just as though he was going to take another smear, and the surface of the cervix would be painted with iodine solution before the colposcope was used to examine it. A small amount of tissue might be removed for examination in the histology department. If this was necessary, Sally could expect to bleed for a few hours afterwards as the cervix contains many blood vessels. Throughout the procedure, the doctor explained what was happening and two biopsies were taken. Sally was asked to return for the results ten days later.

Coping with stress

Although nervous about having colposcopy, Sally had not waited long for her appointment and had been warned that the smear test result might be falsely positive. She was now aware that at least two patches of abnormal tissue had been detected, and became so anxious at the possible implications that she experienced great difficulty continuing normal life at home with her three young children. Her husband was away at sea so she did not receive a great deal of support, and she avoided discussion with her mother and sister because she knew their concern would reinforce her own. Knowledge that the cells might only be pre-cancerous or the very earliest stages of cancer and could be removed by a straightforward surgical procedure ceased to be reassuring during the long days at home alone.

The word 'cancer' conjures up so many fears and negative expectations in the public mind that it has come to be regarded as synonymous with a painful and untimely end. Sally had absorbed these ideas and the recent more positive information given at the hospital failed to contend with her deep-rooted fears.

As the days passed, it occurred to Sally that, if smear tests occasionally turn out to be inaccurate, this might also be true of other investigations. She was never conscious of making the decision to avoid her appointment, but when the day came it seemed imperative to help her sister, who was redecorating the house, and the need to contact the hospital slipped from her mind.

The sister working in the Gynaecology Department arranged for a second appointment to be sent and, as Sally had not contacted the clinic, she informed the health centre. The result was a visit from the health visitor who had developed a good relationship with the family over a period of several years. At first Sally argued that a mistake must have been made as she had no symptoms and was feeling quite well, then she became fatalistic, saying that if she really had cancer she was bound not to recover. However, the health visitor was able to persuade her that no good would come of refusing to hear the colposcopy results, and arranged to accompany Sally to the clinic.

Women employ a variety of different coping strategies when confronted with stressful life events. Some find out everything possible about a problem, others manage to hide their fears even to themselves (*repression*), keep very busy to avoid worrying or rationalise that in the end everything will turn out for the best. Sally's coping strategy was *denial*, which, if allowed to continue, would not have been in her best interests. These psychological defence mechanisms, first described by Freud, are still helpful as a way of giving insight to unexpected and sometimes unpredictable behaviour in people who otherwise behave rationally.

Treatment for early cervical cancer

If the woman has evidence of early malignancy, the cells may be destroyed by laser either in the Outpatient Department or, if growth is a little more extensive, under general anaesthesia. Conservative treatment is performed wherever possible, especially in young women who have not yet completed their families. Once CIN III is established, a cone biopsy may be performed. Specific nursing care is shown in Care Plan 12.2 (page 314).

Tumours of the body of the uterus

The uterus is the site of several very common benign tumours. Polyps can grow inside the uterine cavity or on the cervix (see Chapter 1) or the woman may develop fibroids (see Chapter 7). The endometrium can also be affected by malignant neoplasms which, if not detected in time, can seriously endanger life.

■ Charlotte Scott disliked going to the doctor and, apart from her pregnancies and a time in her forties when she experienced heavy vaginal bleeding, she managed to avoid it. Her doctor had said that she had fibroids and the bleeding could be alleviated by hysterectomy, but Charlotte did not want to have an operation and, as fibroids are oestrogen-dependent, her menorrhagia resolved after the menopause.

Charlotte was now 68 and it was many years since she had experienced vaginal bleeding. At first she was puzzled when blood began to stain her underclothes, especially as it was bright red and sufficient to require sanitary protection. She thought she had haemorrhoids and, as far as possible, ignored what was happening.

Charlotte's grand-daughter Julie was startled when Charlotte asked her to purchase sanitary protection and asked why it was required. Julie was an extremely health conscious young woman who knew from all that she had read about women's health that *any* vaginal bleeding experienced by a post-menopausal woman should be investigated *at once*. She realised that Charlotte should see a doctor to find out exactly where the blood was coming from, and accompanied her to the health centre and, the following week, to an appointment with the gynaecologist.

Charlotte needed a great deal of persuasion before she would submit to pelvic examination. A uterine mass was palpated and the cervix felt hard due to secondary deposits of the tumour. The nurse who helped prepare Charlotte for physical examination noticed that her blood pressure was elevated, and when Charlotte's urine was tested it contained glucose.

Endometrial carcinoma: aetiology, incidence and risk factors
The body of the uterus can be affected by *sarcoma*, a fast growing and rapidly invasive tumour of connective tissue, and by *carcinoma of the endometrium*.

Endometrial carcinoma is more common and outlook is better, perhaps because the thick myometrium prevents rapid spread to other pelvic organs. Aetiology is unknown but there is a definite link with excessive oestrogenic stimulation, so post-menopausal women receiving hormone replacement therapy must be carefully

Care plan 12.2 (Roper, Logan and Tierney: Activities of Living model)

Name: Sally Carder

Treatment/position: Post-operative care and rehabilitation following cone biopsy. Selective problems identified

Activity of Living	Date of Assessment	Assessment	Problems	Goal	Nursing Intervention	Evaluation
Maintaining a safe environment	20.02.89 2 pm	Returned from theatre. Vital signs stable and within normal limits. Skin warm, well perfused. Vaginal loss nil. Conscious. Oriented. Vaginal pack *in situ:* pack acts as a pressure dressing on the vascular cervix, reducing blood loss and risk of haemorrhage. (If bleeding occurs from the cervical wound it may be necessary to suture bleeding points in theatre under anaesthetic)	(1) Haemorrhage from cervical wound site (potential) (2) Hypovolaemic shock (potential) (3) Pain (potential)	(1/2) Prevent/ recognise haemorrhage/shock. Summon medical help promptly (3) Anticipate/ prevent pain	(1/2) Monitor vital signs half hourly for six hours then 12 hourly if stable. Thereafter monitor four hourly. Observe for signs of restlessness, distress. Monitor vaginal loss (3) Provide analgesia if there are no signs of shock or bleeding – opiate analgesics lower blood pressure, a dangerous effect in the event of severe bleeding (1/2) Bedrest until pack is removed – to prevent pack becoming dislodged	23.02.89 2 pm Vital signs stable. No vaginal loss. Says she is uncomfortable in bed, but has no pain

| Maintaining a safe environment | 28.02.89 2 pm | Condition stable. Vaginal pack to be removed (medical instruction) | (1) Pain when pack is removed (potential)
 (2) Shock/haemorrhage from fresh blood loss when pack is removed (potential)
 (3) Anxiety anticipating uncomfortable nursing procedure (actual)
 (4) Secondary infection of cervical wound from normal vaginal organisms once sterile pack is removed (potential) | (1) Prevent pain
 (2) Recognise signs of shock/bleeding and summon medical aid promptly
 (3) Provide explanations reassurance
 (4) Monitor for signs of infection | (1) Give opiate analgesia one hour before removal of pack is planned. Explain what procedure will entail and how long it will take
 (2) Monitor vital signs and vaginal loss half hourly for four hours. Summon medical aid if necessary. Explain to Sally that she must remain in bed until it is certain that no bleeding will occur from the internal wound
 (3) Explain that some stale blood may drain from the internal wound site as the pack is removed, but this is normal and does not indicate fresh bleeding.
 (4) Take temperature four hourly. Observe amount, character and odour of vaginal loss. Provide sterile | 23.02.89 2 pm
 Analgesia given. Pack removed, vagina draining moderate amounts of old, dark blood. No signs of haemorrhage or incipient infection. Sally has sat in a chair for half an hour but says she feels tired |

Activity of Living	Date of Assessment	Assessment	Problems	Goal	Nursing Intervention	Evaluation
					sanitary towels. Ask Sally to use towels, not tampons, when she goes home, and for her next period	
Elimination	20.02.89 2 pm	Indwelling urethral catheter *in situ*, draining freely. Fluid balance chart in progress. *Rationale:* pressure of vaginal pack on bladder will prevent micturition	Urinary tract infection (potential)	Prevent urinary tract infection	Monitor fluid intake. Sally should drink at least two litres of clear fluid daily. Monitor amount and character of urinary output. Give catheter care and perineal toilet. Remove catheter as soon as vaginal pack is no longer necessary and check that Sally is able to pass urine. Send catheter specimen for bacteriological monitoring	23.02.89 8 pm Catheter removed. 300 ml urine passed *per urethrum*. No evidence of urinary tract infection
Working and playing	20.02.89	Three children. Husband at sea. Visits disabled	(1) Does not understand need to	(1/2) Sally will realistically appreciate	(1) Discuss effects of surgery (2) Explore sources of	23.02.89 Surprised at how tired and weak she feels.

	mother daily. Works part-time as nursing auxiliary. Does not plan to return to work until she has had a holiday	reduce current levels of activity during rehabilitation (actual) (2) Tiredness/reduced mobility after surgery (potential)	effects of surgery and make plans for child-care and help in the home on discharge	help for childcare and housework	Knows this is to be expected despite absence of visible wound. Sister will stay for one week to help in house and look after children. Husband will then be on leave
Expressing sexuality	23.02.89				25.02.89
	Sally has three children and takes oral contraceptives. She and her husband are not planning to have more children. She is 35 and smokes ten cigarettes daily. Says she is worried in case surgery will affect sexual relations	(1) Effects of oral contraceptives long-term (actual). NB age and cigarette consumption (2) Concern about effect of surgery on sex life (actual)	(1) Solution to contraceptive problem acceptable to Sally and her husband (2) Will understand effect of cone biopsy on sexual activity	(1) Discuss contraception (2) Discuss effects of cone biopsy	Sally and her husband will explore more permanent forms of contraception with fewer health risks now their family is complete. Sally knows that removal of cervical tissue should be without effect on sexual relations once tissue has healed and bleeding/discharge has stopped (should take about six weeks). She knows that

Activity of Living	Date of Assessment	Assessment	Problems	Goal	Nursing Intervention	Evaluation
						cone biopsy can increase risk of miscarriage, but is not concerned about this. *Rationale*: incompetent cervix after wedge removal of tissue, risk increasing with amount removed

Orem's self care model (1985) has been used here to show its effectiveness in an acute care situation. The need for information and advice about issues concerning longer term recovery at home and contraception could easily be overlooked unless a comprehensive framework is also required for providing holistic care. Sally's social situation is discussed in some depth in Chapter 1. How well does Orem's model identify the difficulties associated with Sally's present lifestyle? How realistically could a nurse in hospital help Sally tackle these?

monitored. Women continue to secrete small amounts of oestrogen from the adrenal cortex after the menopause and, in some, it may be sufficient to stimulate development of endometrial carcinoma. There is also increased risk for women who have oestrogen-secreting tumours of the ovary. Incidence is higher in obese, hypertensive women, especially those with diabetes mellitus. The precise relationship is difficult to determine since obese women have an increased tendency to develop *Type 2 (adult onset) diabetes* as they grow older in any case.

Endometrial carcinoma is traditionally regarded as a disease of women in their late 60s, but there is increasing evidence of its occurrence in slightly younger women, possibly because oestrogens are now so liberally prescribed as contraceptives and hormone replacement therapy. Formerly found mainly in nulliparous women, its incidence is now increasing among those who have had children although it is still less common than cancer of the ovary or cervix (see Table 12.2).

Investigations

■   Charlotte was admitted to the gynaecology ward to have an endometrial biopsy. This took place in theatre under general anaesthesia, in view of Charlotte's age, anxiety and possible extent of her disease. Her blood glucose levels confirmed that she was mildly diabetic, although this could probably be controlled by diet. Even when she had settled into the ward, her diastolic as well as systolic blood pressure was elevated and hypertensive drugs were prescribed.

Charlotte was admitted several days before surgery for these additional investigations to be performed as the results would influence treatment and aftercare. Away from familiar surroundings she was frightened, sometimes confused and heavily reliant upon Julie, who was also distressed, to explain events to her.

Treatment
Treatment of endometrial carcinoma depends on the stage of the disease (see Table 12.5).

■   Examination under anaesthesia and histology results showed that Charlotte had progressed to Stage 3 on the International System of Classification, with invasion of the other reproductive structures, though not of the bladder or rectum. Her prognosis was therefore very poor. Under these circumstances, the most effective treatment is radiotherapy coupled with palliative surgery if this may help control symptoms. Charlotte was not in discomfort except for bleeding, so the treatment of choice was radiotherapy. In other cases, where surgery may still be of benefit, doctors and nurses may have to face the

Table 12.5 International staging system, treatment and survival rates for endometrial carcinoma

Stage	Extent of disease	Probable treatment	Five year survival rate
0	Histological appearance suggests cancer, but is not conclusive	Total hysterectomy and bilateral salpingo-oöphorectomy with pre-operative radiotherapy to reduce the size of the tumour	80%
1	Cancer is confined to the body of the uterus		
1a	Cavity length of uterus is 8 cm or less		
1b	Cavity length of uterus is more than 8 cm		
2	Cancer has extended to the cervix	Wertheim's hysterectomy and radiotherapy	50%
3	Cancer has extended to other pelvic organs (ovaries, uterine tubes, lymph nodes) excluding the bladder and rectum	Radiotherapy; palliative surgery may be possible	Very poor
4	Cancer has invaded the bladder, rectum and/or organs outside the pelvis	Radiotherapy	Very poor

Note: Progestogens may be given at all stages of treatment because they help reduce growth of the tumour.

difficult ethical dilemma of not giving *active* treatment to women who do not want it.

Radiotherapy

Ionising radiation causes damage to living cells (Tiffany 1979). The aim of radiotherapy is to destroy those cells which are malignant while causing minimal damage to healthy cells which will then be able to recover and regenerate. As radiation passes through tissue some of its energy is transferred to the cells, causing ionisation and chemical changes, ultimately leading to cellular destruction. The target of radiation-induced damage is DNA, so maximal effect occurs during the phase of the cell cycle when mitosis occurs (see Fig. 12.3).

Cellular damage may be:

- *Partial* – the cells mutate, giving rise to abnormal daughter cells when they divide.
- *Total* – the cells either die altogether or are so badly damaged they remain unable to divide.

Normal cells undergo repair more rapidly than malignant ones and, with repeated treatments, the tumour will gradually be destroyed. However, neither malignant or normal cells can withstand the total destruction that ionising radiation can inflict, explaining many of the side effects associated with radiotherapy. Cell destruction is known to follow one of three different patterns:

- *Immediate death* (within approximately two hours) due to irreversible damage to DNA. Immediate cellular destruction accounts for the early side effects of radiotherapy.
- *Delayed cellular damage*, following mutation of DNA in affected cells. Limited cell function is possible until mitosis, then ceases as division is no longer possible. Delayed cell damage accounts for the longer term side effects of radiotherapy. Cells which undergo frequent divisions are affected within 24 hours (skin, bone marrow, gut endothelium) but in others damage may not become apparent for weeks or months.
- *Natural cellular death* – exposure to radiation causes the formation of 'giant cells' which continue to function normally but eventually degenerate because they have lost the capacity to divide.

If healthy parts of the body are to remain undamaged by radiotherapy, the patient must receive a carefully calculated amount of radiation called the *fractionated dose* and healthy tissues must be protected as far as possible during treatment.

Psychological care
Although there are many accounts in the literature of the psychological impact of cancer and radical surgery, remarkably little has been written about coping with radiotherapy (Eardley 1986). This is surprising in view of the number of people who undergo treatment, especially since it has been available for many years and is now increasingly replacing radical surgery. Eardley's literature review revealed that many patients appeared remarkably uninformed about the nature of their treatment, including safety aspects, and had exaggerated misconceptions of expected side effects. A classic early study by Peck and Borland (1977) suggested strongly negative attitudes, reflecting a belief that surgery had 'failed' or was not possible owing to extensive malignant spread. From these findings, it would appear that patients and their families need to be told about the nature of radiotherapy, highlighting exactly what it is meant to achieve. They may benefit if warned about possible side effects in advance, especially if they appreciate that these can be reduced or prevented by nursing interventions (see Table 12.6). Unless they are given the opportunity to express their fears, women may worry needlessly.

Methods of radiotherapy
There are three possible methods of administering radiotherapy – plesiotherapy, teletherapy, and unsealed sources. These are sometimes used in combination.

Plesiotherapy
The radioactive source is positioned either directly inside the tumour or inside an applicator as close to it as possible. In the case of endometrial cancer, the radioactive source is usually *caesium* inserted into the uterine cavity while the patient is anaesthetised. Repeated insertions of about 24 hours duration are necessary at intervals of several weeks to allow normal cells to recover. After the caesium has been inserted the patient returns to the ward, so all staff must be aware of the hazards of radiation

Table 12.6 Complications of radiotherapy to the pelvic area

Complications	Nursing intervention
Early complications	
Vaginal inflammation	Local hygienic measures – use of the mildest possible, unscented soap, wash with warm water and pat dry with soft towel
Irritation of the bladder mucosa and cystitis	Encourage clear fluids with a high pH (lemon barley) to avoid infection. Measure intake and output to ensure adequate hydration
Proctitis, diarrhoea, tenesmus, bleeding	Good hygiene, application of barrier cream to protect perianal skin if necessary, record episodes of bleeding. Give steroid suppositories (anti-inflammatory effect) and anti-diarrhoeal agents as prescribed
Nausea	Small, attractive meals, mouthcare, anti-emetics as prescribed
Longer term	
Ovulation failure in pre-menopausal women	Reassurance that although periods will cease local steroid treatment can be given to prevent other menopausal effects
Vaginal atrophy	Depends on whether the woman is sexually active. Full discussion and the use of vaginal lubricants advised
Fistula formation between vagina and bladder or rectum	This is extremely rare and may take up to two years to develop. Surgical repair and nursing care are discussed in Chapter 11
Skin reactions	Good local skin care and hygiene advised to continue for years after treatment

both for their own protection and to explain the reasons for precautions to the patient and her relatives.

Certain safety measures are taken:

- A special 'after-loading' technique permitting the radiotherapist to insert applicators containing a dummy source into the best possible position, followed by an X-ray check. The radioactive source itself is then inserted.
- Isolating the patient once the source is in position. Although a single room is desirable, it should not be forgotten that thin partition walls in modern buildings offer little protection against ionising radiation.
- Positioning lead screens between the patient and nurses or visitors, so that as many radioactive particles as possible are absorbed.
- Carefully timing treatment and handling and checking of the source when it is

removed and returned to its lead container. This normally takes place on the ward, and the procedure may be performed by a nurse.

- Monitor badges worn by all staff to indicate the amount of radiation to which each is exposed. Regular checking is necessary to ensure that safety limits are not exceeded.
- Regular meetings of the hospital Radiation Safety Committee and updating of its policies.

■   Women requiring caesium insertion were admitted to Charlotte's ward quite often, and the Senior Nurse in charge of the Unit had been invited to be a member of the Radiation Safety Committee. She arranged teaching sessions for all new staff and learners on the ward to ensure they were fully conversant with its policies and procedures. In particular she was concerned to ensure the following:

- That patients and relatives were aware of the need for safety precautions, especially the restriction of visiting times, and know how to summon a nurse quickly if they needed help during the period of isolation.
- That patients knew that the rest of the body was exposed as little as possible to ionising radiation (packing between the source and the vaginal walls helps to protect the bladder and rectum unless they too are affected by the tumour).
- That patients knew they would receive analgesia before the source was removed and that this procedure would take only a few minutes.

Charlotte found the experience of plesiotherapy distressing – it was difficult for the nurse to explain why neither she nor Julie was able to remain in the room for long.

Teletherapy (external beam radiotherapy)

An external source some distance from the patient is specifically focused onto the tumour from the following:

- A *linear accelerator* (conventional source);
- A *cobalt 60 unit* producing gamma rays;
- A *betatron unit* emitting beams of high energy electrons and neutrons.

Treatment takes place in a room with special protective walls and a door-locking device which prevents the apparatus operating until the lock is engaged. Staff must leave before treatment begins, but can observe the patient through a protected window.

Although teletherapy is painless and each session usually quite short, patients may feel apprehensive at the prospect of being alone beneath imposing apparatus, especially when they know that elaborate safety precautions are provided for others.

Claustrophobia may be increased because unaffected parts of the body are shielded and the patient is instructed not to move.

Unsealed source
This method, no longer much in use, involves the injection of a liquid radioactive source (often colloidal gold) into the peritoneal cavity. Removal is unnecessary because radioactive emissions rapidly decline (sources with a short half life are used) so risk to the rest of the body and to other people is not great, although the use of lead screens is advised.

Terminal care
If endometrial cancer is detected early, prognosis is favourable but, for those in whom the disease has advanced, the outlook is poor.

Dawning knowledge that they have cancer is viewed by most people as stressful (Peck 1972, Hinton 1973). For many years, it was believed that individuals should be spared the truth. In consequence, relatives and nurses in everyday contact with the patient found it difficult to carry on as normal, especially when it became evident that the individual was aware of the nature of the diagnosis without being explicitly told. Often the stress of *not* knowing must have been even more difficult to bear. This situation is now changing, although it is apparent that people vary in their desire for information. Spencer Jones (1981), reporting discussions with over 200 cancer patients, claims that approximately half wanted full information about diagnosis and prognosis. Of the remainder, half again indicated that they were aware of the nature of their disease, although they did not want to discuss it. The results of another study showed that even those without any desire to learn details of their prognosis wished to be given information about treatment (Reynolds *et al.* 1981). Attempts have been made to identify the characteristics of patients who wish to be fully informed. Prognosis alone does not appear to be a powerful determinant, but younger patients generally seek most information (Cassileth *et al.* 1980).

Nurses, the health care professionals in closest and most continuous contact with the patient, are in many ways the best placed to pick up cues and identify the needs of the individual: it is tragic for people to face terminal illness alone because nobody will allow then to discuss their fears, and equally tragic to force on people information for which they have no desire.

■   Radiotherapy reduced the size of Charlotte's tumour and helped to control the development of other symptoms, but malignancy was already advanced and she was eventually admitted for terminal care. Julie told the nurses that her grandmother had not discussed the nature of her illness with the family, although she had spent some time 'putting her affairs in order'. She appeared to realise that she was gravely ill, but she did not broach the subject with anyone in the hospital. Her desire for privacy was therefore respected and the model on which her nursing care was based was that developed by Roper *et al.* (1981): see Care plan 12.3, page 325).

Care plan 12.3 (Roper, Logan and Tierney: Activities of Living model)

Name: Charlotte Scott

Treatment/condition: Carcinoma of the uterus. Terminal support and care

Assessment and care plan:

Activity of Living	Date & Time of Assessment	Assessment	Problems	Goal	Nursing Intervention	Evaluation
Providing a safe environment	20.02.89	Charlotte has been admitted to the side room of the same ward to which she had previously been admitted. Her condition has clearly deteriorated. She is nursed in bed as her ability to move is now restricted, and this is the most comfortable alternative. Charlotte is sometimes confused, but not restless. She does not pose a threat to her own safety (see also 'Mobility')	Deterioration of general condition. Can provide no self-care	Provide all physical and psychological care necessary for Charlotte and her family in a supportive environment	Provide help with all ALs, as below	23.02.89 All care has been provided and documented as below
Communication	20.02.89	*From previous admission*: Charlotte realises that she is gravely ill, but has never displayed any interest in learning her	(1) Drowsy, confused. Not able to speak coherently (actual)	(1) Anticipate Charlotte's needs as far as possible (2) Encourage her family to	Charlotte's care is planned so that her family are able to spend as much time with her as possible. Time is spent with	23.02.89 It is often difficult to understand what Charlotte is asking for, but she remains peaceful most of the

Activity of Living	Date & Time of Assessment	Assessment	Problems	Goal	Nursing Intervention	Evaluation
		prognosis or diagnosis, although she has previously asked for information about treatment (radiotherapy) and its expected side effects 20.02.89 Is drowsy and confused at times. She is not able to speak coherently, but does not appear to be in distress. Her family is very distressed, especially her granddaughter Julie	(2) Family distressed (actual). Charlotte does not appear to be aware of their distress	spend time with her and express their emotions	her and efforts are made to understand what she says	time, especially when family members are present. The family appreciate recognition of their need for privacy and feel able to ask the nurses any questions they wish
Breathing	20.02.89	Breathing laboured. Tendency to Cheyne-Stokes respiration. Rate – 22 breaths/minute. Cannot expectorate	(1) Laboured breathing. Cannot expectorate (actual) (2) Chest infection (potential) (3) Narcotic drugs given for pain relief may depress respiratory	(1,2,3) Charlotte will be nursed in a comfortable position, turning her from side to side so that pulmonary secretions will drain (4) Explanations of her condition	(1) Position Charlotte so that respiratory secretions drain and respiratory effort is minimised (2) Turn Charlotte hourly to help respiratory secretions drain and to aid pulmonary ventilation	23.02.89 Charlotte shows signs of hypostatic pneumonia on medical examination, but this does not appear to add to her discomfort

			Problems	Goals	Nursing actions	Evaluation
			centre (potential)	will be provided to Charlotte and her family	(3) Monitor respiratory rate and depth (4) Provide full explanation of nursing actions to Charlotte and her family	
			(4) Distress of family (actual)			
Eating and drinking	20.02.89	Charlotte's appetite has disappeared. She will sometimes accept a little soup brought by her family, but it is otherwise difficult to persuade her to drink	(1) Loss of appetite (actual) (2) Weight loss (potential) (3) Dehydration (potential) (4) Sore, dry, infected mouth (potential) (5) Distress for Charlotte's family (actual)	(1,2,3) Persuade Charlotte to accept small amounts of food and sips of fluid (3) Avoid painful dehydration (4) Keep her mouth moist and infection-free (5) Explain and provide comfort to her family	(1,2) Ask Charlotte if she wishes to eat – mention suitable (soft) food and provide in small amounts (1,3) Offer sips of fluid often (every half hour). Ask family what she especially likes to drink (4) Observe condition of oral mucosa. Offer mouthwashes. Provide mouth care with soft toothbrush. Clean dentures (5) Discuss the situation with Charlotte's family. Allow them to show distress	23.02.89 Charlotte will accept sips of fluid, but refuses to eat. Her mouth is moist and she is in no apparent discomfort. Her family feel distress but accept the situation

Activity of Living	Date & Time of Assessment	Assessment	Problems	Goal	Nursing Intervention	Evaluation
Elimination	20.02.89	Bowels last opened 16.02.89. Grand-daughter says that Charlotte has been constipated. Loss of urinary continence (scant amounts, dark and concentrated, passed intermittently)	(1) Constipation (actual) (2) Urinary incontinence (actual) (3) Urinary tract infection (potential)	(1) Alleviate constipation (2) Control urinary incontinence and maintain dignity (3) Prevent development of urinary tract infection	(1) Give enema (small dis-posable) to relieve constipation. Monitor bowel actions daily (2) Observe whether alleviation of constipation helps to reduce urinary incontinence. Try to establish when urinary leakage occurs and offer bedpans. If regime fails, re-evaluate and consider catheterisation with Foley catheter (3) Send urine specimen for bacteriological screening. (Bacteriological screening is	20.02.89 Enema moderately successful 22.02.89 Catheterised, as urinary incontinence remains troublesome 23.02.89 Catheter draining concentrated urine (500 ml daily). Result of bacterio-logical screening – mixed bacterial growth

necessary to identify the infective organism even if it is not in the best interests of the affected patient to receive treatment, as cross-infection could occur to others on the same ward)

Activity of living	Date	Assessment / problems	Objectives and nursing actions	Nursing actions	Date	Evaluation
Personal cleansing and dressing	20.02.89	Hygiene poor. Charlotte has not allowed her granddaughter to assist with personal needs. Incontinent of urine. Dark, offensive vaginal discharge. Unable to wash and dress herself (1) Poor hygiene – refuses help from family (actual) (2) Urinary incontinence – see 'Elimination' (3) Vaginal discharge (actual)	(1) Provide help with hygiene. Be aware that in the past Charlotte has disliked receiving such help from other people, and that it is important for her dignity to be respected (2) Arrange for medical investigation and treatment for vaginal discharge	(1) Bedbath (2) Provide sanitary protection. Monitor vaginal bleeding (appearance, number of pads per day). Send high vaginal swab to Bacteriology Laboratory (3) Perform vulval toilet two hourly	23.02.89	Accepts help with personal hygiene from nurse.

Activity of Living	Date & Time of Assessment	Assessment	Problems	Goal	Nursing Intervention	Evaluation
Controlling body temperature	20.02.89	Axillary temperature 36.5°C. Has always 'felt the cold' (previous assessment). Is not complaining now	Tendency to feel cold (potential)	Will feel warm and comfortable	Be aware of Charlotte's tendency to feel cold. Check that she is comfortable every time she is turned (hourly)	23.02.89 Charlotte has remained comfortable. She has not complained of feeling cold
Mobilising	20.02.89	Charlotte is too weak to walk or stand unaided. She needs help to turn in bed. She has small broken areas of skin over her sacrum (1 cm diameter), involving the superficial tissue. Both her elbows are red	(1) Lack of mobility (actual) (2) Broken skin over sacrum (actual) (3) Red elbows (actual)	(1) Ensure comfortable position in bed (2,3) Prevent deterioration of Charlotte's pressure areas and avoid further pressure sores	– Turn every hour – Nurse with bedcradle and pressure-relieving devices as appropriate – Monitor pressure areas when turned (size, depth, amount of inflammation) – Dress sacral sores with transparent polyurethane dressing (op site) and observe condition daily	25.02.89 No further pressure sores. Condition of sacral sore unchanged. Needs to be reminded of the need to move every time she is turned, as she sometimes resents this
Working and playing	20.02.89	*From previous admission:* Widowed for 20 years. Brought up three grandchildren when her daughter divorced. All have now left home, except for	Charlotte is withdrawing from the world. This represents a problem for her family, rather than herself	(1) Charlotte's family will express their feelings (2) Allow Charlotte to enjoy the	(1) Give the family the opportunity to express their fears (2) Encourage Charlotte's visitors to sit	23.02.89 Charlotte's family and friends from church visit daily. She seems contented for them to sit with her. Conversation

Activity	Assessment	Problem/need	Goal	Nursing action	Evaluation
	the youngest (Julie), still at college. Charlotte has not worked outside the home since she married. She likes to read, watch television and has been involved in church activities all her life 20.02.89 Charlotte is no longer able to get around the house. She has lost interest in all recreational activities		time remaining to her as much as possible	with her and read to her	and diversion do not appear necessary
Expressing sexuality 20.02.89	*From previous admission:* Charlotte has been widowed for many years. She has two children and three grandchildren. Her grandaughter says that she has always been reluctant to discuss sexual matters with anyone, and her dislike of visiting the GP when symptoms first appeared may have delayed diagnosis and treatment. She will never discuss 'personal problems'	(1) Does not welcome help with personal needs (actual); see 'Personal cleansing and dressing') (2) Inability to look after herself will affect normal feminine appearance (potential)	(2) Help Charlotte look as much like her usual self as possible	(2) Comb hair in usual style, dress Charlotte in her own nightdresses, use her favourite scented soap, talcum powder and perfume	23.02.89 Charlotte's family express their appreciation of the efforts made to help preserve her dignity and the recognition that she always liked to look 'respectable' and 'nice'

Activity of Living	Date & Time of Assessment	Assessment	Problems	Goal	Nursing Intervention	Evaluation
		20.02.89 Vaginal bleeding (see personal cleansing and dressing)				
Sleeping and resting	20.02.89	*From previous admission*: goes to bed at 11 pm, rises at 7 am. Not a good sleeper. Often gets up in the night 20.02.89 Drowsy and confused. Resents rousing to be turned. Receiving diamorphine 5 mg intramuscularly every four hours. This appears to be controlling pain	(1) Resentment at rousing for nursing actions (actual) (2) Pain (potential) (3) Pain may interfere with sleep (potential)	(1) Will receive explanations and reassurance concerning nursing intervention (2,3) Pain will be controlled	(1) Explain the reason for every nursing intervention, saying exactly what will happen (2,3) Give analgesia as prescribed and monitor effectiveness	23.02.89 Charlotte's pain appears to be controlled. She spends much of the time sleeping despite hourly turning, and accepts the need for this
Dying	20.02.89	*From previous admission*: Charlotte knows that she is gravely ill, but has not asked for explicit information concerning	(1) Family's distress (actual) (2) Family's lack of knowledge about how	Charlotte and her family will be given the opportunity to express their fears	(1) Observe use of words indicating need to express fears for self and family. Answer questions	20.02.89 Charlotte's granddaughter has asked if this is likely to be her last admission, and the

prognosis or diagnosis. Her granddaughter says she never mentions this

20.02.89
Charlotte has not discussed her prognosis with anyone, but her granddaughter says that several weeks ago she 'put her affairs in order'. Her family are distressed. No-one is sure how much Charlotte knows about her condition, or wishes to know

much Charlotte knows about her condition or wishes to know (actual)

honestly
(2) Respect Charlotte's need not to talk about dying or her future

situation has been explained
23.02.89
Charlotte died peacefully. Her granddaughter and her primary nurse were with her

---

The model by Roper et al. (1985) was used to plan care effectively for Charlotte and her family, highlighting the many areas where physical and psychological care were required. Two major problems encountered were pain control and pressure area care. Many people would argue that pain should be measured on a scale (visual analogue scale, pain thermometer). If you have not yet encountered these methods of pain assessment it might be helpful to obtain further information from your library. How successfully do you think such scales could be used for Charlotte? There are also a number of scales and measuring devices to assess susceptibility to pressure sore development. Obtain some information about these and determine Charlotte's susceptibility during the terminal stage of her illness. How realistically could pressure sores be prevented in this situation?

Tumours of the uterine tubes

Benign cysts may develop in the broad ligament close to the uterine tubes, but malignancy is rare. Research studies have been few and aetiology is unknown. Women who present with tumours of the uterine tubes are usually in their fifties and their main complaints are of pain and vaginal discharge. These non-specific symptoms, coupled with the rarity of the disease, mean that diagnosis is usually late and prognosis is not generally good. Treatment involves hysterectomy, bilateral salpingo-oöphorectomy and removal of any affected lymph nodes, followed by radiotherapy.

Ovarian tumours

Several types of ovarian malignancy are known (see Table 12.7), but the most common is carcinoma (neoplastic change of connective tissue). Approximately 80 per

Table 12.7 Ovarian tumours

Name	Histological origin	Malignant/ benign	Appearance	Other
Mucinous cystadenoma	Epithelium surrounding ovary	Benign	Cyst filled with thick fluid	Usually large. May occur at any age. Common
Mucinous cystadenocarcinoma	Epithelium surrounding ovary	Malignant	Cyst filled with thick fluid and solid areas of malignancy	Uncommon
Serous cystadenoma	Similar to epithelium lining uterine tube	Benign	Cyst filled with serous fluid	20% of all ovarian neoplasia. Often bilateral
Serous cyst-adenocarcinoma	Epithelium	Malignant	Cysts and invasive papillary projections	60% of all ovarian cancers. Bilateral in about 50% of cases. Ascites always present
Brenner tumour	Epithelium	Benign	Fibrous, sometimes with mucus-filled cysts	Most common in older women
Fibroma	Ovarian stroma (connective tissue). May arise from theca	Malignant/ benign	Resembles fibroids	Most in older women 4–5% of all ovarian neoplasia
Dysgerminoma	Germ cell tumour	Benign or malignant– grade of malignancy variable	Smooth, ovoid and rubbery. Solid	Commonest in women under 30. Sometimes bilateral

Table 12.7 (con't.)

Name	Histological origin	Malignant/ benign	Appearance	Other
Cystic teratoma/ dermoid cyst	Germ cell tumour	Benign, but may undergo malignant change	May contain skin, teeth, hair, bones and fibrous tissue. Filled with yellow thick sebaceous fluid	Often bilateral, quite common, especially in women under 30 years
Solid teratoma	Germ cell tumour	Benign, but very often undergoes malignant change	Solid tumour	Usually occurs at an earlier age than dermoids, often in childhood
Gonadoblastoma	Germ cell tumour	Benign, but may undergo malignant change	Solid tumour	Associated with women who have genetic abnormalities (see Chapter 14)
Yolk sac tumour	Germ cell tumour	Highly malignant	Structure is very variable	Rare. Affects children and young adults
Krükenberg tumour	Secondary carcinoma of the ovary. Primary is usually in the stomach, and clinically silent.	Malignant. Most women die within a year of diagnosis	Bilateral, large, smooth tumour	Affects 30–40 age group
Hormone producing tumours				
(a) Oestrogen secreting	Theca of ovary	Benign or malignant	Solid	Rare. May cause precocious puberty in children, post-menopausal bleeding or irregular menses throughout the reproductive years. Breasts and uterus enlarge
(b) Androgen secreting	Variable	Malignant in 20% of cases	Solid or cystic	Rare. Less than 1% of all ovarian neoplasia. *Period of defeminisation is followed by period of masculisation

* Defeminisation includes atrophy of breasts, loss of fat on hips, atrophy of genitalia, oligomenorrhoea, then amenorrhoea. Masculisation includes development of male hair distribution, hirsuitism, deepening of voice, enlargement of clitoris and flattened breasts

cent are primary tumours of the ovary itself, while the remainder represent secondary invasion of malignancy elsewhere in the genital tract, breast, stomach or large intestine. Often metastases become large while the primary tumour remains small and therefore difficult or impossible to locate. In most ways metastases behave like primary growths and are histologically the same.

Carcinoma of the ovary

Ovarian carcinoma was once considered uncommon but improved diagnostic techniques now indicate that it may be more widespread than any other malignancy of the female genital tract (see Table 12.1). Incidence may previously have been underestimated because tumours had become so widely disseminated by the time of diagnosis that the site of the primary could not be identified. Unfortunately early diagnosis, on which success of treatment depends (see Table 12.8), often still tends to be delayed because the tumour grows insidiously deep inside the pelvis.

■   Elizabeth Fox was referred to the gynaecologist with a history of lassitude and ill-defined abdominal pain. Elizabeth was 56 and had experienced the menopause several years previously. At first she was unable to accept her doctor's

Table 12.8 International staging, treatment and five year survival rates for cancer of the ovary

Stage	Extent of disease	Treatment	Five year survival rate
1	Limited to ovaries		
1a	One ovary affected. No ascites		
1b	Both ovaries affected. No ascites.	Surgery	60–70%
1c	One or two ovaries affected with evidence of ascites	Surgery and chemotherapy	
2	Extension to other pelvic organs		
2a	Spread to uterus/uterine tubes No ascites		
2b	Spread to other pelvic tissues No ascites	Surgery and chemotherapy	40–50%
2c	Spread to other pelvic tissues with ascites		
3	Extension to small bowel, with metastases to the peritoneum	Extensive surgical resection and chemotherapy	5–10%
4	Distant metastases (liver and lungs)	Extensive surgery possibly including colostomy, chemotherapy, perhaps palliative radiotherapy	None

concern. She attributed her gradually increasing girth to 'middle age spread' and had felt comforted by the assurances of Ralph, her husband, that she was still attractive.

The gynaecologist suspected that Elizabeth had a malignant growth and, to help confirm diagnosis and plan treatment, it was necessary for her to undergo two further investigations – *ultrasonography* (see Chapter 4) and *computerised axial tomography* (*CAT scanning*). Both are non-invasive, sparing the patient diagnostic laparotomy.

Investigations and treatment

The presence of a malignant ovarian tumour can be detected by pelvic and abdominal examination. Ovarian carcinoma is generally accompanied by *ascites* (fluid filled with malignant cells) and the bowel tends to float on top of the fluid. Tapping the top of the swelling with the fingers produces a full percussion note, but over the flanks of the abdomen percussion is resonant. Benign tumours are never accompanied by ascites, so they do not elicit these signs.

Computerised axial tomography

■   The nurse in the Outpatient Department who arranged Elizabeth's appointment informed her that the CAT scan is free of side effects and little special preparation is required. She explained that the scanner would take repeated X-rays at high speed (about 300 films within five seconds) while the X-ray source rotated around her body. The films would be used to build up pictures showing a cross-section through the pelvis at different levels. Most centres advise patients to follow a low residue diet for two days before the investigation (Booth 1983). There are no contraindications for CAT scans and no complications. The patient is asked to lie on a couch running through the middle of the machinery and the X-ray equipment surrounds the tunnel, separated by metal.

Elizabeth felt rather claustrophobic during the test as the equipment looked imposing and she had to lie in one position, but she was able to drive herself home. She had heard about CAT scanning through charitable appeals on behalf of the local hospital, and she had been told by the gynaecologist that she probably had an ovarian cyst of some kind.

Several weeks passed between Elizabeth's initial visit to the gynaecologist and her return to obtain the results. This gave her the opportunity to think what the possible diagnosis might be and to discuss it with Ralph. Elizabeth felt that she would never have been subjected to so many tests so quickly unless there was a chance of something seriously wrong. She made up her mind from the beginning that she wanted to be told the truth.

The gynaecologist was honest. Elizabeth had an ovarian malignancy (Stage 2C) which had spread to the other pelvic tissues. The most effective treatment would be *Wertheim's hysterectomy* (see Chapter 7) to remove as much malignant tissue as possible, followed by intensive chemotherapy. The effectiveness of treatment would be checked a few months later by 'second look' laparotomy to decide whether chemotherapy should be repeated and to remove any malignant recurrence.

Elizabeth and Ralph were shocked. At first they thought that Elizabeth was bound to die anyway and could not see the point of chemotherapy, especially as they had heard so many negative things about it. However, survival rate for women who have reached Elizabeth's stage of the disease is now 28–50 per cent (Barker and Wiltshaw 1981) and occasionally complete remission has been achieved.

Elizabeth and Ralph required a great deal of information which could not be provided all at once as it would have overwhelmed them. They also needed reassurance but not false hope, for there is no guarantee that this treatment regime, the best currently available, will be completely successful for every woman.

Chemotherapy

Cytotoxic drugs exert their effects by damaging the genetic material of cells so they can no longer divide. All cells are affected but, as with radiotherapy, normal cells repair faster and more effectively than malignant ones.

Traditionally, cytotoxic drugs have been classified according to the system shown in Table 12.9, depending on mode of action. However, research conducted in the 1970s suggested that some cytotoxic drugs damage cells most reaily at particular stages in the cell cycle (*phase specific drugs*), while others appear to exert their effects throughout the entire cell cycle (*cycle specific drugs*). This more recent method of classification is shown on Table 12.10. No effect is exerted by any cytotoxic agents in the GO phase. The most effective drug regime reported by Barker and Wiltshaw (1981) for ovarian carcinoma is Cisplatin (cisdiamminedichloroplatinum) and chlorambucil. Both are cycle specific.

Most cytotoxic drugs currently used are maximally effective on solid tumours when the total number of malignant cells present is relatively small. Chemotherapy is therefore most often employed as adjuvant therapy once as much malignant tissue as possible has been removed. Increasing knowledge of cell kinetics and the development of many new cytotoxic agents influences method of administration.

Cytotoxic drugs: methods of administration

At one time, when it was thought that malignant cells divided more rapidly than normal ones, patients generally received a single cytotoxic agent continuously. This has now been almost entirely superseded by combination chemotherapy where more than one agent is given simultaneously. The particular combination is selected so that the drugs destroy cells by different mechanisms. Toxicity to normal tissues is therefore controlled. For example, Compound A may disrupt regeneration of gut endothelium, as well as cancer cells, but may not have a very marked effect on bone marrow.

Table 12.9 Traditional classification of cytotoxic drugs and their mechanisms of action

Drug	Method of action	Side effects
Adriamycin	Antimitotic antibiotic; cycle specific	1. Gut toxicity 2. Cardiotoxicity (chest pain, palpitations) 3. Bone marrow suppression 4. Stomatitis
Cyclophosphamide	Alkylating agent. Its chemical structure contains an alkyl group ($-CH2$) which combines with cellular DNA to alter its structure and destroy normal function. The cell cannot divide. Cycle specific	1. Bone marrow suppression 2. Alopecia (dose related) 3. Gut toxicity 4. Irritation to bladder lining – chemical cystitis
Methotrexate	Anti-metabolite. It is taken up by the cell nucleus in mistake for chemically similar metabolites (folic acid in this particular case) and binds to nuclear enzymes, rendering them non-functional. Cell growth is halted. Phase specific	2. Gut toxicity 2. Severe stomatitis 3. Bone marrow suppression
Vincristine	Vinca alkaloid. Appears to disrupt mitosis. Precise mode of action unknown. May also halt DNA replication at S phase of cell cycle. Phase specific	1. Leucopenia but otherwise not particularly toxic to bone marrow 2. Alopecia 3. Gut toxicity 4. Stomatitis 5. Peripheral neuropathy 6. Constipation (neuropathy to nerves supplying gut)
Fluorouracil	Antimetabolite for uracil, an important component of the genetic material (RNA). Cycle specific	1. Gut toxicity 2. Bone marrow suppression 3. Alopecia 4. Stomatitis 5. Skin reaction, especially in strong sunlight 6. Discolouration of the veins with continued use
Phenylalanine mustard (mephalan)	Alkylating agent; cycle specific	1. Alopecia 2. Gut toxicity 3. Extreme lethargy 4. Severe bone marrow suppression – very high risk of infection if given in high doses
Cisplatin	Binds to DNA and inactivates it, but not by alkylation. Precise action unknown. Cycle specific	1. Neurotoxic 2. Nephrotoxic 3. Gut toxicity 4. Bone marrow suppression 5. Alopecia
Chlorambucil	Alkylating agent; cycle specific	1. Bone marrow suppression

Table 12.10 Kinetic classification of cytotoxic drugs

Cycle specific	Phase specific
Actinomycin D	Asparaginase
Adriamycin	Bleomycin
Busulphan	Cytosine arabinoside
Chlorambucil	Methotrexate
Cyclophosphamide	Procarbazine
5 Fluorouracil	Vinblastine
Mithramycin	Vincristine
Mitomycin–C	
Phenylalanine mustard	
Nitrogen mustard	
Thiotepa	
Cisplatin	

Compound B may be more toxic to bone marrow, depressing blood cell counts more significantly, but not producing gastro-intestinal symptoms. From Table 12.8 it can be seen that although cisplatin and chlorambucil both exert undesirable side effects, these differ. Symptoms experienced are likely to vary between one person and another.

■   Elizabeth had a number of worries about the effects of chemotherapy, especially on her appearance. Her care plan (Care plan 12.4, page 341) was drawn up using the model developed by Roper *et al.* (1983) as, during the intravenous administration of cisplatin, Elizabeth was physically unwell. (Chlorambucil was given orally and continued after she went home.)

Although Elizabeth stayed in hospital overnight to receive intravenous chemotherapy, the doses were intermittent, and she was able to go home after each administration.

Intermittent chemotherapy
Work by Skipper's team (1964) resulted in three important discoveries, eventually leading to the concept of intermittent chemotherapy:

- Cytotoxic agents destroy a fixed percentage of the total cells present. They do *not* kill a set number of cells.
- If the dosage of the cytotoxic agent is increased, the percentage of cells destroyed will likewise increase.
- Normal cells, though sustaining the same damage, recover more rapidly than malignant ones so the population of malignant cells will diminish more swiftly than that of normal cells.

Care plan 12.4 (Roper, Logan and Tierney: Activities of Living model)

Name: Elizabeth Fox

Treatment/condition: Cytotoxic chemotherapy for carcinoma of the ovary

Assessment and care plan:

Activity of Living	Date & Time of Assessment	Assessment	Problems	Goal	Nursing Intervention	Evaluation
Maintaining a safe environment	20.02.89	Elizabeth is receiving chlorambucil orally (10 mg daily for 14 days every month) and is to receive her second intravenous dose of cisplatin (20 mg) overnight in hospital. The first treatment took place four weeks ago when Elizabeth experienced severe nausea and vomited several times despite receiving anti-emetics and sedation	(1) Neutropenia and increased risks of infection – effect of chlorambucil (actual) (2) Anaemia – effect of chlorambucil (potential) (3) Dehydration from vomiting (potential) (4) Renal damage – effect of cisplatin (potential) (5) Thrombocytopaenia – effect of	(1) Prevent infection (2) Give iron supplements as prescribed (3) Control vomiting (3,4) Prevent dehydration (5) Alleviate symptoms associated with thrombocytopaenia (bleeding)	(1) Precautions against cross-infection (2) Give iron supplements as prescribed. Monitor tolerance (3,4) Monitor fluid balance. Give anti-emetics as prescribed and monitor effectiveness (5) Examine skin and mouth for signs of bleeding • *Teach Elizabeth to look for and recognise signs of infection and bleeding when she goes home*	23.02.89 Elizabeth's white and red cell counts do not appear to have deteriorated further since admission. She has not developed infection and is not in negative fluid balance. Vomiting has been troublesome during treatment. She knows that between 7–14 days after treatment the drugs will exert maximal effect on her bone marrow, so that blood cell and platelet counts will be at their lowest, and that she must report any bleeding or infection to her doctor at once. She can list the symptoms to

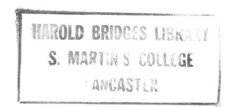

Activity of Living	Date & Time of Assessment	Assessment	Problems	Goal	Nursing Intervention	Evaluation
			chlorambucil and cisplatin (potential)			look for. She knows that she must not take aspirin as this prevents blood clotting
Communicating	20.02.89 2 pm	Looks apprehensive and says she is afraid of treatment because she knows it will make her sick. Her husband, who is also anxious, says that she has become increasingly distressed over the past few days	Extreme anxiety concerning side effects of treatment (actual)	Reduce anxiety to controllable levels before treatment commences at 8 pm	(1) Give honest explanations about probable side effects and their treatment. Include husband in explanations (2) Give anti-emetics (metoclorpropamide) *before* treatment commences and explain that this will be repeated regularly as long as nausea persists (3) Describe other nursing measures that may help reduce nausea and vomiting (4) Reinforce teaching about the delayed effects of drugs after discharge: • risk of infection (bone marrow	20.02.89 2 pm Has settled into ward and says she feels less anxious. 20.02.89 10 pm Intravenous chemotherapy has commenced following earlier administration of anti-emetics (9 pm). Elizabeth is drowsy. Nausea is mild. 23.02.89 2 pm Ready to leave hospital. Has experienced some nausea and vomiting throughout treatment but says she is now feeling much better. Feels side effects were less severe because of the practical and emotional support

Activity	Date	Assessment	Problem	Goal	Nursing intervention	Evaluation
					suppression); • bleeding/poor healing thrombo-cytopaenia). Make sure Elizabeth knows what to look for and what action to take	offered by the nurse and her husband
Breathing	20.02.89 2 pm	Restless. Respiratory rate: 22 breaths/minute. Rhythm regular. Skin cool but well perfused	(1) Anxiety due to anticipation of side effects of treatment (actual) leading to: (2) Hyperventilation (actual)	Elimination of anxiety. Return of respiratory rate to normal limits (14–20 breaths per minute)	(1) Give explanations of possible duration of nausea and vomiting, and of interventions which may help reduce it, including anti-emetics (2) Monitor respiratory rate four hourly. Teach deep breathing exercises	20.02.89 Elizabeth is practising slow, deep breathing. Her respiratory rate is 20 breaths per minute
Eating and drinking	20.02.89 2 pm	Weight 56 kg. Height 5' 6". Has regained 1 kg of weight lost since first admission	(1) Reluctance to take oral fluids due to nausea (potential). NB Cisplatin is nephrotoxic and diuresis must be maintained throughout treatment to	(1) Reduce nausea (2) Emphasise role of diet in tissue recovery – high in protein and calories	(1) Give anti-emetics before treatment starts and regularly thereafter and monitor effectiveness. Give sedation as prescribed. (2) Discuss diet. A light meal (soup, toast) before treatment may help prevent nausea	23.02.89 Anti-emetics and sedation given as prescribed. Elizabeth managed to sleep throughout much of the time treatment was in progress. A light meal (soup, toast) before treatment helped to prevent nausea this time

Activity of Living	Date & Time of Assessment	Assessment	Problems	Goal	Nursing Intervention	Evaluation
			(2) Anorexia due to nausea (potential)	prevent renal damage		
Eliminating	20.02.89 2 pm	Elizabeth has no problems with the process of elimination, but once treatment commences she will vomit and will need to empty her bladder frequently because of the intravenous infusion	(1) Vomiting (potential) (2) Need to empty bladder frequently while in bed receiving intravenous fluids (potential)	(1) Vomiting – see ALs above. (2) Offer bedpans frequently. Monitor fluid balance. Avoid dehydration	– Prompt disposal of vomitus and urine – Management of IVI – Maintenance of fluid balance chart – Administration of anti-emetics as prescribed – Mouth care, with soft toothbrush, taking care not to damage the oral mucosa (risk of bleeding: see 'Providing a safe environment')	23.02.89 2 pm Elizabeth is not in negative fluid balance. Her mouth is clean and moist. Nausea has subsided
Personal cleansing and dressing	20.02.89 2 pm	On admission: well groomed. Knows that during treatment she will be in bed, wearing nightclothes. Anticipates	Anticipates feeling uncomfortable and unattractive during treatment (potential)	Elizabeth's feelings of unattractiveness will be minimised	– Frequent bedbaths, changes of bedclothes and nightdress – Prompt removal of excreta – Encourage use of cosmetics, perfume	21.02.89 Treatment is in progress. Elizabeth says she feels clean and comfortable 23.02.89 Says that consideration of personal needs

Activity	Date	Assessment	Problem	Goal	Nursing action	Evaluation
		looking 'a mess' while nauseated				helped to maintain dignity during treatment
Maintaining body temperature	20.02.89 2 pm	Oral temperature 36.9°C. Feels cold and shivery. Attributes this to apprehension	Feels cold and shivery	Will feel warm and comfortable	Allow Elizabeth to voice her fears. Provide extra blanket or local source of heat for comfort if required	20.02.89 4 pm Elizabeth feels warmer and says she is comfortable
Mobilising	20.02.89 2 pm	On admission: no problems. Will be in bed during chemotherapy, movement restricted by the intravenous infusion	(1) Sore, inflamed pressure areas (potential) (2) Deep vein thrombosis (potential) (3) Tiredness may restrict activities after treatment, when Elizabeth goes home (potential)	(1) Will not develop pressure sores (2) Will not develop deep vein thrombosis (3) Will accept reduced level of functioning during recovery at home	(1) Remind Elizabeth to move at least hourly when awake. Give careful skin care (2) Encourage leg exercises previously taught by physiotherapist (3) Explain the effects of the drugs over a longer term – that they will make Elizabeth feel tired	23.02.89 Has not developed pressures sores or deep venous thrombosis. Knows that she will feel more tired than usual when she goes home, but feels able to accept help and support from husband
Working and playing	20.02.89 2 pm	From previous admission: housewife. Does typing and book-keeping for husband's business. Other help arranged	Increased tiredness (effects of drugs) will reduce activity when Elizabeth goes home (potential)	Elizabeth will understand and accept the effects of the drugs	Teach Elizabeth about the effects of the drugs and their likely duration	23.02.89 Grateful to be going home. Glad she does not have to face housework. Knows that she will feel tired, but can cope with this

Activity of Living	Date & Time of Assessment	Assessment	Problems	Goal	Nursing Intervention	Evaluation
		since diagnosis. Always has paid help two mornings a week to help with housework				
Expressing sexuality	20.02.89 2 pm	Tearful. Upset because she has noticed some hair loss (effect of cisplatin). Thinks further treatment will make it worse. Dreads treatment as she will vomit, feel tired and look unattractive	Effect of treatment on body image (actual)	Elizabeth will express her fears to her nurse and husband	– Allow Elizabeth to discuss her fears – Discuss hair loss (which is not marked) and ways of disguising it with a new hairstyle	23.02.89 Fears expressed. Problems of hair loss discussed. Elizabeth will arrange for her hairdresser to visit her at home to experiment with new hairstyles. She believes that anti-cipating the side effects of treatment is probably worse than actually experiencing them
Sleeping and resting	20.02.89	Usually goes to bed at 11 pm. Not sleeping well since illness. Knows she will receive sedation during treatment. Accepts that 'Hospital is not a good place	None			

					23.02.89 Elizabeth and her husband have discussed their future honestly. This treatment is complete and Elizabeth is tired, but feels that this time things did not go too badly. With the support of her husband she feels able to undergo further chemotherapy in future if necessary, and that it will be worthwhile
				– Allow Elizabeth and her husband to voice their fears – Encourage her to participate in her treatment by promoting motivation to undergo intravenous administration of her drugs, and to strive for recovery	
			Elizabeth and her husband will express their fears and grief		
		Afraid that treatment will not be successful (actual)			
for sleeping'. Can rest when she gets home	20.02.89 2 pm	Tearful. Afraid that if treatment does not work she will die soon. Husband distressed			
Dying					

Some people would be surprised at the use of Roper, Logan and Tierney's (1985) model in this care plan as it focuses on the activities of living rather than self care, which would appear more appropriate for a relatively young woman in hospital for a short period, very strongly motivated to participate in her own care. However, during the period when cytotoxic drugs were administered, Elizabeth's activities of living were severely disrupted and she was highly dependent on her nurse for physical care and psychological support, hence its use is justified. Perhaps this situation suggests that there can never be a single 'correct' approach to care, but several different ones. Sometimes one model will be more appropriate than another, at other times the model may be chosen arbitrarily. The situation should not exist where nurses use different approaches for the same patient, as this could result in confusion and needs being overlooked.

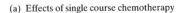

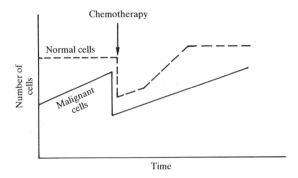

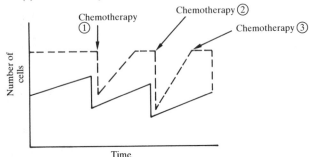

Figure 12.10 Comparison of single and multiple courses of chemotherapeutic agents.

As a result of Skipper's work, and other related discoveries, new treatment regimes have evolved in which high doses of combination chemotherapy alternate with periods of rest, allowing normal cells to recover. The effectiveness of a typical regime incorporating three different agents, compared to a single agent given over the same period of time, is indicated in Fig. 12.10.

Although malignant cells are destroyed, they can never be completely eradicated and, unless administration is repeated, the tumour would eventually begin to grow again (see Fig. 12.10a). When multiple course chemotherapy is given (see Fig. 12.10b), the first dose affects normal and malignant cells in the same way but, with repeated administration, the percentage of malignant cells decreases further. Treatment may continue until all signs of the tumour disappear.

When a patient is receiving intermittent high dose chemotherapy, recovery of normal cells must be carefully monitored – sufficient time must be allowed to lapse between each administration. If the drugs are given too closely together there may be an undesirably large decrease in the population of normal cells, resulting in side effects severe enough to kill the patient. On the other hand, an excessively long interval between administration may result in loss of therapeutic effect by allowing malignant cells to reach pre-treatment levels.

Many cytotoxic drugs are given intravenously. This may form part of the extended role of the nurse in some hospitals or departments, while in others the doctor is responsible for administration, helped by the nurse. Cytotoxic drugs are powerful agents, capable of severe tissue damage: all nurses handling them must be aware of the safety procedures operating in their hospital. Guidelines for safe practice have been outlined by the RCN (1987) and by numerous other authors in more specialist journals (Trester 1982, Walter 1982, Dodd and Mood 1981).

Benign tumours of the ovary
The ovary is affected by a wide variety of different cysts and solid tumours and, as Table 12.5 shows, many are non-malignant.

■   Anna Judge lived with her parents and worked in a department store. She was a clothes-conscious young woman who became distressed when her friends teased her about her figure. Anna had always been reasonably slim, but she worried a lot about her abdomen protruding and was horrified to find that her jeans were becoming increasingly difficult to fasten. She connected this with constipation, a problem which she found increasingly troublesome. However, Anna's mother thought she was exaggerating, especially as she already regarded Anna as a worrier concerning her figure. Anna dismissed her growing discomfort and went to work as usual, but was more tired than normal. The summer weather arrived and to her chagrin she noticed that all her light clothing, purchased the previous year, looked and felt tight. Anna's self-esteem was damaged. She felt unattractive and disinclined to buy anything new to wear. She was troubled by vague abdominal discomfort which she felt should be relieved when she unfastened her clothing, although it was not. She did not associate her pelvic symptoms with her periods, as they remained regular, but she became increasingly tearful and disinclined to go out.

The Occupational Health Nurse noticed that Anna looked unwell during a visit to her department. It was a hot day and Anna needed little persuasion to take a break. She told the nurse that she had a dragging pain in her abdomen, and was found to have an elevated temperature and pulse rate. Anna went home early, having made an appointment to see her GP. She found this distressing, as she was subjected to a pelvic examination, asked about her menstrual history and whether there was any chance she might be pregnant. Far from dismissing her problems the GP made arrangements for Anna to be seen in the gynaecology clinic without delay.

Anna dreaded her hospital appointment, especially as her mother, now shaken, insisted on accompanying her. Anna was nervous about the physical examination which she knew must be repeated, and did not want to face questions about pregnancy in front of her mother. In the event, she found she had worried needlessly. The sister in the Clinic explained what would happen when Anna saw the doctor and, in response to Anna's queries, reassured her that she would be given as much privacy as possible and covered with a blanket when she was lying on the examination couch. Women of all ages may dislike the prospect of pelvic examinations and, if their first experiences are insensitively handled, they may delay seeking help another time. The sister tactfully suggested that Mrs Judge might like to have a cup of tea while Anna was seeing the doctor.

Benign ovarian tumours can occur at any age, although the chances of malignant change increase as the woman grows older. There are many different kinds (Table 12.5) but, apart from distinguishing between benign and a possibly malignant tumour, it is not possible to obtain much further information on clinical examination.

■   Bimanual pelvic examination suggested that Anna had a large tumour of the left ovary, and the diagnosis was confirmed by ultrasonography (see Chapter 4). She was reassured that the tumour was almost certainly benign because:

- Benign ovarian tumours are more common than malignant ones, especially in young women. (Those developing in childhood are usually aggressively malignant, though fortunately, rare.)
- If a tumour has grown large, it is not likely to be malignant because the effects would be detrimental before reaching this stage.
- Although it was causing discomfort, the tumour was not giving rise to the severe, referred pain generally associated with advanced malignant growth.

Small ovarian tumours are usually asymptomatic. Symptoms caused by larger ones are mainly due to pressure as they grow and can result in the following:

- Constipation, if pressure is exerted on the bowel;
- Frequency from forward pressure;
- Respiratory embarrassment if a very large cyst exerts upward pressure;
- Varicose veins through pressure on the veins supplying the legs.

The other side effect commonly associated with ovarian cysts is *torsion*. Unless the cyst is firmly anchored into position its pedicle is likely to become twisted (see Fig. 12.11) so blood supply is interrupted, and there may be bleeding into the tumour itself or the pelvic cavity, setting up local irritation. Pain, vomiting, fever and tachycardia will be experienced during torsion. Low grade pyrexia and pelvic pain may be due to subacute torsion, with the pain subsiding as the pedicle untwists.

In cases of acute torsion, the woman may be suddenly admitted to hospital. Laparoscopy may be necessary to rule out other gynaecological and surgical emergencies (pelvic inflammatory disease, ectopic pregnancy, appendicitis, intestinal obstruction, diverticulitis). Cystic ovarian tumours sometimes rupture spontaneously or

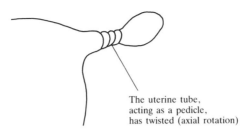

The uterine tube,
acting as a pedicle,
has twisted (axial rotation)

Figure 12.11 Torsion of an ovarian cyst.

during surgical intervention but, unless the escaping fluid contains malignant cells, this does not result in additional complications.

■ Anna wanted to know why her GP had questioned her so persistently about pregnancy. The gynaecologist explained that on palpation the pedicle of an ovarian cyst feels rather like the growing uterus at about sixteen weeks gestation, and women have sometimes been incorrectly diagnosed. Co-existent ovarian cysts often become noticeable for the first time during pregnancy.

Treatment of benign ovarian cysts
Although most ovarian tumours are benign, they must be surgically removed and subjected to histological examination because ovarian malignancy carries an extremely poor prognosis. In most cases benign tumours can be shelled out of the ovary (*cystectomy*), leaving functional tissue, and this is the treatment of choice, especially in young women. If there is more extensive damage to the ovary all (*oöphorectomy*) or part (*ovariotomy*) may be removed, especially if the woman is post-menopausal. Women must be reassured before surgery that only a small amount of ovarian tissue is necessary to maintain normal endocrine function, and that fertility is usually unimpaired if one ovary remains, providing there are no pelvic adhesions.

Nursing care

■ Anna was admitted to the gynaecology ward to have a laparotomy and removal of the ovarian cyst. Routine pre- and post-operative care are the same as for other major gynaecological operations. Anna's pre-operative nursing assessment revealed two problems, one emotional, the other a physical problem.

Surgery and self concept

■   Anna was concerned that the scar would damage her appearance. This fear is probably more widespread among patients than nurses acknowledge. Black (1982) found that surgeons were more concerned with avoiding physical complications than achieving good cosmetic results, and that choice of suturing material depended more on tradition and personal preference than on the results of evaluative performance studies. The results of Black's small study suggested that, although male patients and older women were more concerned with making an uneventful recovery, younger women were seriously distressed at the appearance of their wounds.

Anna's nurse was able to provide reassurance by explaining that the operation would be performed via a Pfannenstiel incision which would be invisible once her pubic hair had grown. If a wound is disrupted by infection, the cosmetic result is less good, but infection is unlikely to supervene in young, generally fit, adults, especially if the wound does not require drainage. Anna could help herself by actively performing post-operative exercises and regaining mobility as swiftly as possible with the help of adequate analgesia. This helps reduce hospital stay, minimising the chance of secondary wound infection from the hospital environment.

Anna's other problem was constipation. It was necessary for her to have an enema pre-operatively, a procedure which she found uncomfortable and embarrassing. Although Anna accepted the need for this nursing intervention because it had been fully explained, the experience of herself as dependent, ill, and in need of assistance with personal functions did nothing to bolster her damaged self-esteem. Nurses who work with women in *any* age group must remain aware of the effect that this invasion of privacy can have, but young women having their first introduction to hospital care perhaps deserve special consideration. The introduction of the nursing process has done much to eliminate the old care routines which were so demoralising (women queuing outside the treatment room to be shaved for theatre, for example) although it has increased the stress of nurses who now get to know and identify with their patients more closely. This possibility is always greater when the nurse on the gynaecology ward is caring for women in a similar age group to her own.

References

Barker, G.H. and Wiltshaw, E. (1981) 'Randomised trial comparing low-dose cisplatin and chlorambucil with low-dose cisplatin, chlorambucil and doxorubicin in advanced carcinoma', *Lancet* 1, pp. 747–9.

Black, J.J. (1982) 'A stitch in time', *Nursing Times* 78 (17), pp. 709–11.

Booth, J.A. (1983) *Handbook of Investigations*, London: Harper and Row.

Borley, D. (1985) 'Women at risk of cervical cancer', *Senior Nurse* 3 (2), pp. 17–18.

Brannigan, J. and McCullough, A. (1987) 'Setting up a vulval clinic', *Nursing Times* 83 (14), pp. 30–32.

British Medical Association (1986) *Cervical Cancer and Screening in Great Britain*, London: Chameleon Press.

Cancer Research Campaign (1986) *Facts about Cancer*, London: Cancer Research Campaign.

Cassileth, B. *et al*. (1980) 'Information and participation preference among cancer patients', *Annals of Internal Medicine* 92, pp. 832–6.

Clarke, C.A. (1987) *Human Genetics and Medicine*, London: Edward Arnold.

Dodd, M.J. and Mood, D.W. (1981) 'Chemotherapy: helping patients to know the drugs they are receiving and their possible side effects', *Cancer Nursing* 4 (4), pp. 311–18.

Doll, R. and Peto, R. (1981) *The Causes of Cancer*, Oxford: Oxford University Press.

Eardley, A. (1986) 'Radiotherapy: what do patients need to know?' *Nursing Times* 82 (16), pp. 24–6.

Elkington, J (1986) *The Poisoned Womb*, London: Pelican.

Goodman, M. (1984) 'Caring for laser vulvectomy patients', *Nursing Mirror* 159 (3), Clinical Forum i–v.

Griffiths, R. (1983) 'Smears: are we ready to pay the price?' *Health and Social Services Journal* 18 August, pp. 983–6.

Harsanyi, Z. and Hutton, R. (1983) *Genetic Prophecy: Beyond the Double Helix*, London: Paladin Granada.

Hinton, J. (1973) 'Bearing cancer', *British Journal of Psychology* 43, pp. 105–13.

HMSO (1985) *Mortality Statistics: Cause. England and Wales 1984*, London: HMSO.

HMSO (1986) *Cancer Statistics: Registrations. England and Wales 1983*, London: HMSO.

Mitchell, J. (1984) *What is to be done about Illness and Health?*, London: Penguin.

OPCS *Mortality Statistics. Review of the Registrar General on deaths by Cause, Sex and Age in England and Wales 1964–1985*, London: HMSO.

Orem, D.E. (1985) *Nursing Concepts and Practice*, 3rd ed. New York: McGraw-Hill.

Parkin, D.M. *et al*. (1985) 'Cervical cancer', *British Journal of Obstetrics and Gynaecology* 92, pp. 150–7.

Peck, A. (1972) 'Emotional reactions to having cancer', *Cancer* 22, pp. 284–99.

Peck, A. and Borland, J. (1977) 'Emotional reactions to radiation treatment', *Cancer* 40, pp. 180–4.

Petot, H.C. (1986) *Fundamentals of Oncology*, 3rd ed. New York: Marcel Dekker.

Pridan, H. and Lilienfield, A. (1971) 'Carcinoma of the cervix in Jewish women in Israel 1960–1967: An edpidemiological study', *Israel Journal of Medical Science*, 7, pp. 1465–70.

Reynolds, P. *et al*. (1981) 'Cancer and communication: information given in an oncology clinic', *British Medical Journal*. 1, pp. 1449–50.

Roper, N. *et al*. (1981) *The Process of Nursing*, Edinburgh: Churchill Livingstone.

Roper, N., Logan, W.W. and Tierney, A.J. (1985) *The Elements of Nursing*, 2nd ed., Edinburgh: Churchill Livingstone.

Royal College of Nursing, Department of Nursing Policy and Practice (1987) *Drug Administration: A Nursing Responsibility*, London: RCN.

Skipper, H.E. et al. (1964) 'Experimental evaluation of potential anti-cancer agents', *Cancer Chemotherapy Reports* 35, pp. 3–11.

Spencer-Jones, J. (1981) 'Telling the right patient', *British Medical Journal* 2, pp. 291–2.

Spriggs, I.A. and Husain, O.A.N. (1977) 'Cervical smears', *British Medical Journal* 1, pp. 1516–18.

Tiffany, R. (1979) *Cancer Nursing. Radiotherapy*, London: Faber.

Trester, A.K. (1982) 'Nursing management of patients receiving cancer chemotherapy', *Cancer Nursing* 5 (3), pp. 201–10.

Trevathan, E. *et al.* (1983) 'Cigarette smoking and dysplasia and carcinoma *in situ* of the uterine cervix', *Journal of the American Medical Association* 250, pp. 499–502.

Walter, J. (1982) 'Care of the patient receiving anti-cancer drugs', *Nursing Clinics of North America* 17 (4), pp. 607–29.

Wolfendale, M. *et al.* (1983) 'Abnormal cervical smears: are we in for an epidemic?' *British Medical Journal* 287, pp. 526–8.

Yule, R. (1984) 'Screening for prevention', *Nursing Mirror* 159 (13), pp. 37–9.

13   The Breast and Breast Disease

Breast cancer is the most common malignancy affecting women in the UK, where its incidence is greater than anywhere else in the Western world (DHSS 1987). Every year approximately 24,000 new cases are diagnosed and over 15,000 women die, making it the most common cause of mortality among women during middle age. Aetiology and effective methods of prevention remain obscure although development of the disease is believed to reflect Western lifestyle, especially patterns of child-bearing and lactation. Approaches to treatment have changed over the years but with little impact on life expectancy (Baum 1981). However the psychological effects of breast cancer and the effect of treatment on body image and feminine self-esteem are well documented (Maguire, 1980, Krause 1987).

Women with breast disease are treated by general surgeons and admitted to general rather than gynaecology wards. However the nurse, in her capacity as a health educator, has many opportunities to advise women about the care of their breasts (Marks-Maran and Pope 1985). This is especially important for those receiving oral contraceptives or hormone replacement therapy in view of possible links between oestrogen and breast cancer. Any abnormalities should be reported at once.

Breast self-examination

It was argued by Hobbs (1973) over ten years ago that before women would submit to regular breast self-examination and screening they must be convinced on two counts:

- The importance of early treatment for breast disease;
- The large number of benign cysts detected in comparison to malignant neo-plasms (see Table 13.1).

This may not be fully appreciated by nurses working in hospital wards as women with non-malignant breast disease are so often treated as outpatients. Some health professionals argue that breast self-examination is of only limited value, because two thirds of those with malignant lesions will eventually die of their disease, while others believe that it can actually be harmful by acting as a continual reminder of a disease that may never develop (Holmes 1987). However, the evidence of the Forrest Report (DHSS 1987) strongly indicates that women may benefit from regular screening, especially if it takes place in a supportive atmosphere.

Table 13.1 Benign diseases of the breast

Name	Pathology	Treatment
Mastitis – acute	Acute inflammation. Usually accompanies lactation. Staphylococcal infection, sometimes followed by abscess formation	Antibiotics. Rest. Drainage of abscesses
Mastitis – chronic	Following acute mastitis. Chronic infection and blockage of the ducts. May lead to cyst formation as the infected material builds up in the obstructed ducts (ductal ectasia)	Surgical excision of obstructed ducts
Fibroadenoma	Small benign solid tumour, usually in young women	Surgical excision
Cystadenoma	Benign tumour filled with fluid	Aspiration or surgical excision
Papilloma	Benign tumour formed from part of the duct system. Dicharge from the nipple is common, sometimes bloodstained	Surgical excision of the tumour and associated ducts

Before they become expert at breast self-examination, women must be taught the normal anatomy and physiology of the breasts, emphasising the natural monthly changes accompanying the menstrual cycle. As this topic is likely to provoke anxiety, special attention must be paid to individual needs for information otherwise effective learning will not be possible.

■   When Ingrid Almond started to take oral contraceptives she was invited to a self-help group to learn about breast examination. The group was organised by two nurses, one from the family planning clinic, the other from the health centre of the college where Ingrid was a student. At the group meeting, a number of myths were exploded: size of the breasts is not influenced by massage, creams or exercise, although exercise may improve shape and correct posture enhances the figure. Anxiety about appearance is common in view of the sexual and reproductive significance of the bosom historically and the current trend of using the breasts to market a wide range of consumer products. A large clear diagram was used to demonstrate the external and internal appearance of the breasts (see Fig. 13.1).

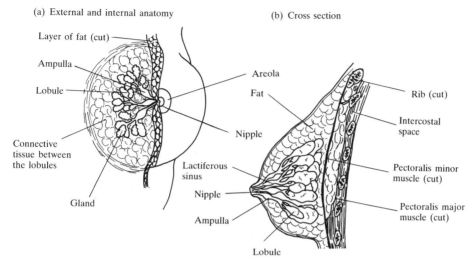

(a) External and internal anatomy

Layer of fat (cut)

Ampulla

Lobule

Connective
tissue between
the lobules

Gland

(b) Cross section

Areola

Fat

Nipple

Lactiferous
sinus

Nipple

Ampulla

Lobule

Rib (cut)

Intercostal
space

Pectoralis minor
muscle (cut)

Pectoralis major
muscle (cut)

Figure 13.1 The breast.

Structure and function of the breasts

The left breast (*mammary gland*) is usually a little larger than the right. Both are separated from the underlying pectoral muscles by a layer of connective tissue. The nipple is situated just below the centre of each and, like the surrounding *areola*, is pigmented. This effect is most marked during pregnancy when the areola enlarges. It returns to normal size when lactation ceases, but never returns to its original colour. The shape of the nipple is variable in response to sexual stimulation and temperature change through contraction of its muscular fibres. There is also some natural variation in size and shape between women.

Each breast is a greatly developed sebaceous gland consisting of alveolar (*racemose*) glandular tissue, fibrous tissue and fat organised into approximately 20 lobes separated by suspensory ligaments (Cooper's ligaments). These help to maintain position. Each lobe consists of lobules of lactiferous tissue with ducts converging towards the nipple, where they unite. Just before opening onto the nipple surface, the ducts dilate to form sinuses which provide reservoirs for milk during lactation.

The breasts are subject to considerable change throughout the woman's lifetime (see Fig. 13.2). Before puberty they are very small but are stimulated to develop by oestrogen, the hormone which maintains their condition and appearance throughout the reproductive lifespan of the woman. At the menopause, waning oestrogen levels cause the breasts to atrophy, and cyclical changes cease. When a woman is in her fifties, glandular tissue is gradually replace by fibrous and adipose tissue but, with increasing age, some of the fat may be lost. In the late sixties and seventies, the breasts may became wrinkled and droop.

Development of glandular tissue and extra fat causes the breasts to enlarge during pregnancy and lactation. Throughout pregnancy oestrogen, released from the

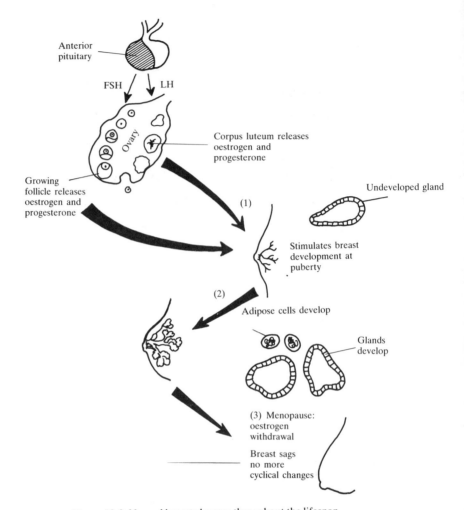

Figure 13.2 Normal breast changes throughout the lifespan.

placenta, stimulates the ducts to grow and branch, with the deposition of fat in between. Progesterone makes the lobules grow and stimulates development of the secretory cells. As pregnancy reaches term, *prolactin* – a hormone secreted by the anterior pituitary – helps progesterone to stimulate further glandular development and promotes lactation. Milk is secreted continuously after parturition but must be ejected from the alveoli of the glands where it collects into the ducts before the baby can obtain it. The 'let down' reflex is stimulated when the baby sucks. Nerves acting on the hypothalamus cause the release of *oxytocin*, a hormone, which stimulates the tightening of special cells with contractile properties (*myoepithelial cells*) around the alveoli. Milk is then ejected.

Although breasts reach their greatest development during pregnancy and lactation, they prepare for pregnancy each month when progesterone, released from the corpus

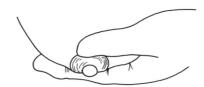

Figure 13.3 Checking the nipples for discharge.

luteum, promotes development of the alveoli and lobules. Just before menstruation the breasts swell, partly due to secretory development, partly because blood supply increases and extra fluid is retained in the subcutaneous tissues. Many women complain that their breasts feel sore or 'heavy' before menstruation. Temporarily they may feel lumpy.

All these changes are normal. Women examining their breasts before menstruation may mistakenly believe they have detected a lump. To avoid unnecessary anxiety, the breasts should be examined at the *end* of menstruation when they are less sensitive to hormonal fluctuations.

Detecting abnormalities

Much can be learned by looking at the breasts. At the beginning of the examination, the woman should view them in a mirror. The following abnormalities might be revealed:

- Dimpling or an inverted nipple resulting from an underlying lesion pulling the skin inwards;
- Inflammation or infection indicated by patches of redness or, occasionally, by discharge from the nipples (see Fig. 13.3).

A prosthesis can be used to demonstrate how to detect a possible lump by palpation. The need for systematic examination must be emphasised, feeling each breast in turn with the pads of the fingers (as these are more sensitive than fingertips) and working in a circular motion until all tissue has been palpated (see Fig. 13.4). Diagrams can be used to demonstrate the position in which abnormalities are most readily detected (see Fig. 13.5).

Women may be anxious about false alarms – they may want to know what a lump would actually feel like. The nurse can demonstrate this using a practical tip (Stanway and Stanway 1982). Women may be instructed to close one eye before placing a fingertip on the eyelid. When the finger is moved gently, the eyelid can be felt sliding over the underlying eyeball. This is the sensation when a harmless cyst is felt. She can then ask the woman to notice how easily they can pick up the eyelid and pull it away from the eyeball. Next she can ask them to place their fingertips on the ends of their noses, demonstrating that this time the skin will not move because it is tethered firmly to the underlying structures and cannot be lifted. A serious lump feels like this because it is attached to the tissue beneath. She should emphasise the need to go to

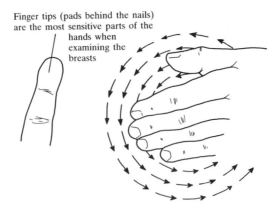

Finger tips (pads behind the nails) are the most sensitive parts of the hands when examining the breasts

Figure 13.4 Systematic examination of the breasts.

the doctor at once if any abnormality is detected, reassuring them that, once they have become familiar with their breasts, they will be less likely to worry unnecessarily.

There is evidence that women can learn breast self-examination techniques if they are provided with written material (Turner *et al.* 1984), but a study by Marty *et al.* (1983) among 219 women indicated that attitudes were more positive, and compliance enhanced if they were able to participate in programmes combining discussions, demonstrations and guided practice.

Benign cysts are commonly detected: about 55 per cent of women referred to a breast clinic can be expected to have a benign condition and, for a further 30 per cent, it is likely that no abnormality will be detected at all (Chetty 1980). This evidence is supported by the results of trials conducted on a larger scale in other countries (Verbeek *et al.* 1984). Far from causing unnecessary anxiety, some authors believe that one of the main benefits of regular breast self-examination is reassurance that all is well (Practitioner 1982).

Breast tumours

Investigating breast lesions and risk factors

■ Ingrid, convinced of the value of a healthy lifestyle, examined her breasts every month. With a little practice she soon became accustomed to their texture and was confident that she would detect any change.

Some months later Ingrid felt unusually fatigued after swimming. Her breasts seemed heavy and uncomfortable. It was then that she felt the lump.

Arrangements were made by Ingrid's GP for her to be seen at the Breast Clinic of the local hospital.

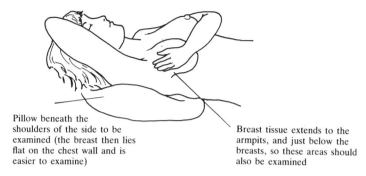

Pillow beneath the shoulders of the side to be examined (the breast then lies flat on the chest wall and is easier to examine)

Breast tissue extends to the armpits, and just below the breasts, so these areas should also be examined

Figure 13.5 Suggested position for palpating the breasts in self examination.

The main pre-disposing factor to breast malignancy is age. Although malignancy occurs in young women, its incidence is seven times greater among those aged 50–54 than for women in their early thirties or younger, and mortality is over twelve times as likely (DHSS 1987, Annexe 5). It has been suggested on the evidence of the Forrest Report that women over 50 are likely to benefit from regular screening, while further evidence of its effectiveness in young age groups is still wanting. Studies are continuing in the UK, Canada and Sweden. The frequency with which screening should be repeated has yet to be established although it has been suggested that repeated radiological examinations may slightly increase the risk of breast cancer in women who might not otherwise have developed it. The benefit of attempting to screen those over 65 is also questioned since it is known that far fewer women in this age group find breast examination acceptable (Tabar et al. 1985). However, breast tissue is technically easier to examine with increasing age because it is less dense owing to a higher ratio of adipose to glandular substance.

One of the problems of organising a major screening programme for the detection of breast cancer, apart from cost, is the lack of risk factors (other than age) which lead to development of the disease. The following definitions of women at risk have been described in the literature (Dupont and Page 1985) but occur in only 25 per cent of those affected:

- Those for whom one malignant breast lesion has already been detected;
- Those who are nulliparous or who have had their first baby after 30 years of age;
- Those who experience an early menarche and a late menopause – risk seems to increase with the years of hormonal fluctuations associated with the menstrual cycle;
- Those who have familial incidence of breast cancer, especially if their mothers were affected;
- Those whose diets include a high proportion of fat.

There is little doubt that susceptibility to breast cancer is associated with Western lifestyle, especially repeated menstrual cycles due to delay in childbearing and suppressed lactation, but cause and effective means of prevention remain obscure. The

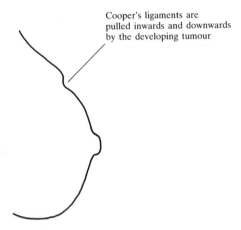

Cooper's ligaments are
pulled inwards and downwards
by the developing tumour

Figure 13.6 Dimpling of breast skin.

success of screening programmes depends on the natural history of the disease, which
is described below.

The natural history of breast cancer

Although malignant changes can occur in any part of the breast, they are most frequently detected in the left upper quadrant, and over 90 per cent arise in the lactiferous ducts (*intra-duct adenocarcinomas*). Neoplastic change begins in the secretory
cells of the alveolar glands or epithelial cells lining the lactiferous ducts. This represents the pre-invasive stage of the disease (see Chapter 12) in which malignancy is
locally confined. Spread to other sites begins at a very early stage in the development
of breast cancer, however, both locally and as *metastases*.

Local spread (infiltrating intraduct adenocarcinoma)
Infiltration may occur in a number of ways:

- Along Cooper's ligaments, pulling them downwards to form a dimple visible on
  the surface of the breast (see Fig. 13.6);
- Along the lactiferous ducts, eventually causing shrinkage and nipple inversion
  (see Fig. 13.7);
- Inwards towards the chest wall, tethering the tumour to underlying muscles and
  ribs;
- Outwards through the substance of the breast towards the overlying skin, resulting in the formation of an open, ulcerating lesion (*fungation*) if neglected.

Infiltration over a wide area without fungation causes oedema and the appearance
of numerous small dimples on the skin surface, which has been compared to the pitted
surface of orange skin (peau d'orange appearance). These visible changes explain the
abnormalities which women are taught to recognise when they examine their breasts.

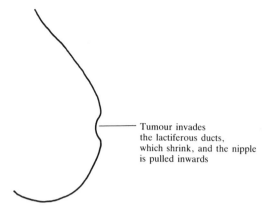

Tumour invades
the lactiferous ducts,
which shrink, and the nipple
is pulled inwards

Figure 13.7 Inverted nipple.

Metastases

As most malignant lesions develop in the upper outer quadrant of the breast, the lymphatic vessels draining this area and, to a lesser extent, the local blood vessels play an important part in subsequent development by carrying malignant cells to distant sites including the following:

- Axillary lymph nodes;
- Bone;
- Liver;
- Brain.

Although breast cancer is notorious for its ability to disseminate early, rate may vary between one woman and another and factors influencing spread have yet to be identified. Research in this sphere is vitally important; if more was known, larger numbers of women could perhaps be spared the trauma of aggressive surgery. Currently it is believed that as many as 80 per cent of breast cancers too small to detect clinically may already be invasive, but that those under 1 cm in diameter are less likely to have formed metastases.

Evidence suggests that screening programmes provide effective means of identifying early signs of malignancy (Verbeek 1984, Tabar 1985). Shapiro *et al.* (1982), screening 31,000 women as part of a health insurance plan for New York employees, found that subjects over 50 years of the age had singificantly reduced changes of mortality compared to the same numbers of matched but unscreened controls. As the study progressed and diagnostic procedures became more refined, evidence of early, non-invasive disease became increasingly apparent among younger women. Screening female staff in a large retail company gave a detection rate of 4.8 cases per 1,000 women over 35, rising to 8 per 1,000 for those over 50. With such early diagnosis, five-year survival rate reached 100 per cent (Hutchinson and Tucker 1984). However, results of another study published the same year provide fewer grounds for optimism (Fentimen *et al.* 1984). These authors suggest that once disease has begun to progress metastases may recur after very long time intervals. Their twenty year follow-up study revealed that only 20 per cent survived without recurrence, and that it was difficult to identify women likely to escape further disease as tumour size and degree of axillary lymph node involvement did not appear to provide reliable indicators of outcome.

Mammography and xeroradiography

Mammography involves X-raying the breast tissues. The related technique of xero-radiography is also an X-ray but the processing and appearance of the films differ. However, the procedure for both is the same and the chances of identifying a lesion without giving false negative or positive results is higher than for other methods (95 per cent). Hence mammography was identified as the most valuable screening technique currently available by the authors of the Forrest Report (DHSS 1987).

Women on whom mammography is being performed will need to be aware of the following procedures:

- They will be asked to remove all their clothes above the waist and sit in front of the X-ray machine.
- One at a time the breasts will be placed gently on a ledge, with an X-ray plate positioned beneath.
- A small dose of radiation will be passed through each breast onto the X-ray plate while it is held in position by the machine.
- The procedure may be uncomfortable but not painful.
- Once the films have been developed and checked to ensure they are of a satisfactory standard, they will be free to dress and leave the clinic.

Methods of detection and screening

The same techniques are used to screen women routinely for the presence of suspicious breast lesions, and to provide more information if a woman or her GP has detected a lump. They include ultrasonography, thermography and mammography.

Increasingly, screening and subsequent investigations are taking place in specialist clinics where members of a team (surgeon, radiologist, technician, nurse) are able to combine expertise. It is vital for nurses working with women to recognise that, although routine screening inevitably causes anxiety, those having investigations for a lump that has already been detected are likely to experience considerably greater stress.

Ultrasonography
Ultrasonography (see Chapter 4) has two great advantages:

- It is non-invasive, and
- Painless.

On the negative side it does not, at the present time, appear to be a particularly reliable method of detecting breast cancer during routine screening and so is not widely used. Techniques vary considerably in those units where it is employed.

Thermography

Thermography, the most recently developed technique of the three described here, is designed to measure skin temperature over the breast. Malignant lesions can be detected because they tend to generate more heat than surrounding tissue (1–2°C difference).

Unfortunately, thermography detects only 70–80 per cent of breast cancers and may sometimes give false positive results in the presence of their inflammatory conditions (Moskowitz *et al.* 1976). It is most valuable if used in conjunction with other techniques, but again women can be reassured that it is painless and non-invasive.

It is helpful for women to know in advance what investigations will involve. The nurse may explain the procedure as follows:

- Thermography involves taking photographs of the breasts under special conditions to provide information about the state of their tissues.
- When the woman attends the clinic, she will be asked to remove all her clothes from the waist upwards and sit in a cubicle with her arms above her head.
- The cubicle is set at a cool constant temperature (about 20°C).
- After approximately ten minutes, she will be called into an adjoining room where her breasts will be photographed with an infra-red camera.
- The entire procedure will take no more than fifteen minutes and, once the films have been developed and found to be of a satisfactory standard, she will be free to leave.
- Results will probably be available a week later, when the radiologist and surgeon have seen the films.
- The woman may find it reassuring to have a partner or friend accompany her to the clinic when results are expected.
- Sometimes other investigations may be performed to help confirm diagnosis.

■ Ingrid found her visit to the breast clinic most stressful because of the other women waiting anxiously for tests and results. One woman was in tears. The distress of other patients is known to be among the most anxiety-provoking aspects of hospital life, as is undergoing an investigation or treatment (Wilson-Barnett 1979). People cope with stress in different ways, some helpful, others said to be maladaptive because they may generate additional damage to the health of the individual (smoking, drug or alcohol abuse). Ingrid was fortunate, for her coping strategies were of a more positive nature, and she had a great deal of support from her social network.

Biopsy and histological examination

Although the nature of a breast tumour and likelihood of malignancy are to some extent evident on the basis of skilled clinical examination, cancer cannot be ruled out until some cells have been sent to the histology department for analysis. Cells can be obtained in several ways:

- Aspiration from a fluid-filled cyst (usually benign).
- Biopsy from a solid tumour (which may be benign or malignant).
- Excision of the lump.
- Tissue removed during more extensive surgery.

Several years ago it was fashionable for the woman to be taken to theatre for the biopsy which was then examined in the histology department while she was still anaesthesised ('frozen section' technique). Depending on the result, she might awaken to find that she had had only a minor operation or that her whole breast had been removed. Recognition of the severe stress placed on the woman and her family has caused this technique to fall from favour. It is now considered better for the woman to be given some time to adjust to her diagnosis and the need for surgery, even if this means having two anaesthetics and two separate operations. It is often possible for a small piece of the affected tissue to be removed under local anaesthesia.

■   When Ingrid returned to the clinic, she was relieved to hear that no further lumps had been detected and that a fine needle biopsy would be performed under local anaesthetic.

The procedure for a fine needle biopsy under local anaesthetic is as follows:

- Local anaesthetic is injected into the skin overlying the cyst.
- When the injection has taken effect, some fluid is withdrawn via a larger needle, then sent to the histology department for analysis.
- The wound is small, requiring only the protection of an elastoplast dressing which can be soaked off later in the bath.
- If, contrary to expectation, the lump proves solid, inserting the needle will cause no harm, but a slightly different technique may be employed to obtain some cells for histology.

Treatment of breast cancer: recent advances

Nurses responsible for patient/client teaching are likely to be asked about treatment for breast cancer. The main idea to emerge from the literature today is that no nurse or doctor can afford to have fixed ideas about the 'best' approach to treatment because much depends on the extent of the disease, the woman as an individual (including her age and general health), and her feelings about the disease and its treatment.

Several approaches presently exist, often used in combination:

- Surgery;
- Radiotherapy;
- Chemotherapy;
- Hormone manipulation;
- In some centres yttrium needles may be inserted into the lesion, acting as a local radioactive source.

It is vital that the nurse knows which treatments her patients are undergoing so that she can explain what each will entail, anticipate possible problems and plan nursing interventions.

It is also important for nurses to know why a particular approach to treatment has been selected; many women are affected, and many will encounter others with the same diagnosis and may wonder why the same information and treatment have not been provided.

Each of the four main methods of treatment is described below, but a more detailed account is beyond the scope of this book and further reading may be found in the references at the end of this chapter. The general principles of radiotherapy and chemotherapy are discussed in Chapter 12.

Surgery

Mastectomy, the primary treatment for breast cancer still most frequently undertaken, has been employed since Roman times, and the types of operation performed today are influenced by former practice. Traditionally, breast cancer was viewed as a local disease and it was thought advisable to excise as much of the affected tissue as possible to prevent dissemination. This led to radical and mutilating operations in which all breast tissue, lymph nodes, underlying pectoral muscles and even ribs were removed in an effort to prevent local spread. Wide excision meant that many women were unable to wear a prothesis to hide their disfigurement and, in some specialist centres, plastic surgery was performed. However, increasing knowledge of early neoplastic behaviour pointed to a disease that could not be viewed as local or discrete since size of the primary tumour does not appear to be closely related to possible extent of metastatic spread or prognosis, once it is no longer pre-invasive. Radical surgery, first described by Halsted in 1890, is less often performed today in favour of more conservative techniques.

As long ago as 1842, Symes suggested that by the time clumps of malignant cells have reached the axillary lymph nodes there seems little to prevent further spread to more distant sites, as metastases might remain undetectable for a very long period. However, it is only quite recently that other surgeons have concurred. Increasing readiness to perform more conservative operations has been influenced by the development of a clinical staging system which helps to classify the extent of disease (see

Table 13.2). Unfortunately, the results of clinical trials have not suggested that any particular technique or surgical procedure is superior to another, either in halting spread or increasing life expectancy, but more moderate views have resulted in fewer mutilating operations being performed on women who already have extensive disease. For these the aims of treatment are to reduce symptoms and to enhance quality of life – palliation rather than cure. Simple mastectomy may still have a place in the care of these women, however, as it may prevent local spread and fungation.

■   Jane Bishop worked in the High Street branch of a large chain store which offered employees a comprehensive health screening programme, and her breast lump was detected during a routine check. Jane was 39 years old and had no previous history of benign breast disease. She had not worried about breast examinations, regarding them as routine, and was shocked when arrangements were made for her to go to a Breast Clinic.

On clinical examination, the tumour appeared to be a solid mass tethered to the underlying tissues and, after investigations, was staged at T2b (between 2–5 cms diameter, attached to underlying tissue). Jane's axillary lymph nodes were palpable.

Jane was admitted to a general surgical ward to undergo simple mastectomy. On admission she was accompanied by her husband, Martin, who told the nurse that Jane's mother was staying to look after their three children. The tutor attached to the ward helped the learners to identify a number of problems for Jane (see Care plan 13.1 on page 370). Orem's Model (1980) was used to plan care.

Radiotherapy

At the present time women who have breast cancer may be given radiotherapy for one of three distinct purposes:

- As primary treatment instead of surgery. Its aim may be curative (small, non-invasive tumours) or palliative.
- As an adjunct to local excision to destroy any remaining malignant cells.
- As palliative treatment to relieve pain from metastases.

The oncologist arranged for Jane to receive radiotherapy as adjuvant treatment to try and prevent metastases, and the aim was for cure. Jane received *teletherapy* (see Chapter 12) as an outpatient as she did not want to be separated from her family any more than necessary. Her hospital stay had been short (five days) and she was still worried about many aspects of her disease and treatment when she came for her first appointment. A review of the literature has shown that recently discharged patients do not always receive all the information and reassurance they require even though physical nursing needs are met (Gould 1984). In some cases this may be due to poor

Table 13.2 TNM staging for breast cancer

Stage	Appearance
T0	Tumour not palpable
T1	Tumour 2 cm or less. No fixation to other tissues
T1a	Not attached to underlying muscles
T1b	Tumour attached to underlying muscle
T2	Tumour more than 2 cm but less than 5 cm, not fixed to underlying tissues
T2a	Size as above, not attached to underlying muscles
T2b	Fixed tumour, size as above, now attached to underlying muscles
T3	Tumour more than 5 cm in diameter
T3a	Tumour more than 5 cm not attached to underlying muscles
T3b	Tumour more than 5 cm attached to underlying muscles
T4	Tumour of any size with skin ulceration *or* fixed to chest wall
	Nodes
N0	Axillary nodes not palpable
N1	Axillary nodes palpable, but not fixed to skin
N1a	Axillary nodes palpable, but do not appear to contain tumour
N1b	Axillary nodes palpable and appear to contain tumour
N2	Nodes greater than 2 cm fixed to one another and to underlying tissues
N3	Involvement of supraclavicular lymph nodes
	Metastases
M0	No distant metastases apparent
M1	Distant metastases apparent

Care plan 13.1 (Orem's Self Care model)

Name: Jane Bishop

Treatment/condition: Mastectomy

Universal Self Care Requisites	Therapeutic Self Care Requisites	Self Care Agency	Self Care Deficits	Nursing Systems	Nursing Agency	Future
Maintain sufficient intake of oxygen	At risk of respiratory infection following anaesthesia. Post-operative breathing exercises four hourly	Adequate pain control to permit chest movement. Understands rationale for breathing exercises. Physiotherapist visiting	None at present. Prophylactic action required	Supportive	Monitor pain control. Monitor temperature four hourly for early evidence of infection. Reinforce breathing exercises	Self caring
Maintain sufficient intake of water	Unable to drink. Has intravenous fluids for 24 hours	Anticipated nausea following anaesthesia for first six hours post-operatively	IV fluids required for first 24 hours post-operatively	Monitor patency of IV line	Check patency four hourly and monitor IV site for inflammation	Self caring
Maintain sufficient intake of food	Nutritious diet, enriched with vitamin C, increased calories and increased protein for tissue repair and recovery	Anorexic. Does not feel like eating at present. *Causes:* – nausea – hospital food – anxiety – depression *Usual weight:* 56 kg, appears slightly built. Is	Intake diminished at present. Needs information for suitable diet at home	Supportive/educative	Explore reasons for present anorexia. Explore usual eating patterns. Suggest alterations that will deviate from usual pattern but still be nutritious and healing/supporting	Will need assistance especially during planned radiotherapy treatments, but this should be

		not aware what constitutes a well-balanced, nutritious diet				temporary
Care associated with elimination	At risk of temporary constipation related to post-operative opiate analgesia	Usual pattern is daily (morning). Able to ambulate to manage own toilet needs	None at present. At risk of constipation	Supportive	Monitor daily bowel movement. Encourage mobility and high fibre diet	
Maintain balance between activity and rest	Temporary fatigue related to major surgical procedure. Continuing fatigue related to: – radiotherapy – travelling for daily radiotherapy – depression	States she is very tired. Not sleeping well. Awake at night because she is: – worried about the future – experiencing discomfort in suture line. Upon discharge will have to care for home and three young children	Unable to rest related to pain and worries. Will need to plan for management of activities at home and adequate rest	Partially compensatory/ supportive	(1) Evaluate wound pain management, especially at night (2) Explore and encourage the expression of concerns especially in relation to self concept and her relationship to Martin, her husband (3) Break down household responsibilities into smaller components and explore extra support after discharge and during radiotherapy. Will require assistance with transport during radiotherapy therefore explore resources	Once through this intense period, should be fully self-caring. She does appear to cope poorly with stress and worry

Universal Self Care Requisites	Therapeutic Self Care Requisites	Self Care Agency	Self Care Deficits	Nursing Systems	Nursing Agency	Future
Maintain a balance between solitude and social interaction	Temporary fatigue. Cancer diagnosis may lead to social withdrawal. Diminished social contact during radiotherapy (lack of energy, time)	Withdrawn. Jane does not want to discuss her illness or treatment with her husband, friends who visit or with other women on the ward. She prefers to sit in the day room alone. Jane says she finds discussion of her situation painful. She worries that she will be unable to resume her previous role of 'good' and competent wife and mother	Altered family relationships. Altered social relationships	Supportive	(1) Provide time to explore feelings about having cancer, having a mastectomy and radiotherapy. This will give her a safe opportunity to share this with a neutral supportive person before she can share with family (2) She may benefit from meeting other women through the Mastectomy Association (3) Set realistic targets to support understanding of recovery and assist to appreciate that recovery is gradual (4) These reactions take time to work through. She will need continuing support following discharge. *Resources available:* –Breast specialist	

– District nurse
– Radiotherapy nurse
– Cancer counsellor
(5) Explore Martin's concerns and feelings about diagnosis and mastectomy. Evaluate his need for support

| Prevent hazards to life, well-being and functioning | At risk of infection at wound site. At risk of limitation of movement of right shoulder. At risk of lymphoedema and potential complications. Planned radiotherapy of chest wall will result in temporary inflammation | Wound site inflamed, tender and oozing due to probable haematoma and infection. Besides discomfort to Jane, there is concern because if healing of wound is delayed, radiotherapy may also be delayed. Discomfort may also be related to muscle stiffness and stiffened shoulder. Jane is reluctant to perform exercises under supervision of physiotherapist. Is not aware of risk of lymphoedema and potential problems related to it – swelling, infection | Impaired wound healing. At risk of diminished movement of right shoulder. Is unaware of lymphoedema and associated problems | Supportive/ educative | (1) Wound care (2) Provide time to discuss concerns about physical functioning. Explore normal activities with physiotherapist that could be substituted for formal exercises, e.g. hair brushing, putting on necklace. Provide presence during these activities for support. Evaluate daily (3) At an appropriate time – *not now* – but before discharge explain physiology of axillary lymph system (function and structure) and disruption to normal functioning due to | Wound should heal completely. Movement of right shoulder should be equal to other shoulder. There may be compromise in lifting capacity. May experience swelling of right arm |

Universal Self Care Requisites	Therapeutic Self Care Requisites	Self Care Agency	Self Care Deficits	Nursing Systems	Nursing Agency	Future
					mastectomy. Discuss implications of lymphoedema and susceptibility to infection and care that is required to prevent problems and minimise complications	
Promote normalcy	Altered body image with an impact on self concept	Jane feels she will never be 'normal' again. She does not want to look at wound or initiate discussions about it. She is reluctant to discuss plans for the future, including radiotherapy and arrangements to have prosthesis fitted. She has large breasts and feels lop-sided, needing encouragement to handle the temporary prosthesis that has been provided	Has not incorporated in an adaptive way her changed self. Has difficulty thinking past the present situation, e.g. cannot understand 'how women continue to lead active useful lives after mastectomy' or that a well fitting prosthesis will hide her loss	Supportive	(1) Encourage expression of feelings (bereavement) and fears. Reassure that these are reasonable and expected concerns. Do not rush (2) Offer to help contact Mastectomy Association (3) Discuss referral to Breast Specialist nurse (4) When changing dressing, if possible stand mastectomy side so that mastectomy is between nurse and Jane. Make positive comments if possible	Concerns about the adjustments Jane will have to undergo following discharge. She will need planned support which should begin immediately

Problem	Assessment		Nursing intervention
			about incision during dressing change, e.g. inflammation being contained or reduced
Threat of shortened life. Prognosis at this time is unknown	Coping style, as evidenced during this admission, has been to deny problems. However, within the context of an established relationship has began to express her feelings and fears regarding mastectomy. She states she is unwilling to discuss these issues with her husband and mother. Husband wants to talk about these concerns and has done so with ward sister	Coping style is not flexible and may not be effective to deal with future changes. Currently not able to use support of family effectively	Supportive — (1) Jane will need on-going support after discharge. Explore who is available and acceptable to Jane. Introduce support within the relatively safe (known) environment of hospital to help bridge transition between hospital/home/radiotherapy treatment centre (2) Discuss with consultant the prognosis so the exploration of realistic issues can be planned, i.e. roles of wife and mother, return to work, social relationships
Uncertainty related to: (a) unknown future (b) new experiences in new settings	Withdrawn and has expressed feelings of helplessness ('Anything you want, nurse. It doesn't matter...')	Depressed and not willing to involve herself in care. Has difficulty in viewing the future positively	Supportive — (1) Needs time to work through what is happening. Invite exploration of what she is feeling and what she perceives as the future. She will require on-going support

Universal Self Care Requisites	Therapeutic Self Care Requisites	Self Care Agency	Self Care Deficits	Nursing Systems	Nursing Agency	Future
					(2) Locate attractive mastectomy visitor with children to discuss prosthesis and common problems (3) Break down care into small units where improvements can be easily identified. Explore acceptable input into care. Reinforce the influence on outcome of self care – i.e. increased movement in arm, improved healing	

The psychological trauma associated with a diagnosis of breast cancer and mastectomy demand that the nursing model chosen should provide a framework for identifying and tackling emotional problems as well as physical ones. How effectively does Orem's model (1985) used here achieve this during early recovery, then later, planning for discharge? Two models – Roper (1985) and Orem (1985) – have been used in this book. But others exist, and may be equally, if not more, appropriate in some of the situations described. A textbook concerned with models of nursing may help you to identify other suitable approaches for Jane and her family. You could write a care plan based on one of these. Justify your choice.

communication between community and hospital staff, or between wards and departments of the same hospital. Jane was fortunate because her case was co-ordinated by
a team (oncologist, nurses in the ward, Breast and Radiotherapy Department) who
believed that the woman and her family should be considered the most important
members of the team. Jane had visited the Radiotherapy Department before she left
hospital to meet the nurses and to see the equipment, which can look very imposing
to the person receiving treatment. She had been given the following information:

- Radiotherapy destroys the axillary sweat glands, so normal odour in this area
  would be lost.
- Contrary to popular belief, washing the irradiated areas gently with warm water
  and drying with a soft towel will *not* result in rashes or soreness. Soaps and
  scented products should be avoided.
- She might not feel nauseated (the gut is not irradiated) but would almost certainly feel tired because of the combined effects of treatment and daily travel to
  the department.

The nurse in the Radiotherapy Department warned Jane about problems she might
encounter, but pointed out that not all women would develop them:

- Anorexia;
- Dry cough due to inflammation of the mucosa lining the respiratory tract;
- Breathlessness due to inflammation of the pulmonary tissues;
- Limited arm movements accompanied by oedema.

Lymphoedema can be a problem for women who have had extensive surgery involving removal of the axillary lymph nodes, as drainage of tissue fluid from the area
will be impeded. However, the extent to which it persists does not appear to have
been well documented in the literature (Marks-Maran and Pope 1985). Women may
find exercises taught by the physiotherapist helpful, but must accept that fluid will
begin to collect again if these are discontinued.

Chemotherapy

Traditionally, chemotherapy was not considered suitable for breast cancer because it
was viewed as a local disease and hormone manipulation was attempted as a means of
controlling metastases. However, a number of cytotoxic agents are now used (see
Table 13.3) although their side effects are distressing, particularly to women who
have already been subjected to mutilating surgery. Table 12.8 indicates some of the
problems faced by women undergoing chemotherapy.

Several of the drugs commonly employed in the treatment of breast cancer cause
alopecia. Hair loss may be reduced for some, though unfortunately not for all women,
by cooling the scalp before intravenous administration (Anderson 1981).

Chemotherapy for breast cancer is most likely to be effective when the total number of tumour cells is small. It is therefore most commonly used as adjuvant therapy,
usually after surgical excision.

Table 13.3 Cytotoxic drugs commonly used to treat breast cancer

---

Adriamycin
Cyclophosphamide
Methotrexate
Vincristine
5–Fluorouracil
Phenylalanine mustard – used in high doses
   in conjunction with bone marrow
   transplant in some
   centres

Hormone manipulation

Many hormones influence breast tissue. The effects of oestrogen and progesterone have already been described (see page 357). Table 13.4 shows the effects of others released mainly from the pituitary.

Hormone manipulation has been used as a method of controlling breast cancer for many years, but is regarded as palliative rather than curative. Its aim is to slow the disease process, improving quality of life, although not necessarily prolonging it. It is not suitable for every woman, and those who do *not* appear to respond well fall into the following categories:

- Rapidly growing tumours, with metastases developing soon after primary diagnosis;
- Middle-aged, perhaps because hormone levels are naturally in a state of flux at this time;
- Secondary deposits in the liver; bony metastases seem more responsive.

Approaches to treatment vary according to whether the woman is pre- or post-menopausal.

Pre-menopausal women
Natural oestrogens are prevented from stimulating breast tissue by one of two possible means:

- Irradiating the ovaries;
- Surgically removing the ovaries.

Oestrogen withdrawal is more abrupt following surgical removal, and women must be warned that they will experience sudden menopausal symptoms (see Chapters 9 and 12). Radiotherapy to destroy the ovaries is usually attempted when the woman is unfit for further surgical intervention as the levels of circulating oestrogen decline more slowly (over a period of about six weeks). Menopausal symptoms appear gradually.

Table 13.4 Hormones affecting breast tissue

Posterior pituitary	Anterior pituitary
1. Oxytocin – stimulates milk release on suckling ('let down reflex')	1. Oestrogen – stimulates breast growth
	2. Progesterone – stimulates development of breast ducts and secretory tissue
	3. Adrenocorticotrophic hormone (ACTH) – stimulates adrenal cortex to release steroid hormones which affect all tissues, including the breasts. Essential to life
	4. Thyroid stimulating hormone (TSH) – stimulates thyroid gland to release thyroxine and tri-iodo thyronine, which regulates basal metabolic rate of all tissues, including the breasts
	5. Growth hormone (GH) – responsible for the promotion of all tissue growth, including breast tissue. Unless adequate levels of thyroxine are present, GH will not function properly
	6. LH and FSH – influential because they control the release of oestrogen and progesterone
	7. Prolactin – stimulates milk production

Post-menopausal women

After the menopause, plasma oestrogen levels are very low, but small amounts are released by the adrenal cortex. Oestrogenic stimulation of breast tissue may be prevented by adrenalectomy or the administration of a drug, aminoglutethmide, which blocks oestrogen production in the adrenal cortex. Irrespective of the method, the woman must receive corticosteroid hormones also released by the adrenal cortex which are essential to life.

Recent advances in treatment and care

Breast tumours are influenced by oestrogen because their cells contain specific receptors for the hormone (see Chapter 1). This enables oestrogen to act on tumour cell

DNA to make the tumour grow. Anti-oestrogens are synthetic drugs able to attach themselves to the same receptors, blocking the entrance of oestrogen, but are too dissimilar to stimulate tumour growth. Trials with the anti-oestrogenic agent tamoxifen suggest that disease may be effectively controlled if therapy begins immediately after mastectomy or in the early stages of pre-invasive development. This offers a ray of hope for women whose futures are shadowed by the possibility of recurrence. Not all is gloom. Clinical trials to explore the effectiveness of different methods of treatment continue and it is now possible for many women to have breast reconstruction with silicone implants at the time of mastectomy or a few weeks later (Miller *et al.* 1977).

Meanwhile, more attention is being paid to the psychological effects of the disease on women and their families. As nurses become increasingly willing to incorporate the findings of reasearch studies into their care more women will benefit and many of these studies are now being undertaken by nurses themselves. A recent investigation by Eardley (1988), for example, has clearly demonstrated the benefits of providing written information for people who are to undergo radiotherapy.

Resources

Booklets on breast self-examination are obtainable from:

The Health Education Authority
78 New Oxford Street
London WC1

The Mastectomy Association
36 Harrison Street
London WC1H 8JG

The Women's National Cancer Control Campaign
1 South Audley Street
London W17 5DQ

The Marie Curie Memorial Foundation Fund
28 Belgrave Square
London

References

Anderson, J. (1981) 'Scalp hypothermia in the prevention of doxorubicin-induced alopecia' In: Tiffany, R. (ed.) *Cancer Nursing Update*, London: Ballière-Tindall.
Baum, M. (1981) *Breast Cancer – The Facts*, Oxford: Oxford University Press.
Chetty, U. *et al.* (1980) 'Benign breast disease and cancer', *British Journal of Surgery* 67, pp. 789–90.
DHSS (1987) *Breast Cancer Screening (The Forrest Report)*, London: HMSO.

Dupont, W.D. and Page, D.L. (1985) 'Risk factors for breast cancer in women with pro-liferative breast disease', *New England Journal of Medicine* 312, pp. 146–51.

Eardley, A. (1988) 'Patients' worries about radiotherapy: evaluation of a preparatory booklet', *Psychology and Health* 2, pp. 79–89.

Fentiman, I.S. *et al.* (1984) 'Which patients are cured of breast cancer?' *British Medical Journal* 2, pp. 1108–11.

Gould, D.J. (1984) 'Time to explain', *Nursing Mirror* 158 (8), pp. 20–2.

Hobbs, P. (1973) 'Applied research in teaching breast self-examination', *Health Education Journal* 32, pp. 47–51.

Holmes, P. (1987) 'Examining the evidence', *Nursing Times* 83 (31), pp. 28–30.

Hutchinson, J. and Tucker, A.K. (1984) 'Breast screening results from a healthy working population', *Clinical Oncology* 10, pp. 123–8.

Krause, K. (1987) 'Responding to breast cancer', *Nursing Times* 83 (10), pp. 63–6.

Maguire, P. *et al.* (1980) 'The effects of monitoring the psychiatric morbidity associated with mastectomy', *British Medical Journal* 281, pp. 1454–6.

Marks-Maran, D.J. and Pope, B.M. (1985) *Breast Cancer Nursing and Counselling*, Oxford: Blackwell.

Marty, P.J. *et al.* (1983) 'An assessment of 3 alternative formats for promoting breast self-examination', *Cancer Nursing* 6, pp. 207–12.

Miller, S.H. *et al.* (1977) 'Breast reconstruction following mastectomy', *Australian Operating Room Nurses' Journal* 25 (5), pp. 945–9.

Moskowitz, M. *et al.* (1976) 'Lack of efficacy of thermography as a screening tool for minimal stage 1 breast cancer', *New England Journal of Medicine* 295, pp. 249–52.

Orem, D. (1980) *Nursing – Concepts of Practice*, New York: McGraw-Hill.

Shapiro, S. *et al.* (1982) 'Ten to fourteen years effects of breast cancer screening on mortality', *Journal of the National Cancer Institute* 69, pp. 349–55.

Stanway, A. and Stanway, P. (1982) *The Breast*, London: Granada.

Tabar, L. *et al.* (1985) 'Reducation in mortality from breast cancer after mass screening with mammography', *Lancet* 1, pp. 829–32.

The Practitioner (1982) Whole Issue, 226, pp. 1371–1437.

Turner, J. *et al.* (1984) 'Does a booklet on breast self-examination improve subsequent detection rates?, *Lancet* 2, pp. 337–8.

Verbeek, A.L.M. (1984) 'Reduction of breast cancer mortality through mass screening with modern mammography' (First Results of the Nijmegen Project. 1975–1981), *Lancet* 1, pp. 1222–4.

Wilson-Barnett, J. (1979) *Stress in Hospital*, Edinburgh, London: Churchill Livingstone.

14   Abnormalities of the Reproductive Tract

Most nurses are keenly aware of the important of body image to self esteem. This chapter, focusing on abnormalities of the reproductive tract, has been included despite the rarity of these conditions because of its interest to nurses who work in fertility clinics and in specialist gynaecology wards where corrective plastic surgery may be undertaken when a patient has an abnormality involving the genital tract. Evans (1977) argues the need for an holistic approach to nursing intervention, encompassing the following:

- Physical care;
- Psychological care;
- Social care;
- Psychosexual counselling.

Mazur (1983), emphasising the vital importance of counselling to young people and their families, points out the need for congenital defects to be detected early so that all concerned have some opportunity to come to terms with the situation. However, this is not always possible.

■   Ruth and Roger Freeman, married for three years, had been trying to start a family. Investigations revealed that Roger's semen contained no sperm at all (*azoospermia*). On the basis of clinical examination, the doctor suspected that Roger might have *Klinefelter's syndrome*, a rare abnormality of the sex chromosomes inevitably associated with sterility. Arrangements were made for chromosome analysis to be conducted, using a sample of Roger's blood. The cells examined are leucocytes.

Sex determination

Sex is genetically determined at fertilisation. Tissue cells of a normal human being contain forty-six chromosomes which carry DNA inherited from one generation to the next. DNA controls the cell's activity and is responsible for its unique appearance and behaviour. All the cells of the same individual contain the same identical DNA, but activity varies between one cell and another. Thus, some of the DNA in any cell at

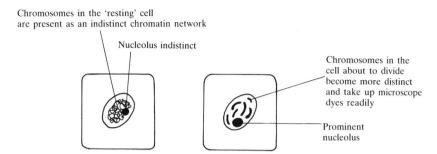

Chromosomes in the 'resting' cell are present as an indistinct chromatin network

Nucleolus indistinct

Chromosomes in the cell about to divide become more distinct and take up microscope dyes readily

Prominent nucleolus

Figure 14.1 Chromosome appearance in dividing and resting cells.

a particular time will be temporarily or permanently 'switched off', explaining why cells in different tissues look and behave differently (see Chapter 12).

The slender, thread-like chromosomes are inside the nucleus but can only be seen clearly at the time of cell division, and even then only if the cell is treated with special microscope dyes (see Fig. 14.1). When chromosome analysis is performed, cells are grown in a tissue culture. At the point of cell division they are treated with a drug called colchicine which arrests further activity. Photographs of the chromosomes taken at this point are enlarged, cut out and lined up in order of diminishing size, to form a *karyotype* (see Fig. 14.2).

The forty-six chromosomes can be arranged in pairs, which geneticists call *homologous* pairs. Twenty-two of the pairs are similar in both males and females and, within each homologous pair, the partners are identical. The remaining pair constitutes the sex chromosomes. In genetic females there are two X sex chromosomes which are alike. However, in genetic males there is one large X chromosome as in

A female karyotype would have two X chromosomes and no Y

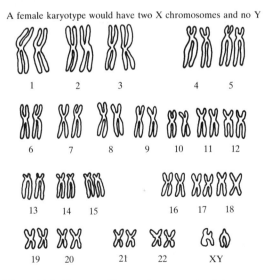

Figure 14.2 The normal human karyotype (male).

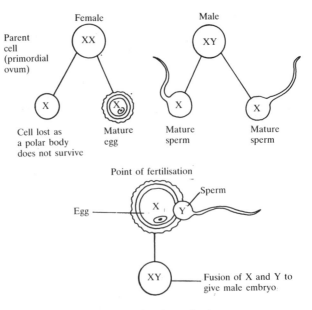

Figure 14.3 Sex determination.

females and a much smaller Y chromosome. Genetic females are thus designated XX, while genetic males are designated XY.

Eggs and sperm differ from all the other cells in the body by containing only twenty-three chromosomes each – exactly half the usual number. Special divisions of the cell nucleus take place when they are formed, ensuring that each sex cell receives only *one* chromosome from each homologous pair of the parent (*meiosis*). This means that all eggs carry only one X chromosome from the mother, while 50 per cent of sperms carry an X chromosome and the other 50 per cent carry a Y chromosome (see Fig. 14.3). When the egg and sperm fuse at fertilisation, there will again be forty-six chromosomes, including two sex chromosomes. The particular combination of sex chromosomes will determine the sex of the child.

Genetic abnormalities

Sometimes genetic abnormalities occur when sperm and eggs develop. An extra chromosome may become incorporated into a sex cell by accident or it may be missed out altogether. (Sometimes just part of a chromosome may be repeated or deleted.)

Occasionally a sperm or egg may incorporate an extra X chromosome. These sex cells are capable of fertilisation, but the resulting embryo will have three sex chromosomes – XXY if the child is a male. This is Klinefelter's syndrome. Physically the individual is a male, although the testes do not grow much at puberty. Facial hair always remains scanty and the pubic hair has a feminine distribution. In some men feminine contours may be apparent (breast tissue and curved hips) and there may be some degree of mental retardation, although this is certainly not always the case. Adults often lead normal married lives, realising that all is not well only when they attempt to start a family.

Nothing can be done about the sterility, inevitable with Klinefelter's syndrome. Added to this, there is the difficulty of explaining the nature of the genetic defect to the individuals concerned. Extreme sensitivity is necessary when deciding how much and when to tell, because of the possible damage that may be dealt to the body image of *both* partners. Throughout this book emphasis has been placed on communicating with patients and clients so they can become genuine partners in their own care. There are cases, however, when some people may be happier not knowing *all* the facts and when the absence of complete knowledge may not interfere with the outcome of their treatment. Nurses and doctors must become very well acquainted with the people whose best interests they are trying to serve; as well as providing opportunities for exchange of information, they also need to judge when a particular individual might be happier if some knowledge is withheld, either on a temporary or a permanent basis.

■ Tissue culture and chromosome analysis take several weeks so Ruth and Roger had made a number of visits to the clinic before diagnosis was confirmed. Before their next appointment a meeting was arranged among the staff, who agreed that from their behaviour they seemed a happily married couple, stable and mutually supportive. Their chief concern was Roger's feelings about being unmanly, which had come to light during nursing assessment when he was asked about any particular concerns associated with fertility investigations. It was known, however, that Roger and Ruth had a genuine desire for children and had already stated that they would definitely wish to adopt if the tests were unfavourable.

When Ruth and Roger returned to the clinic, they were told that Roger had a condition carried on one of his chromosomes which meant that he would remain unable to father a child.

The couple left the clinic too distressed to ask questions, but several weeks later they telephoned the sister and asked for an appointment. They wanted practical help about approaching an adoption agency. They remained in touch with the clinic, later adopting two children, but expressed no desire to be given further information about Roger's 'chromosome problem' and did not attempt to seek information from any other source.

Other congenital problems of the reproductive tract

Turner's syndrome

Turner's syndrome is another chromosomal abnormality, this time affecting the female. Women with Turner's syndrome have only one X chromosome, so genetically

Table 14.1 Features of Turner's syndrome (XO)

1. Normal intelligence
2. Congenital malformation of the aorta (coarctation)
3. Small stature
4. Failure of ovarian development – the ovaries are present as streaks of connective tissue
5. Absent secondary sexual characteristics unless treated
6. Characteristic webbed appearance of the skin covering the neck

they are XO. The typical features of Turner's syndrome are shown in Table 14.1. These children are more easily identified because of their short stature, so chromosome studies can be conducted before puberty. This is important because hormone therapy can be used to stimulate development of the uterus and breasts, and menstruation can sometimes be induced, depending on the state of ovarian development. Pregnancy is not possible, however, because the uterus is not sufficiently developed.

Chromosome analysis of fetal tissue after spontaneous abortion sometimes shows that the baby would have had Turner's syndrome. It appears that the maternal tissues can recognise genetic abnormality and the pregnancy is prevented from continuing.

Non-genetic problems

Not all congenital problems are genetic in origin. Some may be caused by maternal infection (Morgan-Capner and Griffiths 1984) while others may result from drugs taken during pregnancy. The organ systems affected are those developing at the time of exposure to the noxious agent and the reproductive tract of the fetus may sometimes be damaged. Women given the synthetic hormone Stilboestrol to prevent morning sickness gave birth to daughters who developed carcinoma of the vagina (normally a rare disease) as they reached puberty (Elkington 1986). The dangers of taking drugs during pregnancy are now well documented and women are no longer given hormones to treat threatened abortion, although this was once the fashion. Evidence from biologists working with animal embryos has demonstrated that developing tissues are genetically programmed by the activity of DNA on the chromosomes to behave in a prescribed fashion as each new stage is reached. Interference, particularly by hormones, may upset the normal progression of events and permanent damage may occur.

H-Y antigen

Although sex is determined genetically by the sex chromosomes, further development as a normal male or female will proceed according to presence or absence of a chemical called *H-Y antigen*.

Table 14.2 Causes of indeterminate gender

Condition	Cause	Main clinical features
Testicular feminisation	Insensitivity of the male fetus to testosterone	The individual is XY and has testes, but development proceeds along female lines, except that menstruation does not occur
Adreno-genital syndrome	Enzyme deficiency in a genetic female so that excess androgens are released instead of oestrogens	Enlarged clitoris and fused labia with a single orifice. The baby soon becomes ill because the enzyme pathway producing cortisol is also disrupted and there is salt and fluid depletion. Biochemical investigations are necessary to confirm diagnosis
Chromosome mosaics	Genetic; some cells of the individual are XX, some XY	Hermaphroditism, because the XX cells promote ovaries to develop and the XY cells promote testicular development. Great variety is seen in the structure of the external genitalia

Stimulus to release H-Y antigen comes from the Y chromosome. In the male, H-Y antigen causes the primitive gonads (developing sex organs) to release testosterone at a very early stage of development. This promotes formation of the male genitals. In the absence of the Y chromosome, female reproductive organs develop with apparently no further triggering stimulus. The female is thus the 'basic' sex, and failure of a genetic male to release adequate amounts of testosterone or inability of the tissues to respond to it may cause a genetic male to develop a feminine appearance. Congenital abnormalities, including problems of indeterminate gender, may therefore be hormonal in origin. Further information is provided in Table 14.2. However, in many cases the cause is unknown, and even when problems are apparent from childhood, little treatment can be attempted until puberty.

Indeterminate gender

■ June and Gary Jackson had been looking forward to the arrival of their second baby, but they knew at once that something was wrong. The midwife who examined the baby was not sure whether it was a boy or girl.

Table 14.3 Gynaecological problems encountered in childhood

1. Infective and inflammatory conditions, usually affecting the vagina
2. Neoplastic diseases, sometimes resulting in precocious puberty
3. Congenital abnormalities of the reproductive tract, possibly including intersex conditions

Gynaecological disorders in childhood are rare, so expertise in dealing with them is not easily found. Problems fall into three main categories, shown in Table 14.3. Estimates of the rate of congenital abnormalities of the female reproductive tract vary: according to some authorities they occur once in every 1,000 births, while others believe the rate to be one in every 4,000 (Evans 1977). This wide range may reflect the number of conditions identified as children develop.

When congenital abnormality is apparent at delivery, major emphasis must be placed on psychological support of the family but, at the same time, there is considerable need for help of an immediate and practical nature: parents have to decide at a very early stage how much, if anything, they wish to disclose to other people. Grandparents, friends and other family members, will be keen to see the new baby which, until undressed, may appear perfectly normal.

In most cases of indeterminate gender, the baby will appear to belong to one sex or the other with some degree of deviation, so naming and deciding how the child should be brought up are reasonably straightforward decisions. Problems are more acute in those very rare and tragic cases where the baby does not obviously belong to either sex. If gender is questioned *after* naming when socialisation has already begun, the dilemma is magnified. Attempts to alter the patter of socialisation later than three years of age are believed to cause severe psychological damage. Parents need to consider explanations to siblings as well as to the child affected.

■   From the beginning, June and Gary needed tremendous support from the health care team. Fortunately June Jackson had a good relationship with her health visitor, who called as soon as June came home. She found June tired, through coping with the demands of a new baby as well as her little girl, aged four. The health visitor's initial assessment showed that June was experiencing some difficulty setting priorities to the problems facing the family. Her parents lived in a distant town and her mother, arriving the next afternoon, expected to stay for several days. June had not decided what to tell her. She was more immediately concerned with the reactions of neighbours and perhaps, because the community was close knit in a rural area, she was worried about stories that might be spread to the school her eldest child was soon to attend. The health visitor encouraged her to distinguish between the immediate and differing needs of the grandparents compared to those of more casual acquaintances.

Arrangements had been made for the baby to be seen at a specialist hospital in a distant town. The health visitor was able to point out the value of the expertise of doctors and nurses who had previous experience of families in a similar position. The visit entailed careful planning. Early research by psychologists has shown how rapidly information given to anxious patients and clients may be forgotten or never absorbed (Ley and Spelman 1967). Pamphlets may be helpful to supplement verbal information but may not be directly relevant when a condition is very rare. The health visitor encouraged the couple to think in advance about the questions they would like to ask and to write them down, leaving space for information given during the consultation.

Clinical examination and the results of chromosome analysis revealed that the baby was genetically a girl.

When a new baby is examined, health care professionals may be alerted to problems of indeterminate gender by the following:

- Partial fusion of the labial skin giving the appearance of a scrotum despite the lack of a penis and the presence of a vagina;
- A structure looking either like an enlarged clitoris or an usually small penis;
- Absence or partial absence of the gonads.

The way in which these abnormalities occur is better appreciated given an understanding of the embryological development of the reproductive tract.

Embryological development

Ovaries and testes both develop from paired structures called the primitive gonads which arise from a strip of tissue on either side of the embryo called the genital ridge. The primitive gonad is made up of an inner medulla surrounded by a cortex (see Fig. 14.4). Gender is indistinguishable until the seventh week of embryonic life, when testosterone in the male begins to promote development of the genitals. A testis forms from the medulla of each of the primitive gonads. The cortex of each primitive gonad then atrophies and eventually the testes descend into the scrotum. In females, lacking the influence of testosterone, the cortex of each primitive gonad develops into an ovary and the medulla atrophies. As the ovaries grow they project downwards, ultimately lying adjacent to the developing uterus.

The rest of the reproductive tract develops from paired ducts which develop on either side of the embryo. In males they are called *Wolffian ducts* and in females *Müllerian ducts*.

Figure 14.5 shows that Müllerian ducts begin development as separate entities which fuse at the lower end, forming the uterus and vagina. The upper parts of the

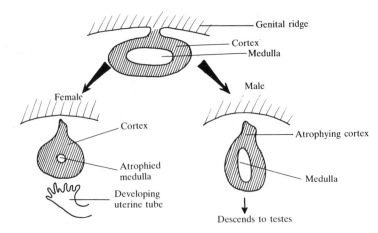

Figure 14.4 The primitive gonads: development of the ovaries and testes in the fetus.

Müllerian ducts remain separate, ultimately giving rise to the uterine tubes. Initially a septum (wall of tissue) separates the cavities at the lower ends of the Müllerian ducts, but later the septum regresses, leaving a single uterine cavity. Further downgrowth of this fused structure results in development of the vagina, which is initially solid becoming canalised later during embryological development. Occasionally the vagina remains solid, so the vulva is not connected to the uterus. This condition,

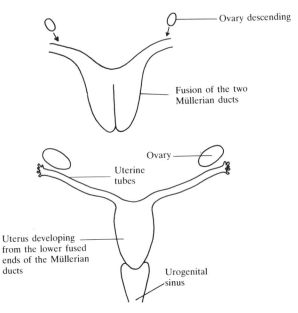

Figure 14.5 Development of the internal female reproductive structures.

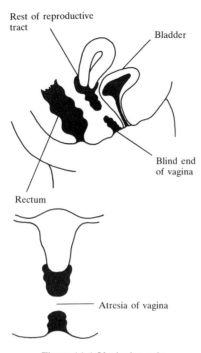

Rest of reproductive
tract

Bladder

Blind end
of vagina

Rectum

Atresia of vagina

Figure 14.6 Vaginal atresia.

which can be corrected by plastic surgery, is called *vaginal atresia* (see Fig. 14.6). In other cases the uterus remains septate or the two halves of the Müllerian ducts fail to unite, giving rise to a bicornuate uterus (Fig. 14.7). This may interfere with future pregnancies and can cause habitual abortion (see Chapter 4).

Development of the male and female external genitals occurs in conjunction with development of the urethra and anus. All open onto an area called the *urogenital sinus* where five swellings become apparent (see Fig 14.8). and are named as follows:

- The genital tubercle;
- The urogenital membranes;
- The anal membrane;
- The labial swellings;
- The urethral fold.

In females the genital tubercle forms the clitoris, but in males it undergoes much greater enlargement, becoming the penis. In females, the two labial swellings grow downwards and encroach on one another, fusing posteriorly to form the labia, but in males fusion is complete giving a scrotum. Figure 14.8 shows the similarity between male and female during early development, indicating how gender may occasionally be ambiguous if some factor, which normally directs tissue differentiation, loses control. Extent of the damage will depend on the degree of interference and it may or may not be associated with a genetic defect.

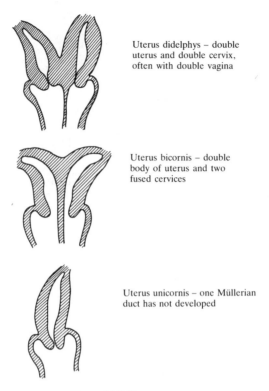

Uterus didelphys – double uterus and double cervix, often with double vagina

Uterus bicornis – double body of uterus and two fused cervices

Uterus unicornis – one Müllerian duct has not developed

Figure 14.7 Bicornuate uterus.

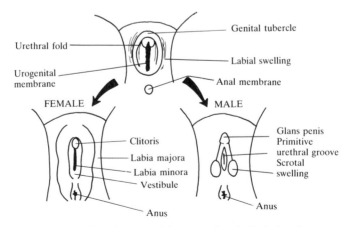

Genital tubercle

Urethral fold

Urogenital membrane

Labial swelling

Anal membrane

FEMALE

MALE

Clitoris

Labia majora

Labia minora

Vestibule

Glans penis
Primitive urethral groove
Scrotal swelling

Anus

Anus

Figure 14.8 Development of the external genitalia (in fetus).

■   Initially, June and Gary felt shocked, but the help of their own health visitor, and prompt referral to a specialist centre, helped them come to terms with their daughter's condition. It was very important for them to establish good relationships with the hospital staff since their daughter will eventually require plastic surgery to reconstruct a vagina, and they will need help to handle the difficult questions she will ask as she grows up. Parents in this situation may experience anger, guilt, depression or denial. They may not wish to discuss the situation with other people because it will then become more 'real', but it is vital to provide some information to the child before puberty, otherwise bitter resentment may be experienced (Evans 1977).

The outcome of reconstructive surgery is often very good (South 1985), and there are other cases where congenital disorders are far less dramatic in their presentation and do not become apparent for several years.

Puberty and the menarche

Gender differs during embryological development mainly because the male secretes testosterone, promoting development of the male primary sexual characteristics. After birth, the testes and ovaries become inactive until the onset of puberty, which on average begins two years earlier for girls compared to boys.

Puberty is the time of greatest sexual differentiation since intrauterine development. Changes take place in the reproductive organs, secondary sexual characteristics, body size and shape (Tanner 1978). There is enormous variation between the ages at which individual girls reach puberty and changes do not occur in the same order for every girl.

For about two thirds of the girls who have taken part in developmental studies the first noticeable change is early development of the breasts, which occurs sometime between 9 and 13, the most typical age being 11 years. In most girls pubic hair begins to grow a little later, followed by the menarche (arrival of the first menstrual period). By this time the uterus and ovaries are approaching adult size, but full reproductive function is not attained with the earliest cycles, which are not only irregular but usually anovulatory (no egg is released although bleeding occurs). The girl, meanwhile, rapidly increases in height and weight, gradually attaining typical feminine contours due to the deposition of fat in the subcutaneous tissues.

Although oestrogen controls all the changes which occur at puberty, the factors which trigger its secretion have yet to be identified. Throughout childhood the hypothalamus does not secrete gonadotrophin releasing factor, so levels of circulating LH, FSH and sex steroids are minimal. As puberty approaches oestrogen begins to be released in gradually increasing amounts, leading endocrinologists to postulate the existence of an unidentified inhibitory factor de-activated as the appropriate time is reached. One of the triggering stimuli may be increase in weight, with the menarche taking place when a certain critical weight has been attained.

There is some support for this theory since menstruation may cease in women who become severely undernourished. Data collected over the last hundred years suggest that, over the Western world, the average age at which girls experience their first period has declined, perhaps due to improved nutrition.

Endocrine disorders may prevent or delay the menarche, but if this happens the other signs and symptoms of puberty fail to appear. The age range of the menarche is so wide in 'normal' girls (11 to 17) that most late developers can be reassured that, from the evidence of height increase, breast development, and appearance of pubic and axillary hair, periods will soon arrive.

■   Lindsay Bridges, aged 15, consulted the school nurse because her periods had not started. The school nurse reassured Lindsay that she would probably soon start to menstruate but nothing happened, although Lindsay sometimes complained of pelvic discomfort. In view of this a visit to the GP was recommended, and Lindsay was referred to a gynaecologist at the local hospital.

When Lindsay and her mother arrived at the clinic they were greeted by the sister, who noticed that, of the two, Mrs Bridges seemed the most anxious. She decided to speak to them separately in case they had any questions to ask before seeing the doctor.

Mrs Bridges was most upset at the thought of her young daughter being subjected to a gynaecological examination. The sister explained that, in girls, it is usual to perform rectal rather than vaginal examination. She also took the opportunity to mention to Mrs Bridges the importance of allowing Lindsay to see the doctor on her own, if she wished, and to be given privacy during the examination. Occasionally menstruation may not 'begin' because the girl is in fact pregnant, a possibility which Mrs Bridges had not apparently considered.

To Lindsay the sister explained that the doctor would perform a full examination, including inspection of the breasts and pubic area, and that rectal examination would be necessary to provide information about the internal reproductive structures. This part of the examination, although uncomfortable, would be over quickly and a nurse would be present throughout. Lindsay's mother could be asked to wait outside if necessary.

The examination suggested that Lindsay had a relatively unusual condition, called *cryptomenorrhoea* (hidden menstruation). The hymen, a membrane partly occluding the vaginal opening, is not perforated, so menstrual flow is unable to escape (see Fig. 14.9) and may give rise to pelvic discomfort. The hymen bulges with the pressure of the blood dammed up behind it and, in more severe cases, there may be abdominal distension and urinary retention. Water is absorbed, so the blood becomes thick and dark. Treatment is by incision and drainage. Lindsay and Mrs Bridges were told that this would be performed as soon as possible under general anaesthetic, but that hospital stay would be short as the procedure is a minor one. The sister emphasised that during recovery personal hygiene would be important, since stale blood is an excellent medium for bacterial growth.

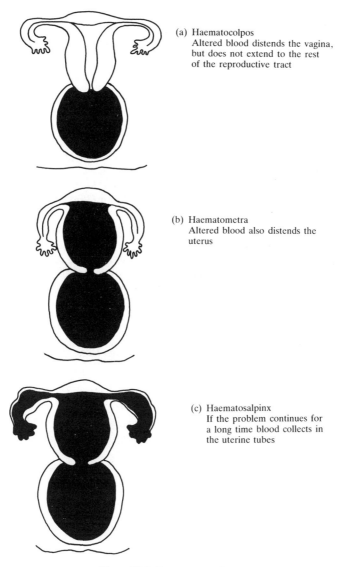

(a) Haematocolpos
Altered blood distends the vagina,
but does not extend to the rest
of the reproductive tract

(b) Haematometra
Altered blood also distends the
uterus

(c) Haematosalpinx
If the problem continues for
a long time blood collects in
the uterine tubes

Figure 14.9 Cryptomenorrhoea.

The onset of menstruation is a significant event in the development of young girls and, despite the discomfort and inconvenience which most experience at some time or another with periods, distress is more likely to be experienced if periods fail to appear through fear of being 'different' from peers (Havens and Swenson 1986). Nurses who work with young women are more likely to encounter the occasional 'late developer' than the unusual conditions described in this chapter, but they can do much to alleviate unnecessary worry, to explain the variable sequence of 'normal' development, and to recognise when and where to obtain expert opinion in those few instances when a genuine problem becomes apparent.

References

Elkington, J. (1986) *The Posioned Womb*, London: Pelican.

Evans, S.K. (1977) 'Supportive care in plastic surgery for congenital absence of vagina: a case presentation', *Journal of Obstetric, Gynaecological and Neonatal Nursing* 6 (4), pp. 31–4.

Havens, B. and Swenson, I. (1986) 'Menstrual perceptions and preparation among female adolescents', *Journal of Obstetric, Gynaecological and Neonatal Nursing* 15 (5), pp. 400–11.

Ley, P. and Spelman, M.S. (1967) *Communicating with the Patient*, London: Staples Press.

Mazur, T. (1983) 'Ambiguous genitalia: detection and counselling', *Paediatric Nurse* 9 (6), pp. 417–22.

Morgan-Capner, P. and Griffiths, G. (1984) 'Foetal and neonatal infection', *Nursing Times* 80 (45), pp. 28–32.

South, G. (1985) 'William's vaginoplasty', *Nursing Mirror* 160 (24), pp. 46–50.

Tanner, J.M. (1978) *Foetus into Man*, London: Open Books.

Underhill, R. (1976) 'Gynaecological problems in children', *Nursing Times* 72 (21), pp. 812–5.

15   Violence against Women: Sexual Crimes

Rape is defined as entry of the penis beyond the labia majora without the woman's consent. The 1976 Sexual Offences (Amendment) Act recognises two categories:

- *Statutory rape* when the girl cannot consent because she is below the legal age (16 years in the UK).
- *Forcible rape* when the woman is made to have intercourse against her will, or when her assailant is reckless as to whether she consents.

Rape is considered a serious crime with a maximum penalty of life imprisonment, although much more lenient sentences are frequently passed. It can only be tried in Crown Court before a jury, and much will rest on whether the woman can 'prove' that consent was not given (Moore 1985). This issue of consent is one of the chief defences against a charge of rape: the assailant pleads that he had intercourse with the woman but at the time believed she consented.

Sexual assault is more loosely defined, and the term has become synonymous with indecent assault, recognised as an offence under the 1956 Sexual Offences Act. From case law it includes forced penetration of mouth by penis, forced penetration of vagina or anus by an object and touching of breasts and buttocks or genitals or forcing the woman to touch in return.

Again girls under 16 years old cannot consent, while for older women consent is an issue. Sexual assault is not regarded as such a serious crime as rape. Maximum sentence is ten years imprisonment, and cases may sometimes be heard in magistrates' rather than Crown Court.

The incidence of sexual crimes is hard to establish. Figures published annually by HMSO suggest that whereas non-sexual violent crimes have risen sharply in recent years, sexual crimes have not tended to increase much, particularly rape, which is not common. However, these incidents are likely to have a devastating effect on victims and have therefore attracted the attention of police, social scientists, feminists and, in recent years, nurses (Hicks 1985). Researchers have been concerned with the psychology of assailants, the sociology and politics of sexual crime and its impact on women, the aspect considered in this chapter.

Evidence that many incidents go unreported is persuasive (Veitch 1980) and it is not difficult to find reasons: women may fear disbelief, especially if they are very young (Schmidt 1981), dislike the idea of police questioning and forensic examination, or experience such distress that they perfer to forget or ignore what has happened. Even if a woman goes to the police she may decide not to press charges because she fears court appearance and cross-examination. This reluctance is unfortunate as the assailant will not be deterred from repeating the same behaviour in future.

A nurse asked for advice by a woman in this position can reassure her of the following:

- Although the police have in the past been criticised for their treatment of rape victims, much has now been done to improve this aspect of police work;
- She is unlikely to be greeted with disbelief as carefully documented evidence collected over the years suggests that very few false accusations are made (O'Reilly 1984);
- The Sexual Offences (Amendment) Act of 1976 stipulates that nothing can be published or broadcast to identify the woman during or after trial, regardless of its outcome.

The nurse's role

Nurses need to be informed about police procedure and after care following sexual crimes for certain reasons:

- They may be confronted by a victim in the A and E department;
- A seriously injured woman may be admitted to hospital following sexual assault;
- They may be asked for information by women who fear attack;
- There is evidence that victims may brood on past incidents, sometimes years afterwards. Today, with emphasis on close, confiding relationships with patients developed through use of the nursing process, nurses may be told about these;
- Because they work shifts, nurses often travel at unsocial hours, and are therefore themselves at risk of assault. Community nurses visiting clients alone are at particular risk (Orr 1988).

Immediate care

Examination and immediate care of the rape victim may take place in one of three places:

- A specially run rape crisis centre. These have been established in a few cities in England, but are more in evidence in the USA than UK.
- The A and E deparment.
- A police station. This is the most usual venue. The examination is usually conducted by a police surgeon (a GP employed on a part-time basis by the police who has been trained in forensic medicine). In hospital, nurses may assist but are unlikely to perform forensic examination, although some have been trained to do so in the USA (Bellack *et al.* 1977 Di Nitto 1986).

In recent years the police have received some criticism about the way in which rape victims are received, and much has been attempted to reduce the ordeal of forensic examination. Experimental training programmes for police recruits have demonstrated that sensitivity and empathy as well as factual knowledge about sexual crimes can be improved (Gottesmann 1977).

Examination involves the following:

- Taking a history;
- General physical examination;
- Vaginal examination;
- Specimen collection to provide evidence if the case is brought to court.

If a nurse is present she can provide emotional support and information about the procedure to the woman:

- She will receive as much privacy as possible and will not be left unattended with the police surgeon, although she must be prepared for specimen collection to take some time (about an hour).
- A full history will be taken of the events leading up to the incident and she will be asked to describe where it occurred to help with police investigations.
- A special kit will be used during the examination. It contains a sheet of brown paper on which the woman will be asked to stand as she undresses so that any particles adhering to her clothing (soil, vegetation, furnishing) can be retained for forensic examination. If she has already changed, this evidence will be lost. Women contacting the police immediately after the incident must be warned not to change or wash.
- Clothing will be further examined for tearing and other signs of struggle and the woman will be asked about any jewellery worn, as it could have damaged the assailant.
- Swabs will be taken from vagina and mouth. Both will be analysed for semen and saliva.
- Physical examination will be performed in addition to inspection of the genital area to identify bruising, lacerations and other injuries. If the woman has been severely injured this may have to take place under general anaesthesia.
- Parings will be taken from her nails as she may have scratched her assailant during a struggle. Injuries may help identification.
- Blood samples will be taken to match any stains on the clothing or person of the assailant.
- The anus will be examined and swabs taken in and outside. Buggery is an offence in law (even between consenting partners).

After the examination the woman will be grateful for a shower and change of clothing. The nurse can help by contacting relatives, arranging transport and discreetly mentioning the need for early pregnancy testing and examination for sexually transmitted infection: neither can be detected immediately. The woman may require further information:

- Advice about post-coital contraception;
- An appointment arranged on her behalf at a Special Clinic;
- Counselling about AIDS. Vass (1987) points out the increasing risk of HIV infection to rape victims.

The woman must be allowed to describe what has happened in her own time and in her own words; routine swabs are taken because it is recognised that some may be unable to discuss oral sex or buggery. Kurdyak (1985), describing her work in a rape crisis centre, acknowledges that while some victims are vocal, frequently aggressive, others may outwardly appear calm. It is also acknowledged that rape can occur within stable relationships, including marriage, and those offering support must recognise that, although the woman will not wish violence to be repeated, she may not want the relationship to end (Orr 1984).

Myths surrounding rape

The public holds certain misconceptions about rape, which is supposedly the fate of flamboyant young women who dress provocatively, may 'ask for what they get' and who are likely to be accosted in dark alleyways by strangers at night. Although women between 14 and 35 years appear more at risk, none are exempt: children as young as two have been raped, as have the elderly (O'Reilly 1984). A study conducted by the London Rape Crisis Centre in 1984 showed that, in a sample of 2,981, a high proportion were attacked indoors and at least half knew their assailants. There was little to suggest provocative behaviour and many crimes occurred in daylight or well-lit streets.

The classic work of Holmstrom, and Burgess (1978) indicates that the rape victim is doubly victimised – by the crime and the reactions of society – and there is unfortunate evidence that nurses may share society's beliefs (Alexander 1980). Experimental studies suggest that nurses' perceptions of victims' behaviour may be coloured by the information they receive about the crime and its circumstances (Damrosch 1981, 1985). Yet in view of the distress already experienced, it seems unjust that women should face stigmatisation by members of a caring profession. On the other hand, sexual crime is a topic likely to evoke strong feelings, especially in members of a predominantly female profession whose working hours and circumstances may place them at risk. It is reasonable that nurses should be offered opportunities to discuss how they might feel when called on to help a rape victim, to consider how they might react themselves in a similar situation and to work through their own feelings. Teaching methods appropriate would include discussions and experiental learning in small groups where 'psychological safety' can be assured.

Rape trauma syndrome

All women are individuals; it is not possible to predict how each will respond in a particular crisis or cope with its aftermath. Nevertheless, it has been possible to

Table 15.1 Grief and bereavement accompanying
the rape trauma syndrome

---

1. *Denial*
   Inability to believe what has happened or to
   discuss the incident, fear of blame and stigma

2. *Anger*
   Hostility, aggression. 'Why should this happen
   to me?' Blame apportioned to others as if they
   could have prevented the incident even though
   this may not be logical

3. *Bargaining*
   Acknowledgement of the event, but
   accompanied by desires to forget it: 'I know this
   has happened but I promise to behave sensibly in
   future, keep indoors, so I do not run risks and
   am not reminded of it'

4. *Depression*

5. *Acceptance*
   The woman comes to terms with what has
   happened, but is able to draw something positive
   from her experience: 'I would not wish what
   happened on anyone, but life goes on, and I can
   cope with what I feel. Perhaps the experience
   has made me wiser'

These stages do not occur consecutively, and some
may be omitted. Time taken to work through the
grieving process may vary

---

adapt the stages of grieving from the *bereavement model* first proposed by Kubler
Ross (1969) to emotional reactions following rape (see Table 15.1). Reviewing the
literature Di Vasto (1985) concludes that predominant reactions include depression,
anxiety, fear and guilt, symptoms which Burgess and Holmstrom (1974) have described as *the rape trauma syndrome*, now measurable by a standardised questionnaire
(Di Vasto 1985).

Much of this research has been conducted in the USA, but in Britain there is growing awareness that the help offered rape victims is fragmented, arbitrary and frequently inadequate. The London Rape Crisis Centre reports between seventy and
eighty calls every week, often made by women some time after the assault, when their
failure to 'forget' their experience prompts them to accept a need for support (Hicks
1985). There is no recipe for helping women to work through their grief, but the
results of a small scale qualitative research study suggest that victims are better able
to cope and return to normal routines if given the opportunity to discuss their feelings
in a supportive atmosphere (Ipema 1979). Non-specialists in this field may not be

able to do much more than listen, provide practical help and know where to refer clients to a specialist agency (Foley 1979) but this will, nonetheless, be a step in the right direction.

References

Alexander, C.S. (1980) 'The responsible victim: nurses' perceptions of victims of rape', *Journal of Health and Social Behavior* 21, pp. 22–33.

Bellack, J.P. *et al.* (1977) 'Improving emergency care for rape victims', *Journal of Emergency Nursing* 3, pp. 32–5.

Burgess, A.W. and Holmstrom, L.L. (1974) 'Crisis and counselling requests of rape victims', *Nursing Research* 23, pp. 196–202.

Damrosch, S.P. (1981) 'How nursing students' reactions to rape victims are affected by a perceived act of carlessness', *Nursing Research* 30, pp. 168–70.

Damrosch, S.P. (1985) 'Nursing students' assessments of behaviourally self-blaming rape victims', *Nursing Research* 34, pp. 221–4.

Di Nitto, D. *et al.* (1986) 'After rape: who should examine rape survivors?' *American Journal of Nursing* 86 (5), pp. 538–40.

Di Vasto, P. (1985) 'Measuring the aftermath of rape', *Journal of Psychosocial Nursing and Mental Health Services* 23 (2), pp. 33–5.

Foley, T.S. (1979) 'Counselling the victim of rape' In: Stuart, G.W. and Sundeen, S.J. (eds.) *Principles and Practice of Psychiatric Nursing*, St. Louis: Mosby, pp. 426–54.

Gottesman, S.T. (1977) 'Police attitudes towards rape before and after a training programme', *Journal of Psychosocial Nursing and Mental Health Services* 15 (12), pp. 14–18.

Holmstrom, L.L. and Burgess, A.W. (1978) *The victim of Rape: Institutional Reactions*, New York: John Wiley.

Hicks, C. (1985) 'Survivor's advocate', *Nursing Times* 81 (9), p. 26.

HMSO (1981) *Criminal Statistics, England and Wales*, London: HMSO.

Ipema, D.K. (1979) 'Rape: the Process of Recovery', *Nursing Research* 28, pp. 272–5.

Kubler Ross, E. (1969) *On Death and Dying*, London: Macmillan.

Kurdyak, A. (1985) 'Rape crisis intervention', *Canadian Nurse* 81 (2), pp. 24–5.

The London Rape Crisis Centre (1984) *Sexual Violence: the Reality for Women*, London: The Women's Press.

Moore, J. (1985) 'Rape: the double victim', *Nursing Times* 81 (19), pp. 24–5.

O'Reilly, H.J. (1984) 'Crisis intervention with victims of possible rape: a police perspective' In: Hopkins, J. (ed.) *Perspectives on Rape and Sexual Assault*, London: Harper and Row, pp. 89–103.

Orr, J. (1984) 'Violence against women', *Nursing Times* 80 (17), pp. 34–6.

Orr, J. (1988) 'We don't need dead heroines', *Nursing Times* 84 (36), p. 22.

Schmidt, A.M. (1981) 'Adolescent female rape victims: special considerations', *Journal of Psychosocial Nursing and Mental Health Services* 19 (8), pp. 17–19.

Vass, T. (1987) 'The growing threat from AIDS to victims of rape and child abuse', *Social Work Today* 18, pp. 8–9.

Veitch, S. (1980) 'The victims who suffer in silence', Report from Birmingham Rape Crisis Centre. *The Guardian* 27.1.1980.

Index